Substance Abuse

A Guide for Health Professionals
2nd Edition

Manuel Schydlower, MD, FAAP
Editor

From the American Academy of Pediatrics,
Committee on Substance Abuse

American Academy of Pediatrics
141 Northwest Point Blvd
PO Box 927
Elk Grove Village, IL 60009-0927

Library of Congress Control Number: 2001132028
ISBN 1-58110-072-8

Quantity prices available on request. Address all inquires to:

American Academy of Pediatrics
141 Northwest Point Boulevard
Elk Grove Village, IL 60007

Suggested citation: [Chapter author]. [Chapter title]. In: Schydlower M, ed.
Substance Abuse: A Guide for Health Professionals. 2nd ed. Elk Grove
Village, IL: American Academy of Pediatrics; 2002:[page numbers]

American Academy of Pediatrics
Committee on Substance Abuse
2001-2002

Edward A. Jacobs, MD, FAAP, Chairperson
Alain Joffe, MD, MPH, FAAP
John R. Knight, MD, FAAP
John Kulig, MD, MPH, FAAP
Peter D. Rogers, MD, MPH, FAAP
Janet F. Williams, MD, FAAP

Liaisons

Gayle M. Boyd, PhD
National Institute of Alcohol Abuse and Alcoholism

Dorynne Czechowicz, MD
National Institute on Drug Abuse

Deborah Simkin, MD
American Academy of Child and Adolescent Psychiatry

Contributors

The editor gratefully acknowledges the invaluable assistance provided by the following individuals who served as contributors and reviewers in the preparation of *Substance Abuse: A Guide for Health Professionals,* 2nd Edition. Their expertise, critical review, and cooperation were essential to the committee's development of recommendations for the prevention, recognition, and treatment of substance use and abuse by children and adolescents.

Every attempt has been made to recognize all those who contributed to *Substance Abuse: A Guide for Health Professionals,* 2nd Edition. The editor regrets any omissions that may have occurred.

Trina Menden Anglin, MD, PhD, FAAP
Maternal and Child Health Bureau/Health Resources and Services Administration, US Department of Health and Human Services
Rockville, MD

Marie E. Armentano, MD
Massachusetts General Hospital
Boston, MA

Gilbert J. Botvin, PhD
Institute for Prevention Research, Weill Medical College, Cornell University
New York, NY

Ira J. Chasnoff, MD, FAAP
Children's Research Triangle
Chicago, IL

George D. Comerci, MD, FAAP
University of Arizona, College of Medicine
Tucson, AZ

Susan M. Coupey, MD, FAAP
Montefiore Medical Center, Albert Einstein College of Medicine
Bronx, NY

Paul G. Fuller, Jr, MD, FAAP
SUNY - Upstate Medical University
Syracuse, NY

J. David Hawkins, PhD
University of Washington
Seattle, WA

Richard B. Heyman, MD, FAAP
University of Cincinnati, College of Medicine
Cincinnati, OH

Edward A. Jacobs, MD, FAAP
Children's Hospital Regional Medical Center,
University of Washington
Everett, WA

Michael S. Jellinek, MD, FAAP
Massachusetts General Hospital
Boston, MA

Alain Joffe, MD, MPH, FAAP
Johns Hopkins University School of Medicine
Baltimore, MD

John R. Knight, MD, MPH, FAAP
Children's Hospital, Harvard Medical School
Boston, MA

John Kulig, MD, MPH, FAAP
Tufts University School of Medicine
Boston, MA

Nancy Neveloff Dubler, LLB
Albert Einstein College of Medicine, Montefiore Medical Center
Bronx, NY

M. Max Quinn, JD
New York, NY

Peter D. Rogers, MD, MPH, FAAP
Ohio State University, College of Medicine and Public Health
Columbus, OH

Walter Rosenfeld, MD, FAAP
Children's Medical Center, Atlantic Health System
Morristown, NJ

Rizwan Z. Shah, MD, FAAP
Blank Children's Hospital, University of Iowa School
of Medicine
Des Moines, IA

Deborah Simkin, MD
American Academy of Child and Adolescent Psychiatry
Washington, DC

J. Ward Stackpole, MD, FAAP
University of Vermont College of Medicine
Burlington, VT

Milton Tenenbein, MD, FAAP
University of Manitoba
Winnipeg, Manitoba, Canada

William E. Wingert, PhD
Lab Corp
Raritan, NJ

Dedication
Substance Abuse: A Guide for Health Professionals, 2nd Edition, is dedicated to all our youth, our most important national treasure and the hope of our future, and to all health care professionals who are devoted to the protection of their health and well-being.

Acknowledgments
The editor extends his gratitude to the American Academy of Pediatrics (AAP) and staff members Karen S. Smith, Manager, Committee on Substance Abuse; Claudia Appledorn, Medical Copy Editor; Jennifer Pane, Senior Medical Copy Editor; Rebecca Marshall, Manager of Section Administration; Rachael Hagan, Division Coordinator; and Bonnie Kozial, Department Assistant and Vera Contreras, Administrative Assistant, Texas Tech University School of Medicine Health Sciences Center at El Paso for their assistance in the preparation of this publication.

Preface

This second edition of *Substance Abuse: A Guide for Health Professionals* is published at the dawn of the 21st century, following extraordinary advances in the health care of children, adolescents, and young adults. Today, substance use and abuse continue to disrupt their health, affect the attainment of developmental tasks, impair identity development, and make it difficult for youth to negotiate the demands of the transition from adolescence to adulthood.[1] Drug use in adolescence is associated with many other risk-taking behaviors and their consequences (sexual activity, sexually transmitted diseases, pregnancy, school failure, injury, suicide, homicide, and motor vehicle crashes) that account for significant morbidity and mortality.[2]

During the last decade of the 20th century, encouraging developments in the area of substance use and abuse included the following[3]:

- a decrease in the rate of alcohol-related motor vehicle crash deaths for people 15 to 24 years of age (21.5 per 100 000 in 1987 to 12.9 per 100 000 in 1996);
- a decrease in the use of alcohol within the past 30 days by adolescents 12 to 17 years of age (33% in 1988 to 19% in 1996);
- a decrease in the prevalence of cigarette smoking by adolescents 12 to 17 years of age (23% in 1988 to 18% in 1996);
- an increase in average age of first use of marijuana (13.4 years in 1988 to 14.4 years in 1996);
- an increase in average age of first use of cigarettes by adolescents 12 to 17 years of age (11.6 years in 1988 to 12.4 in 1996).

As the new century settled in, among adolescents, use increased for a few drugs, stayed steady for many, and decreased for some. However, there is still an unacceptably high proportion of young people who have recently used drugs. The slight downward trend in any illicit drug use among America's adolescents belies an overall enormous cost of drug abuse to society.[4] Latest data reveal that societal costs in 1995 were $110 billion for illegal drugs, $100 billion for nicotine, and $165 billion for alcohol.[5] Drug use by pediatric-aged patients remains a pervasive and extensive problem of significant proportions (Table 0.1).[6-8]

table 0.1 **Prevalence (%) of Recent Use (Within the Past 30 Days) of Substances by Twelfth Graders in the United States[6-8]**

Substance	1988	1990	1992	1994	1996	1998	1999	2000
Alcohol	63.9	57.1	51.3	50.1	50.8	52.0	51.0	50.0
Tobacco	28.7	29.4	27.8	31.2	34.0	35.1	34.6	31.4
Marijuana	18.0	14.0	11.9	19.0	21.9	22.8	23.1	21.6
Cocaine	3.4	1.9	1.3	1.5	2.0	2.4	2.6	2.1
Any illicit drug	21.3	17.2	14.4	21.9	24.6	25.6	25.9	24.9
Inhalants	2.6	2.7	2.3	2.7	2.5	2.3	2.0	2.2
Amphetamines	4.6	3.7	2.8	4.0	4.1	4.6	4.5	5.0
Smokeless tobacco	10.3	---	11.4	11.1	9.8	8.8	8.4	7.6
LSD	1.8	1.9	2.0	2.6	2.5	3.2	2.7	1.6
Hallucinogens	2.2	2.2	2.1	3.1	3.5	3.8	3.5	2.6
MDMA ("ecstasy")	---	---	---	---	2.0	1.5	2.5	3.6
Methamphetamine ("ice")	---	0.6	0.5	0.7	1.1	1.2	0.8	1.0
Rohypnol	---	---	---	---	0.5	0.3	0.3	0.4
Tranquilizers	1.5	1.2	1.0	1.4	2.0	2.4	2.5	2.6
Barbiturates	1.2	1.3	1.1	1.7	2.1	2.6	2.6	3.0
Heroin	0.2	0.2	0.3	0.3	0.5	0.6	0.6	0.7
Steroids	---	1.0	0.6	0.9	0.7	1.1	0.9	0.8
Alcohol used until drunk	---	---	29.9	30.8	31.3	32.9	32.9	32.8

LSD indicates lysergic acid diethylamide; MDMA, 3,4-methylenedioxymethamphetamine.

For yearly updates on trends in drug use by children and adolescents, the health care professional can access the Monitoring the Future Web site at http://www.drugabuse.gov/DrugPages/MTF.html.

The American Academy of Pediatrics (AAP) recognizes that substance abuse is a major concern for all who care for infants, children, adolescents, and young adults. Health care professionals who are in the front lines in the care of patients in these age groups are in an ideal position to determine which young patients are at risk. They can also offer appropriate intervention or treatment counseling to the child or adolescent and his or her family or make a referral to a source where such counseling can be obtained.[9]

A recent conference sponsored by the Office of National Drug Control Policy and the Substance Abuse and Mental Health Services Administration proposed core competencies for involvement of health care professionals in the care of children and adolescents in families affected by substance abuse.[10] *Substance Abuse: A Guide for Health Professionals,* 2nd Edition aims to enhance the capabilities of the health care professional by providing a practical resource and reference for identifying, assessing, treating, or referring young patients who are affected by substance abuse. The chapters of this guide provide the health care professional with a useful reference to determine important clinical aspects related to risk and protective factors, role of the primary care physician, evaluation, use of the laboratory, the referral process, prevention, ethical and legal considerations, specific drugs, tobacco use, perinatal exposure, and dual diagnoses.

The editor is very grateful to all of the contributors for applying their great talents and expertise in the preparation of assigned chapters. In particular, they are recognized with great appreciation for helping to achieve our principal goal of providing the health care professional with a practical guide for use in the care of children, adolescents, and young adults who are vulnerable to or already affected by substance use or abuse. A special thank you goes to the members of the AAP Committee on Substance Abuse for their review and support in the preparation of this publication.

Manuel Schydlower, MD, FAAP, Editor
Texas Tech University, School of Medicine
Health Sciences Center at El Paso, TX

References

1. Center for Substance Abuse Treatment. Screening and assessing adolescents for substance use disorders. Rockville, MD: Substance Abuse and Mental Health Services Administration; 1999. DHHS Publication No. SMA 99-3344

2. Bruner AB, Fishman M. Adolescents and illicit drug use. *JAMA.* 1998;280:597-598

3. Office of Disease Prevention and Health Promotion. *Progress Review. Substance Abuse: Alcohol and Other Drugs.* Washington, DC: US Department of Health and Human Services; 1998:13

4. National Institute on Drug Abuse. Drug abuse cost to society. In: *NIDA Notes.* 1998;13:4 NIH Publication No. 98-3478

5. Waxman N. Center stage: Alan I. Leshner, PhD. *Econ Neurosci.* 2000;2:9

6. Johnston LD, O'Malley PM, Bachman JG. *National Survey Results on Drug Use from the Monitoring the Future Study, 1975-1998. Volume I: Secondary School Students.* Rockville, MD: National Institute on Drug Abuse; 1999. NIH Publication No. 99-4660

7. Johnston LD, O'Malley PM, Bachman JG. *The Monitoring the Future National Survey Results on Adolescent Drug Use: Overview of Key Findings, 1999.* Rockville, MD: National Institute on Drug Abuse; 2000. NIH Publication No. 00-4690

8. Johnston L, O'Malley P, Bachman J. "Ecstasy" use rises sharply among teens in 2000; use of many other drugs stays steady but significant declines are reported for some [press release]. Ann Arbor, MI: University of Michigan, News and Information Services; December 14, 2000

9. American Academy of Pediatrics, Committee on Substance Abuse. Tobacco, alcohol, and other drugs: the role of the pediatrician in prevention and management of substance abuse. *Pediatrics.* 1998;101:125-128

10. Adger H, Macdonald D, Wenger S. Core competencies for involvement of health care providers in the care of children and adolescents in families affected by substance abuse. *Pediatrics.* 1999;103:1083-1084

Table of Contents

Preface viii
    Manuel Schydlower, MD, FAAP

Chapter 1
    Risk and Protective Factors and Their Implications
    for Preventive Interventions for the Health Care
    Professional 1
    J. David Hawkins, PhD

Chapter 2
    The Role of the Primary Care Physician 21
    George D. Comerci, MD, FAAP

Chapter 3
    Evaluation by Interview and Questionnaire 43
    Trina Menden Anglin, MD, PhD, FAAP

Chapter 4
    Scientific Issues in Drug Testing and Use of
    the Laboratory 105
    Walter Rosenfeld, MD, FAAP, and William E. Wingert, PhD

Chapter 5
    The Role of the Primary Care Physician in the
    Referral Process 123
    Paul G. Fuller, Jr, MD, FAAP

Chapter 6
    Preventing the Use of Alcohol, Tobacco,
    and Illicit Drugs 143
    Gilbert J. Botvin, PhD

Chapter 7
    Legal and Ethical Considerations 175
    Nancy Neveloff Dubler, LLB, and M. Max Quinn, JD

Chapter 8
    Specific Drugs 191
    Susan M. Coupey, MD, FAAP

Chapter 9
  Tobacco Use and Abuse 277
  Richard B. Heyman, MD, FAAP

Chapter 10
  Perinatal Exposure to Maternal Substances of Abuse:
  Effect on the Developing Child 293
  Ira J. Chasnoff, MD, FAAP

Chapter 11
  Assessment, Diagnosis, and Treatment of the
  Adolescent With a Dual Diagnosis 307
  Marie E. Armentano, MD, and Michael S. Jellinek, MD, FAAP

Appendix 1
  Self-help and Advocacy Group Resources 325

Appendix 2
  Medical and Medical Specialty Organizations 329

Appendix 3
  Additional Resources 333

Chapter 1

Risk and Protective Factors and Their Implications for Preventive Interventions for the Health Care Professional

J. David Hawkins, PhD

The evaluation, management, referral, and long-term care of the adolescent who is seriously involved in substance abuse are marked by the difficulty of such work, the time and expense of treatment, and the frequency with which best efforts nevertheless result in a poor outcome. Our foremost goal as health care professionals should be to prevent the development of substance abuse by young people before the establishment of patterns of drug use that will be difficult to alter.[1]

Advances in cardiovascular disease prevention provide a model for approaching the prevention of substance abuse. Prospective longitudinal studies of cardiovascular disease identified risk factors for heart disease (family history, smoking, high-fat diet, stress, sedentary lifestyle) and protective factors that decrease or buffer the risk of heart disease (exercise, stress coping skills, healthy eating). Health care professionals have used this information to assess risk of cardiovascular disease in their patients, assessing family, lifestyle, dietary, and smoking histories; measuring blood pressure; and requesting laboratory tests to determine total cholesterol and high-density lipid versus low-density lipid levels. They have used the results of these assessments to advise and prescribe lifestyle changes (exercise, dietary changes, quitting smoking). In the past 30 years, the rate of cardiovascular disease has decreased more than 30% in the United States.[2]

Like cardiovascular disease, substance abuse is a preventable disorder. Current research provides a firm foundation for the health care professional seeking to decrease substance abuse risk among young patients before the appearance of drug use or abuse. The health care professional who cares for children and who knows the risk factors for substance abuse and the protective factors that decrease risk of substance abuse may be able to intervene and avert drug problems before they arise (See Table 2.1, page 25).

The Problem

Before reviewing the risk and protective factors predictive of substance abuse, it is instructive to recognize that currently in the United States, more than 80% of twelfth graders have consumed alcohol, and nearly 50% have used marijuana.[3] In this respect, substance use is widespread by late adolescence, well before alcohol use is legal. The use of alcohol in moderation by adults is socially acceptable and legal. However, starting to drink alcohol during childhood or early adolescence increases risk of later alcohol misuse and drug-related problems.[4]

Substance use is a problem of concern to health care professionals, because it causes harm to the individual or others. Such harm may follow a single event of excessive use or result from prolonged use for a period of years. The use of substances has been associated with motor vehicle crashes,[5] increased suicide risk,[6] sexual behavior resulting in unwanted or unplanned pregnancies or high risk of human immunodeficiency virus (HIV) infection,[7-9] and involvement in violence and crime.[10,11] The continued use of substances during adolescence has been found to negatively affect educational performance and attainment and job stability.[12] Although alcohol and drug abuse and dependence are diagnosable disorders, it is noteworthy that most alcohol-related problems in the United States involve individuals who are not dependent on but who misuse alcohol by drinking to excess on some occasions.[13] More than a third of twelfth graders in the United States reported having been drunk within the past 30 days.[3]

Consistent research evidence indicates that an early age of initiation of alcohol and other substance use is an important predictor of later substance use, abuse, and dependence.[4,14-16] These data suggest that delaying the age of initiation of alcohol use could decrease the use and abuse of alcohol and other drugs.

Research funded by the National Institute on Drug Abuse shows that in 1996, 9.8% of eighth graders and 5.2% of tenth graders reported that they had used alcohol by the fourth grade. Slightly more than 8% of twelfth graders in 1996 reported that they were already drinking alcohol by the sixth grade.

It is important to inform children and their parents that, unless a part of a deeply rooted cultural tradition of moderation, an early age of initiation of drinking is associated with greater risk of alcohol-related problems. Delaying initiation of alcohol use until adulthood is the most healthy choice during adolescence.

During the past 20 years, substance use has shown large fluctuations in prevalence. Rates of use increased in the late 1970s and decreased dramatically through the late 1980s and early 1990s. However, since 1992, rates of alcohol, tobacco, and marijuana use among secondary school students in the United States increased through 1997 before leveling off.[17] To illustrate, the prevalence of lifetime marijuana use among twelfth graders increased from 47.3% in 1975 to a peak of 60.4% in 1979, decreased to 32.6% in 1992, and has since increased to 49.7% in 1999.[3] The prevalence of lifetime cocaine use among twelfth graders increased from 9.0% in 1976 to a high of 17.3% in 1985 but decreased to its 1994 value of 5.9% before increasing to 9.8% in 1999.[3]

Generally, the prevalence of marijuana, cocaine, tobacco, and alcohol use within the past year, month, and day show similar patterns—a prolonged, uninterrupted decrease in the late 1980s and early 1990s followed by a recent increase. Fig 1.1 shows the changing prevalence of substance use within the past 30 days among twelfth graders in the United States since 1975.[3,18,19]

Less is known about the prevalence of substance abuse and dependence among adolescents. In an Oregon high school sample, Lewinsohn et al[20] found a lifetime prevalence of 8.3% for all substance abuse disorders at initial assessment and a lifetime prevalence of 10.8% a year later. The National Comorbidity Study[21] found that the lifetime prevalence of drug dependence excluding alcohol among 15- to 24-year-olds was 9.1% for males and 5.5% for females.

figure 1.1 Trends in substance use within the past 30 days by twelfth graders.[3,18,19]

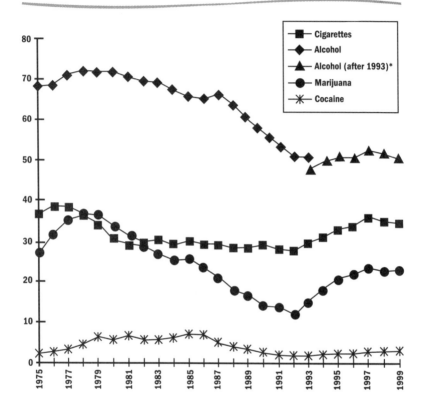

*In 1993, the question text was changed slightly in half of the forms to indicate that a "drink" meant "more than a few sips." Data in the upper line for alcohol came from forms using the original wording, whereas data in the lower line came from forms using the revised wording. In 1993, each line of data was based on 3 of 6 forms (n = 1/2 n). Data for 1994-1995 were based on all forms.

The data are clear. Currently, health care professionals confront high rates of substance use among young people.

Risk Factors for Substance Abuse

Health care professionals who seek to prevent substance use, abuse, and dependence in the children and adolescents with whom they work should use the evidence on predictors of substance abuse. Substance abuse is predicted by multiple biologic, psychologic, and social factors and their interactions.[1,22] Research to understand the interactions of these factors in predicting substance abuse continues. Already, clear evidence is available to guide preventive practice in primary care settings.[23]

Individual Factors

Some children appear to be at greater risk of substance abuse by virtue of their family histories, prenatal and birth experiences, temperaments, and early and persistent displays of problem behaviors.

A family history of alcoholism increases risk of alcoholism in children about 4 times.[24-26] However, less than 30% of children of alcoholics develop alcoholism. There is well-established evidence of genetic transmission of a propensity to alcoholism in males[27,28] and recent evidence of such a transmission in females.[29] Health care professionals should be alert to a family history of alcohol or other drug problems when informing their young patients about their own risk of substance abuse and dependence.

Perinatal complications (including preterm delivery, low birth weight, and anoxia) and brain damage (from infectious disease, traumatic head injury, or prenatal or postnatal exposure to toxins, such as heavy metals, alcohol, tobacco, or cocaine) predispose children to later aggressive behavior and substance abuse.[30,31] Health care professionals who maintain or obtain good birth and trauma histories may see evidence of these risks long before drug use begins. It is important to inform parents and parents-to-be of the risks of alcohol, tobacco, and other drug use during and after pregnancy and of the dangers to their children of toxins in the home.

Some studies suggest that inherited biologic traits and temperaments link genetics and alcohol use behaviors.[24,25,32] High behavior activity level[33] and sensation seeking[34] have been identified as predictors of early drug initiation and abuse. Attention-deficit/hyperactivity disorder in childhood has been found to predict substance abuse disorders in late adolescence, especially when combined with aggressive behaviors or conduct disorders.[35] A pattern of persistent conduct problems, including aggressive behavior in childhood, is an early behavioral predictor of risk of later substance abuse.[36-38]

Health care professionals can help decrease risks for later substance abuse by identifying patients who are experiencing behavioral and attention difficulties in early childhood and treating or referring them and their parents appropriately. Effective referral would include guiding parents to appropriate behaviorally focused parenting resources for skill development in child management.

As children approach adolescence, alienation from the dominant values of society,[39,40] low religiosity,[41,42] and rebelliousness[43-45] predict greater drug use in adolescence. During this period, attitudes favorable to drug use precede the initiation of substance use.[46,47] Health care professionals should begin to assess substance use attitudes and behaviors when they encounter these signals.

As noted earlier, the younger a child is when he or she first initiates the use of alcohol or other drugs, the greater the frequency of drug use,[48] the greater the probability of extensive and persistent involvement in the use of illicit drugs,[44] and the greater the risk of alcohol misuse and drug abuse.[16] Health care professionals should encourage young people to postpone alcohol use until adulthood and to avoid the use of tobacco and illegal drugs for their own health and safety. As discussed later, the adoption of strong norms or standards against drug use appears to inhibit drug use initiation.

Family Factors

As children develop, families affect their drug use behaviors in a number of ways. Drug use by parents and older siblings and permissive parental attitudes toward children's drug use predict greater risk of alcohol and other drug abuse.[49-51] Involving children in parental alcohol or drug using behaviors, such as allowing the child to light a cigarette or to serve a drink to a parent, appears to influence the development of attitudes favorable to drugs and alcohol and to contribute to risk of early initiation of drug use.[52] Early drug use is itself one of the strongest predictors of use, abuse, and dependence. Parents and older siblings can decrease the risks of alcohol and drug abuse in younger children simply by moderating use of alcohol or other drugs in their presence and by not involving children in their own alcohol or drug use behaviors. Health care professionals can help decrease substance abuse risks by ensuring that parents and older siblings know these facts and by encouraging them to act on them.

Parents who are permissive or fail to set clear expectations for their children, who are lax in the supervision of their children, and who are excessively severe and inconsistent in punishing their children increase their children's risk of drug abuse.[53-55] Permissiveness and extremely authoritarian, as opposed to authoritative, parenting practices predict later drug abuse in children.[40,55] Parenting difficulties may be evident in office visits or through conversations with parents, but there is no reason to wait for symptoms. Health care professionals can decrease drug risks in young patients by encouraging parents to learn and practice good parenting skills preventively. Just as participating in childbirth classes helps expectant mothers prepare for having children, providing or referring parents to developmentally appropriate training opportunities in family management skills can result in improved parenting, decreasing the risk of substance abuse.[56]

High levels of family conflict also appear to contribute to risk of higher levels of substance use during adolescence.[57] Studies indicate that children whose parents divorced during their adolescence are more likely to use drugs than are other adolescents.[54,58]

In contrast, positive family relationships appear to discourage the initiation of drug use.[39,59-62] Research has revealed that the quality of mothers' interaction with their children at 5 years of age distinguished children who became frequent users of marijuana by 18 years of age from those who had only tried marijuana.[40] Mothers of children who became frequent users were relatively cold, underresponsive, and underprotective with their children at 5 years of age, giving them little encouragement but pressuring them to perform in tasks.

Parental attitudes, practices, and relationships interact in contributing to risk. For example, low attachment to mother and paternal permissiveness predict movement from low to moderate levels of alcohol and marijuana use.[63] When parents use good family management practices and refrain from involving their children in their alcohol use, these practices inhibit alcohol use among their 15-year-old children, even when adults in the family drink alcohol.[64]

Health care professionals can ensure that parents of young people know the importance of setting clear expectations for not using alcohol or other drugs during childhood and adolescence, the importance of monitoring their children in developmentally appropriate and nonintrusive ways, the importance of consistent and appropriate punishment for violating family expectations, and the importance of providing recognition to young people for living according to healthy standards. Curricula tested for effectiveness in teaching these skills are available.[65-67]

School Factors

School experiences appear to contribute to drug nonuse, use, and abuse. Successful school performance has been shown to be a protective factor mitigating against escalation to a pattern of regular marijuana use and frequent drug use in adolescence.[68,69] Conversely, beginning in the late elementary grades, academic problems have been found to predict early initiation of drug use[70] and greater levels of use of illegal drugs.[71] Achievement problems may result from early behavior problems, learning disabilities, failure of teachers to motivate students, or other causes. Regardless of cause, the experience of not succeeding academically during late childhood appears to contribute to risk of substance abuse. Health care professionals can decrease drug abuse risk by assessing the academic progress of their young patients and suggesting tutoring or other academically focused interventions for young patients who are not making adequate academic progress. As children approach adolescence, those who lose commitment to educational pursuits, as indicated by little time spent on homework, truancy, and a perception that school is unimportant, are at greater risk of drug use in adolescence.[72-74]

Peer Factors
Having friends who drink, smoke, or use other drugs is among the strongest predictors of substance use among youth.[37,41,50,63,75-77]

Contextual Factors
Factors in the broader social environment also affect rates of drug abuse. Patterns of substance use in the neighborhood or community predict individual substance use behaviors.[78] Rates of use are higher in communities where alcohol or other drugs are inexpensive and easily available. Availability and price are influenced by legal restriction or regulation on purchase, by excise taxes, and by market forces. Changes in laws to be more restrictive on alcohol availability (increasing the legal drinking age, increasing excise taxes on alcohol, limiting the number of alcohol outlets) have been followed by decreases in alcohol consumption and alcohol-related fatalities.[79-81]

Broad social norms regarding the acceptability and risk of use of alcohol or other drugs also appear to affect the prevalence of substance use and abuse.[82,83] For example, the inversely proportional relationship between the perceived risk of regular use and prevalence of marijuana use within the past 30 days by twelfth graders is shown in Fig 1.2.[84]

Finally, there is evidence that children who grow up in disorganized neighborhoods with high population density, high residential mobility, physical deterioration, and low levels of neighborhood attachment or cohesion face greater risk of drug trafficking and drug abuse.[85,86] Health care professionals can decrease substance abuse risks in their communities by urging that policies and laws forbidding the sale of alcohol and tobacco to underage individuals are strictly enforced; by communicating strong normative standards to patients and their parents and the public against the use of alcohol, tobacco, or other drugs by children or adolescents; and by participating in groups and coalitions seeking to improve the community.

Protective Factors

There are factors and processes that protect adolescents against substance abuse, even if they have been exposed to multiple risk factors. Individual protective characteristics include a resilient

figure 1.2 Marijuana: trends in perceived availability, perceived risk of regular use, and prevalence of use within the past 30 days for twelfth graders.[83]

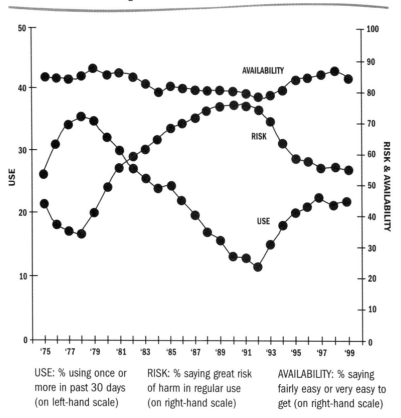

USE: % using once or more in past 30 days (on left-hand scale)

RISK: % saying great risk of harm in regular use (on right-hand scale)

AVAILABILITY: % saying fairly easy or very easy to get (on right-hand scale)

temperament, positive social orientation, and high intelligence and skills.[87] Children who have or develop these characteristics during childhood are more likely to negotiate adolescence without involvement in substance abuse.

Importantly, the development of warm, supportive relationships and social bonds to prosocial adults during childhood appears to inhibit substance abuse as well. This underscores the importance of good parenting skills throughout development. Health care professionals offer childbirth education classes to expectant parents to prevent birthing complications and promote infant health and bonding. Health care professionals can, as a matter of course, link the parents of their patients to appropriate parenting resources across development periods as the patients reach key milestones. At a minimum, this means making pamphlets, brochures, books, or videotapes on parenting available in the office and promoting the importance of keeping family bonds strong throughout development. Some health care professionals offer parenting classes for parents of patients entering adolescence to help them prevent substance abuse problems and promote the healthy development of their children.[23]

Finally, as noted earlier in this chapter, strong norms, beliefs, or behavioral standards that oppose the use of illegal drugs or the use of alcohol by adolescents protect against drug use and abuse.[88] Fluctuations in the prevalence of substance use among adolescents since 1975 reflect changes in levels of social disapproval and risk perceived to be associated with the use of specific substances by young people.[83] Health care professionals are opinion shapers in their communities, especially with respect to matters of health. It is important to advocate abstinence from tobacco and illegal substance use for children and adolescents. With respect to alcohol, the course associated with the least health risk is to delay use until adulthood. Health care professionals should communicate clear norms and standards regarding substances and their use.

Conclusion

Health care professionals who care for children and adolescents can play a critical role in the prevention of substance use and abuse and in early intervention with those patients who have begun to use drugs. Knowledge of those factors that place young people at risk and of those factors that can protect against substance abuse is the foundation for assessment, diagnosis, and preventive action. A healthy, open relationship with children and families and an understanding of normal development allow the health care professional to assess existing and emerging risks for substance abuse across development and across spheres of life. Increasingly, effective approaches for decreasing specific risks and enhancing protection have been identified and tested.[1,22] The potential to intervene before problems arise is the opportunity and obligation of those who care for young people.

References

1. Hawkins JD, Arthur MW, Catalano RF. Preventing substance abuse. In: Tonry M, Farrington DP, eds. *Building a Safer Society: Strategic Approaches to Crime Prevention.* Chicago, IL: University of Chicago Press; 1995:343-427
2. Shine KI. *Presentation to the Committee on the Prevention of Mental Health Disorders.* Washington, DC: National Academy of Sciences; 1994
3. Johnston LD, O'Malley PM, Bachman JG. *The Monitoring the Future National Survey Results on Adolescent Drug Use: Overview of Key Findings, 1999.* Rockville, MD: National Institute on Drug Abuse; 2000. NIH Publication No. 00-4690
4. Hawkins JD, Graham JW, Maguin E, Abbott RD, Catalano RF. Exploring the effects of age of alcohol use initiation and psychosocial risk factors on subsequent alcohol misuse. *J Stud Alcohol.* 1997;58: 280-290
5. Perrine MW, Peck RC, Fell JC. Epidemiologic perspectives on drunk driving. In: *Surgeon General's Workshop on Drunk Driving: Background Papers.* Washington, DC: US Department of Health and Human Services, Public Health Service, Office of the Surgeon General; 1988:35-76
6. Berman AL, Schwartz, RH. Suicide attempts among adolescent drug users. *Am J Dis Child.* 1990;144:310-314

7. Chaiken JM, Chaiken MR. Drugs and predatory crime. In: Tonry M, Wilson JQ, eds. *Drugs and Crime.* Vol 13. Chicago, IL: University of Chicago Press, 1990:203-239

8. Leigh BC, Stall R. Substance use and risky sexual behavior for exposure to HIV: issues in methodology, interpretation, and prevention. *Am J Psychol.* 1993;48:1035-1045

9. Schroeder SA. Substance abuse (president's message). In: *Substance Abuse: The Robert Wood Johnson Foundation 1992 Annual Report.* Princeton, NJ: Robert Wood Johnson Foundation; 1993

10. Fagan J, Browne A. Violence between spouses and intimates: physical aggression between women and men in intimate relationships. In: Reiss AJ Jr, Roth JA, eds. *Understanding and Preventing Violence: Social Influences.* Vol 3. Washington, DC: National Academy Press; 1994:115-292

11. Miczek KA, DeBold JF, Haney M, Tidey J, Vivian J, Weerts EM. Alcohol, drugs of abuse, aggression, and violence. In: Riess AJ Jr, Roth JA, eds. *Understanding and Preventing Violence: Social Influences.* Vol 3. Washington, DC: National Academy Press; 1994:377-570

12. Newcomb MD, Bentler PM. *Consequences of Adolescent Drug Use: Impact on the Lives of Young Adults.* Newbury Park, CA: Sage Publications; 1988

13. Institute of Medicine, Committee on Drug Use in the Workplace. *Under the Influence: Drugs and the American Work Force.* Normand J, Lempert RO, O'Brien CP, eds. Washington, DC: National Academy Press; 1990

14. Kandel DB, Simcha-Fagan O, Davies M. Risk factors for delinquency and illicit drug use from adolescence to young adulthood. *J Drug Issues.* 1986;16:67-90

15. Robins LN. *Synthesis and Analysis of Longitudinal Research on Substance Abuse. Report for the Robert Wood Johnson Foundation.* Princeton, NJ: Robert Wood Johnson Foundation; 1992

16. Robins LN, Przybeck TR. Age of onset of drug use as a factor in drug use and other disorders. In Jones CL, Battjes RJ, eds. *Etiology of Drug Abuse: Implications for Prevention.* Washington, DC: US Department of Health and Human Services, National Institute on Drug Abuse; 1985:178-192

17. Johnston LD, O'Malley DM, Bachman JG. *National Survey Results on Drug Use from the Monitoring the Future Study, 1975-1995: Volume 1, Secondary School Students.* Rockville, MD: National Institute on Drug Abuse; 1996. NIH Publication No. 97-4139

18. Johnston LD, O'Malley PM, Bachman JG. *Trends in Drug Use and Associated Factors Among American High School Students, College Students, and Young Adults 1975-1989.* Ann Arbor, MI: University of Michigan Institute for Social Research; 1991

19. Johnston LD, Bachman JG, O'Malley PM. Drug use rises among the nation's eighth grade students; LSD may be making a come back; twelfth graders showed continued declines in use but a reversal in some key attitudes that have driven the decline [press release]. Ann Arbor, MI: University of Michigan, News and Information Service; April 9, 1993

20. Lewinsohn PM, Hops H, Roberts RE, Seely JR, Andrews TA. Adolescent psychopathology: I. Prevalence and incidence of depression and other DSM-III-R disorders in high school students. *J Abnorm Psychol.* 1993;102:133-144

21. Kessler RC, McGonagle KA, Zhao S, et al. Lifetime and 12-month prevalence of DSM-III-R psychiatric disorders in the United States: results from the National Comorbidity Study. *Arch Gen Psychiatry.* 1994;51:8-19

22. Hawkins JD, Catalano RF, Miller JY. Risk and protective factors for alcohol and other drug problems in adolescence and early adulthood: Implications for substance abuse prevention. *Psychol Bull.* 1992;112: 64-105

23. Hawkins JD, Fitzgibbon JJ. Risk factors and risk behaviors in prevention of adolescent substance abuse. *Adolesc Med.* 1993;4:249-262

24. Schukit MA. Biological vulnerability to alcoholism. *Consult Clin Psychol.* 1987;55:301-309

25. Tarter R. Are there inherited behavioral traits which predispose to substance abuse? *J Consult Clin Psychol.* 1988;56:189-196

26. Merikangas KR, Rounsaville BJ, Prusoff BA. Familial factors in vulnerability to substance abuse. In: Glantz M, Pickens R, eds. *Vulnerability to Drug Abuse.* Washington, DC: American Psychological Association; 1992:75-97

27. Cadoret RJ, Cain CA, Grove WM. Development of alcoholism in adoptees raised apart from alcoholic biologic relatives. *Arch Gen Psychiatry.* 1980;37:561-563

28. Hrubec Z, Omenn GS. Evidence of genetic predisposition to alcoholic cirrhosis and psychosis: Twin concordance for alcoholism and biological endpoints by zygosity among male veterans. *Alcohol Clin Exp Res.* 1981;5:207-215

29. Kendler KF, Heath AC, Neale MC, Kessler RC, Eaves LJ. A population-based twin study of alcoholism in women. *JAMA.* 1992;268:1877-1882

30. Brennan P, Mednick S, Kandel E. Congenital determinants of violent and property offending. In: Pepler DJ, Rubin KH, eds. *The Development and Treatment of Childhood Aggression.* Hillsdale, NJ: Lawrence Erlbaum; 1991:81-92

31. Michaud LJ, Rivara FP, Jaffe KM, Fay G, Dailey JL. Traumatic brain injury as a risk factor for behavioral disorders in children. *Arch Phys Med Rehab.* 1993;74:368-375

32. Blum K, Noble EP, Sheridan PJ, et al. Allelic association of human dopamine D2 receptor gene in alcoholism. *JAMA.* 1990;263:2055-2060

33. Tarter RE, Laird SB, Kabene M, Bukstein O, Kaminer Y. Drug abuse severity in adolescents is associated with magnitude of deviation in temperament traits. *Br J Addict.* 1990;85:1501-1504

34. Cloninger CR, Sigvardsson S, Bohman M. Childhood personality predicts alcohol abuse in young adults. *Alcohol Clin Exp Res.* 1988;12:494-505

35. Gittelman R, Mannuzza S, Smenker R, Bonagura N. Hyperactive boys almost grown up: I. Psychiatric status. *Arch Gen Psychiatry.* 1985;42:937-947

36. Kellam SG, Brown H. *Social Adaptational and Psychological Antecedents of Adolescent Psychopathology Ten Years Later.* Baltimore, MD: Johns Hopkins University; 1982

37. Brook JS, Brook DW, Gordon AS, Whiteman M, Cohen P. The psychosocial etiology of adolescent drug use: a family interactional approach. *Genet Soc Gen Psychol Monogr.* 1990;116:111-267

38. Lewis CE, Robins L, Rice J. Association of alcoholism with anti social personality in urban men. *J Nerv Ment Dis.* 1985;173:166-174

39. Jessor R, Jessor SL. *Problem Behavior and Psychosocial Development: A Longitudinal Study of Youth.* New York, NY: Academic Press; 1977

40. Shedler J, Block J. Adolescent drug use and psychological health: a longitudinal inquiry. *Am Psychol.* 1990;45:612-630

41. Jessor R, Donovan JE, Windmer K. *Psychosocial Factors in Adolescent Alcohol and Drug Use: The 1980 National Sample Study and the 1974-78 Panel Study.* Boulder, CO: University of Colorado, Institute of Behavioral Science; 1980

42. Brunswick AF, Messeri PA, Titus SP. Predictive factors in adult substance abuse: a prospective study of African American adolescents. In: Glantz M, Pickens R, eds. *Vulnerability to Drug Abuse.* Washington, DC: American Psychological Association; 1992:419-472

43. Bachman JG, Johnston LD, O'Malley PM. *Monitoring the Future: Questionnaire Responses from the Nation's High School Seniors.* Ann Arbor, MI: University of Michigan Institute for Social Research; 1981

44. Kandel DB. Epidemiological and psychosocial perspectives on adolescent drug use. *J Am Acad Child Psychiatry.* 1982;21:328-347

45. Block J, Block JH, Keyes S. Longitudinally foretelling drug usage in adolescence: early childhood personality and environmental precursors. *Child Dev.* 1988;59:336-355

46. Kandel DB, Kessler RC, Margulies RZ. Antecedents of adolescent initiation into stages of drug use: a developmental analysis. *J Youth Adolesc.* 1978;7:13-40

47. Krosnick JA, Judd CM. Transitions in social influence at adolescence: who induces cigarette smoking? *Dev Psychol.* 1982; 18:359-368

48. Fleming JP, Kellam SG, Brown CH. Early predictors of age at first use of alcohol, marijuana and cigarettes. *Drug Alcohol Depend.* 1982;9:285-303

49. Johnson GM, Shontz FC, Locke TP. Relationships between adolescent drug use and parental drug behaviors. *Adolescence.* 1984;19:295-299

50. Barnes GM, Welte JW. Patterns and predictors of alcohol use among 7-12th grade students in New York State. *J Stud Alcohol.* 1986;47:53-62

51. Brook JS, Whiteman M, Gordon AS, Brook DW. The role of older brothers in younger brothers' drug use viewed in the context of parent and peer influences. *J Genet Psychol.* 1990;151:59-75

52. Bush PJ, Iannotti R. The development of children's health orientations and behaviors: lessons for substance abuse prevention. In: Jones CL, Battjes RJ, eds. *Etiology of Drug Abuse: Implications for Prevention.* Washington, DC: US Department of Health and Human Services; 1985:45-74

53. Kandel DB, Andrews K. Processes of adolescent socialization by parents and peers. *Int J Addict.* 1987;22:319-342

54. Penning M, Barnes GE. Adolescent marijuana use: a review. *Int J Addict.* 1982;17:749-791

55. Baumrind D. Why adolescents take chances—and why they don't. Paper presented at: Annual Meeting of the National Institute of Child Health and Human Development; 1983; Bethesda, MD

56. Spoth R, Redmond C, Haggerty K, Ward T. A controlled parenting skills outcome study examining individual difference and attendance effects. *J Marriage Fam.* 1995;57:449-464

57. Simcha-Fagan O, Gersten JC, Langner TS. Early precursors and concurrent correlates of patterns of illicit drug-use in adolescence. *J Drug Issues.* 1986;52:157-169

58. Needle RH, Su SS, Doherty WJ. Divorce, remarriage, and adolescent substance use: a prospective longitudinal-study. *J Marriage Fam.* 1990;52:157-169

59. Kim S. An evaluation of ombudsman primary prevention program on student drug abuse. *J Drug Educ.* 1981;11:27-36

60. Norem Hebeisen A, Johnson DW, Anderson D, Johnson R. Predictors and concomitants of changes in drug-use patterns among teenagers. *J Soc Psychol.* 1984;124:43-50

61. Brook JS, Gordon AS, Whiteman M, Cohen P. Some models and mechanisms for explaining the impact of maternal and adolescent characteristics on adolescent stage of drug use. *Dev Psychol.* 1986;22:460-467

62. Selnow GW. Parent-child relationships and single and two parent families: implications for substance usage. *J Drug Educ.* 1987;17: 315-326

63. Brook JS, Cohen P, Whiteman M, Gordon AS. Psychosocial risk factors in the transition from moderate to heavy use or abuse of drugs. In: Glantz M, Pickens R, eds. *Vulnerability to Drug Abuse.* Washington, DC: American Psychological Association; 1992:359-388

64. Peterson PL, Hawkins JD, Abbott RD, Catalano RF. Disentangling the effects of parental drinking, family management, and parental alcohol norms on current drinking by black and white adolescents. *J Res Adolesc.* 1994;4:203-227

65. Kosterman R, Hawkins JD, Spoth R, Haggerty KP, Zhu K. Effects of a preventive parent training intervention on observed family interactions: proximal outcomes from Preparing for the Drug Free Years. *J Comm Psychol.* 1997;25:337-352

66. Catalano RF, Kosterman R, Haggerty K, Hawkins JD, Spoth R. A universal model for the prevention of substance abuse: preparing for the drug (free) years. In: Ashery RS, Robertson EB, Kumpfer KL, eds. *Drug Abuse Prevention Through Family Interventions.* Rockville, MD: National Institute on Drug Abuse; 1998

67. Dishion TJ, Andrews DW. Preventing escalation in problem behaviors with high-risk young adolescents: immediate and 1-year outcomes. *J Consult Clin Psychol.* 1995;63:538-548

68. Kandel DB, Davies M. Progression to regular marijuana involvement: phenomenology and risk factors for near-daily use. In: Glantz M, Pickens R, eds. *Vulnerability to Drug Abuse.* Washington, DC: American Psychological Association; 1992:211-253

69. Hundleby JD, Mercer GW. Family and friends as social environments and their relationship to young adolescents' use of alcohol, tobacco, and marijuana. *J Marriage Fam.* 1987;49:151-164

70. Bachman JG, Johnston LD, O'Malley PM. How changes in drug use are linked to perceived risks and disapproval: evidence from national studies that youth and young adults respond to information about the consequences of drug use. In: Donohew L, Sypher HE, Bukoski WJ, eds. *Persuasive Communication and Drug Abuse Prevention.* Hillsdale, NJ: Lawrence Erlbaum; 1991:133-155

71. Holmberg MB. Longitudinal studies of drug abuse in a fifteen-year-old population: I. Drug career. *Acta Psychiatr Scand* 1985;71:67-79

72. Gottfredson DC. An evaluation of an organization development approach to reducing school disorder. *Eval Rev.* 1988;11:739-763

73. Friedman AS. High school drug abuse clients. In: *Treatment Research Notes.* Rockville, MD: National Institute on Drug Abuse, Division of Clinical Research; 1983

74. Maguin E, Loeber R. Academic performance and delinquency. In: Tonry M, ed. *Crime and Justice: A Review of Research.* Chicago, IL: University of Chicago Press; 1996:145-264

75. Kandel DB. Covergences in prospective longitudinal surveys of drug use in normal populations. In: Kandel DB, ed. *Longitudinal Research on Drug Use: Empirical Findings and Methodological Issues.* Washington, DC: Hemisphere Publishing Corp; 1978:3-38

76. Kandel DB. Processes of peer influence in adolescence. In: Silberstein R, ed. *Development as Action in Context: Problem Behavior and Normal Youth Development.* New York, NY: Springer-Verlag; 1986:203-228

77. Newcomb MD, Bentler PM. Substance use and ethnicity: differential impact of peer and adult models. *J Psychol.* 1986;120:83-95

78. Robins TN. The natural history of adolescent drug use. *Am J Pub Health.* 1984;74:656-657

79. Cook PJ, Tauchen G. The effect of liquor taxes on heavy drinking. *Bell J Econ.* 1982;13:379-390

80. Holder HD, Blose JO. Impact of changes in distilled spirits availability on apparent consumption: a time series analysis of liquor-by-the-drink. *Br J Addict.* 1987;82:623-631

81. Saffer H, Grossman M. Beer taxes, the legal drinking age, and youth motor vehicle fatalities. *Legal Stud.* 1987;16:351-374

82. Vaillant GE. *The Natural History of Alcoholism.* Cambridge, MA: Harvard University Press; 1983

83. Johnston LD. Toward a theory of drug epidemics. In Donohew L, Sypher HE, Bukoski WT, eds. *Persuasive Communication and Drug Abuse Prevention.* Hillsdale, NJ: Lawrence Erlbaum; 1991:93-131

84. Johnston L, O'Malley P, Bachman J. *Monitoring the Future National Survey Results on Drug Use, 1975-1999. Volume I: Secondary School Students.* Rockville, MD: National Institute on Drug Abuse; 2000. NIH publication 00-4802

85. Fagan J. *The Social Organization of Drug Use and Drug Dealing Among Urban Gangs.* New York, NY: John Jay College of Criminal Justice; 1988

86. Simcha-Fagan O, Schwartz JE. Neighborhood and delinquency: an assessment of contextual effects. *Criminology.* 1986;24:667-704

87. O'Dougherty M, Wright FS. Children born at medical risk: factors affecting vulnerability and resilience. In: Rolf J, Masten AS, Cicchetti D, Nuechterlein KH, Weintraub S, eds. *Risk and Protective Factors in the Development of Psychopathology.* Cambridge, England: Cambridge University Press; 1990:120-141

88. Hansen WB, Graham JW. Preventing alcohol, marijuana, and cigarette use among adolescents: Peer pressure resistance training versus establishing conservative norms. *Prev Med.* 1991;20:414-430

Chapter 2

The Role of the Primary Care Physician

George D. Comerci, MD, FAAP

Primary care physicians are in a unique position to play a crucial role in the prevention, identification, and management of the use and abuse of alcohol, tobacco, and other drugs, including prescription drugs. Despite acknowledging this key role, primary care physicians often avoid involvement in the care of patients who abuse drugs. Although their relationship with the young patient, rapport with the family, and position in the community clearly provide the opportunity to intervene, many are reluctant to ask the appropriate questions and fail to take necessary measures to diagnose substance abuse disorders and intervene with patients suffering the consequences of substance abuse.[1]

Many barriers exist for physicians who want to be involved in the diagnosis and treatment of substance abuse.[2] Primary care physicians engage in high-volume and low-encounter time practice styles, resulting in severe constraints on the time available for patient interaction. Overhead expense is a constant factor, and reimbursement usually is inadequate relative to the time and effort required to diagnose substance abuse disorders and confront and work with patients and their families. Because of the positive relationship that exists between primary care physicians and their patients, many are uneasy with this potentially unpleasant area of practice. Because they may have had inadequate training or education in addiction medicine, many primary care physicians believe they do not have the knowledge or skills to meet this seemingly complex and difficult clinical challenge.[3,4]

Primary care physicians often are unaware of the potential for positive outcomes of intervention and good treatment and, therefore, may have a bias against consultation and referral for treatment. Many may not fully appreciate the negative outcomes that result from failure to intervene and, unfortunately, rarely become aware of the negative consequences of a missed diagnosis or of not intervening. Furthermore, most are unaware of the specialized treatment resources available in their communities, are uncertain about how to gain access to such services, and lack the skills necessary to conduct a smooth referral.[5]

Because of the aforementioned barriers and obstacles to involvement of primary care physicians in addiction medicine, it is understandable that primary care physicians may not regularly recognize drug abuse and chemical dependency problems in their practices. Before physicians can be expected to assume their appropriate role in the prevention and management of substance abuse, such barriers must be overcome.

Primary care physicians have a key role in at least 7 areas concerning substance abuse in children and adolescents, including the following:

1. Anticipatory guidance and prevention
2. Diagnosis of substance abuse
3. Intervention and treatment
4. Consultation and referral
5. Family support
6. Education
7. Community action[6]

Anticipatory Guidance and Prevention

Anticipatory guidance is a constant theme in primary care for pediatric patients and their families. Providing counsel about potential problems and their prevention begins with the first prenatal visit and extends through health maintenance visits during infancy, childhood, and adolescence. During such visits, key developmental issues should be addressed at specific critical stages.[7,8] Hence, education of the young person about the use of tobacco, alcohol, and other drugs should begin in childhood, when parental child rearing practices are set and when family standards and values in general are assimilated by the child. Health maintenance visits provide regular opportunities to discuss drug use and prevention with the patient and family (see *Prevention and Intervention*, p 34).

A developmental approach to anticipatory guidance is important, and suggestions for such an approach, including appropriate interview techniques and the use of questionnaires, are covered elsewhere in this manual (see Chapter 3).[9]

Through their counsel, primary care physicians can give a clear message that substance abuse is a subject that can be discussed and that questions about drug use will be welcomed. Regular checkup visits provide the opportunity to educate about drug use, peer pressure to use drugs, and the influence of the media on the young person's attitudes and behavior. Children and adolescents should be encouraged to discuss substance abuse issues with their parents and to share problems that they are experiencing, such as drug use at school or social affairs.

Anticipatory guidance also should be given to parents, especially for the young child and preadolescent. Parents should know that the use of tobacco products, alcohol, and marijuana often begins as early as fourth or fifth grade; that there has been a definite increase in the use of drugs, especially marijuana; and that, compared with their parents, adolescents tend to perceive less associated risk and tend to be less disapproving of drug abuse than children and adolescents were in the recent past (see *Patterns of Substance Use and Abuse*, p 27).[10,11] Parents should be encouraged to examine their own beliefs and practices concerning drugs and should be reminded that their attitudes and practices influence those of their children. Many of today's parents have used drugs themselves, which presents a special dilemma for dealing with drug use by their children. Parents should know that adolescents are especially sensitive to inconsistencies in what parents say compared with what they do (or did).

Anticipatory guidance about substance abuse is not a one-time effort. It should occur at regular intervals during childhood and adolescence.

Diagnosis of Substance Abuse

Inquiries about drug use should be a routine part of every evaluation of the older child and adolescent, regardless of the underlying condition or concern that resulted in seeking care from the physician.[6] Inquiries about drug use are a natural component of a comprehensive health maintenance evaluation. Inquiry into age-appropriate psychosocial functioning, such as school performance and career plans, family and peer relationships, nonacademic activities, behavior, sexual attitudes and practices, acceptance of authority, degree of self-esteem, and ongoing or past intrafamilial or extrafamilial episodes of child abuse, may reveal risk factors for future or present substance abuse (Table 2.1).[6]

To obtain reliable information about drug use, the physician should collect the information in an appropriate setting and use good interviewing skills (see Chapter 3).[12] A useful history-taking tool in the assessment of adolescent health risks is a mnemonic device called the HEADSS exam. HEADSS and its variations incorporate important areas of function or dysfunction in the lives of adolescents, including: **H**ome environment; **E**ducation or **E**mployment; peer and extracurricular **A**ctivities; **D**rugs; **S**exuality; and **S**uicide.[13,14] Information about drug use (as well as other sensitive information, such as sexual activity) should be obtained in privacy. It is unreasonable to expect that an adolescent will be truthful about drug use when such questions are asked in the presence of parents. The adolescent should be assured of some degree of confidentiality if candid responses are expected (see Chapter 7).

Drug screening and testing are valuable diagnostic tools when appropriately selected and properly performed (see Chapters 4 and 7). However, a surreptitiously obtained test can destroy the working relationship between the patient and the physician. The American Academy of Pediatrics (AAP) developed a policy statement on laboratory testing for drugs of abuse as it relates to diagnosis, treatment, or referral by the physician (Table 2.2).[15] A well-obtained history remains the mainstay of diagnosis.

table 2.1 Potential Risk Factors for Substance Abuse[6]

- Paternal or twin alcoholism
- Parental alcohol or other drug use
- Family history of alcoholism
- Family history of antisocial behavior
- Child abuse and neglect (intrafamilial or extrafamilial)
- Parents with poor parenting skills
- Poor relationship with parents
- Drug use by sibling
- Drug use by best friend
- Perceived peer drug use
- Low academic achievement
- Low interest in school and achievement
- Rebelliousness and alienation
- Low self-esteem
- Early antisocial behavior
- Psychopathologic problems, particularly depression
- Negative character traits (eg, frequent lying, lack of empathy, favoring immediate rather than delayed gratification, need to seek sensation, insensitivity to punishment)
- Previous dependence on alcohol or other drugs
- Delinquent behavior
- Low religiosity
- Early alcohol use
- Early experimentation with alcohol and other drugs
- Early sexual activity

---

table 2.2 Testing For Drugs of Abuse in Children and Adolescents

---

- The AAP is opposed to the nontherapeutic use of psychoactive drugs by children and adolescents.

- The appropriate response to suspicion of drug abuse is referral of the child or adolescent to a qualified health care professional for evaluation, counseling, and treatment as needed.

- The role of the primary care physician is one of prevention, diagnosis, counseling, and treatment or appropriate referral for care.

- Voluntary screening may be a deceptive term in that there often are negative consequences for those who decline to volunteer. Parental permission is not sufficient for involuntary screening of the older, competent adolescent, and the AAP opposes such involuntary screening. Consent from the older adolescent may be waived when there is reason to doubt competency or in those circumstances in which information gained by history or physical examination strongly suggests that the young person is at high risk of substance abuse.[16]

- Diagnostic testing for the purpose of drug abuse treatment is within the ethical tradition of health care, and in the competent patient, it should be conducted noncovertly, confidentially, and with informed consent in the same context as for other medical conditions.

- Involuntary testing in a minor who lacks the capacity to make informed judgments may be done with parental permission. Parental permission is not sufficient for involuntary testing of the adolescent with decisional capacity, and the AAP opposes such involuntary testing. Suspicion that an adolescent may be using a psychoactive drug does not justify involuntary testing, and it is not sufficient justification to rely solely on parental agreement to test the patient. Testing adolescents requires their consent unless a patient lacks decision-making capacity or there are strong medical indications or legal requirements to do so.

- Notwithstanding the Supreme Court ruling,[17] students and student athletes should not be singled out for involuntary screening for drugs of abuse. Such testing should not be a condition for participation in sports or any school functions except for health-related purposes. Suspicion of drug use warrants a comprehensive evaluation by a qualified health care professional.

Patterns of Substance Use and Abuse

Patterns of substance use and abuse have changed during the last few decades. The 1980s saw an encouraging overall decrease in the use of illicit substances among adolescents and an increase in the level of disapproval and perceived risk of use among high school and college students. In the early 1990s, there was a reversal of such attitudes and an increase in drug use, especially marijuana, among adolescents, and an earlier age of initiation.[10,11,18] These changing patterns of use and abuse affect the manner in which young people seek care from physicians. During the 1980s, patients were less likely to be seen in an emergency department setting than they were decades earlier. Today, with the increased abuse of amphetamines, designer euphoriants such as 3,4-methylenedioxymethamphetamine (MDMA ["ecstasy"]), and potent forms of heroin, more patients again are being encountered in acute care settings because of the medical consequences of abuse (see Chapter 8). Intentional and nonintentional trauma secondary to injury while under the influence of a substance of abuse continues to be a reason for seeking medical care. Nevertheless, patients with substance abuse disorders are seen more often during routine health maintenance visits, for illnesses unrelated to drug use, or for a behavioral consequence of drug use, such as scholastic failure, oppositional-defiant behavior, or delinquency.

The role of the primary care physician varies depending on the patient's position in the continuum of drug use and abuse. It now is agreed generally that this continuum includes the follow-ing stages: (1) vulnerability and, for a variety of reasons, a high likelihood of experimentation and dependence on drugs[19]; (2) experimentation and knowledge of the effect of drugs on mood; (3) regular use to achieve a euphoric effect; 4) preoccupation with the drugs and the euphoria they produce, multiple drug use, and early dependence; and (5) chemical dependency with severe physical and psychologic consequences of abuse.

Anticipatory counseling of vulnerable and high-risk patients and their parents is most appropriate and useful during early childhood. A patient already involved in experimentation needs the advice of an informed and concerned adult or parent. During this early preabuse stage, a nonjudgmental but authoritative approach is most helpful. Confidential counseling often is preferred.[20] During the later stages of drug abuse, firm intervention is in order. Confidentiality is of less concern, and consultation and referral to a mental health professional, a specialist in addiction medicine, or a drug abuse program is almost always necessary.

It is not the role of the primary care physician to judge or condemn. However, as an important adult in the child's or adolescent's life, as a professional with special knowledge and skill, and as someone who is genuinely concerned about the health and welfare of patients, the primary care physician has a responsibility to provide authoritative information and advice. The physician must be willing to intervene, no matter how unpleasant, time consuming, and difficult the intervention may be.

The physician's reaction to the adolescent's answers when questioned regarding drug use in large part will determine the validity of future responses. If the physician reacts with anger, disgust, dismay, or disapproval, it is unlikely that further interviews will be of any value. If information can be dispensed from physician to patient without conveying alarm, disappointment, or condescension, it is likely that the adolescent will be truthful when queried about his or her drug use. Often, adolescents are eager to have a relationship with a knowledgeable adult with whom to discuss drug use. The primary care physician is an ideal person to fulfill such a role.

The adolescent who is not using drugs should be commended and encouraged to continue avoiding them. When a positive drug history is confirmed, the physician should determine the extent to which drug use interferes with the adolescent's life as well as that of the family. It is risky to attribute the early signs of drug abuse to normal adolescent experimentation and risk taking. Adolescents who use alcohol or marijuana only occasionally and who are not having problems or showing evidence of disruptive behavior should be alerted to associated risks, including motor vehicle crashes, injuries, sexual assault, unplanned pregnancy, sexually transmitted disease, and the potential for future problems. For adolescents who are driving or dating, the physician may suggest that they consider what to do if they become intoxicated away from home or are passengers in a car to be driven by someone who is intoxicated. National efforts and resources to curb such activity should be brought to the attention of the family (Appendix 1).

If drug abuse continues despite adverse physical, psychologic, or social consequences, the physician should intervene. At this point, the adolescent has relinquished the right to confidentiality because of the risk to self or others (see *Confidentiality*, p 33). The intervention may include individual and family counseling by the primary care physician, consultation with a mental health professional skilled and experienced in caring for pediatric and adolescent patients, or referral to a substance abuse specialist or program[21] (see Table 2.3 and Chapter 5). Sometimes, the physician will need the help of the juvenile court or the police to protect the patient, the family, and others.

Certain children and adolescents are at higher risk of abusing drugs than are others. Predictors of substance abuse include peer and family use of alcohol, tobacco, and other drugs; inadequate knowledge of negative consequences and a belief that substance abuse is normal; personality factors and temperament, especially low self-esteem; antisocial behavior and poor academic performance; and a family history of alcoholism, substance abuse, and affective disorders[19] (see Chapter 1). An important task for the primary care physician is to identify patients who have such risk factors. The identification of preexisting or coexisting mental disorders is an important consideration when dealing with substance abuse, because the use of drugs may precipitate psychiatric symptoms, mimic or mask primary psychiatric symptoms, or ameliorate or relieve such symptoms.[22] An underlying psychiatric disorder should be suspected when there is early use of drugs and a family history of chemical dependence and psychiatric disorders. When substance abuse and a psychiatric disorder coexist, optimal management should include the services of a child-adolescent psychologist or psychiatrist.

table 2.3 **Criteria for Treatment and Referral of the Adolescent Involved With Substance Abuse***

Follow-up by the primary care physician
- Primary care physician knowledgeable in these areas
- Drug use intermittent, experimental, and not unusual for age and sociocultural group
- No significant psychopathologic problems
- Function in educational, social, or vocational sphere unimpaired
- Reasonable progress in developmental tasks
- No antisocial behavior

Referral to specialist or outpatient program
- Lack of experience or uncertainty on part of the primary care physician
- Significant drug abuse (frequent or regular, major life concern)
- Psychopathologic problems requiring evaluation and care
- Impaired function in educational, social, legal, or vocational sphere
- In certain instances (eg, when a specialized unit is available), evaluate on an inpatient basis

Referral to intensive inpatient or outpatient drug treatment program
- Compulsive drug abuse
- Impaired function in educational, social, legal, or vocational sphere
- Imminent danger to physical or mental health of patient
- Persistent antisocial behavior
- Outpatient treatment unsuccessful
- Psychopathologic problems requiring behavior control, medication, or both

*Adapted with permission from Millman RB. Treatment and modalities. In: Litt IF, ed. *Adolescent Substance Abuse: Report of the 14th Ross Roundtable on Critical Approaches to Common Pediatric Problems.* Columbus, OH: Ross Laboratories; 1983:63-64.

Patients who have medical complications resulting from their drug abuse or who have coexisting chronic medical conditions should be given special consideration. Likewise, pregnant adolescents and young adults deserve special counseling. All pregnant adolescents should be asked about their use of tobacco, alcohol, and drugs. Pregnant adolescents should be informed about the potential consequences to their offspring.[23] Many adolescents who are unconcerned about the effects of drugs on their own health will respond to counseling when warned about the potential ill effects on the unborn infant.

Intervention and Treatment

Most experimental and occasional use of drugs, particularly tobacco, alcohol, and marijuana, can be managed by the primary care physician (Table 2.3). Although the potential for detrimental effects of such substances to the development of the maturing person should not be minimized, most acute consequences of their use can and at times must be treated without referral or consultation. Minor patients should be reminded that the use of alcohol and marijuana and the purchase of alcohol, tobacco products, and other drugs are illegal.

The adolescent who abuses substances may first receive medical attention as a result of trauma related to intoxication, an acute drug overdose, medical complications of drug abuse (such as cellulitis or hepatitis), or withdrawal symptoms. The physician has a responsibility not only to treat the trauma, acute physiologic compromise, or complication of substance abuse but also to recognize and assess the extent to which drug abuse, episodic or chronic, has led to the circumstance that mandated medical attention. Such recognition and assessment is a prerequisite to a determination of the need for in-office counseling or referral for treatment. It is important to recognize the increased likelihood of drug abuse by adolescents who are depressed, anxious, or suicidal. The skills of the physician for treating the presenting complaint influence subsequent success in addressing underlying issues of substance abuse.

Consultation and Referral

Any use of drugs by a child or adolescent has the potential for serious untoward consequences, but not all drug use necessarily indicates a disturbed youth or one in need of consultation or referral. All drug using children and adolescents deserve a primary care physician who is willing to counsel them about drug use.

Young people who experience major disruptions in their lives as a result of drug abuse need consultation with a mental health, adolescent, or addiction specialist. Those who have had a near tragedy, such as an overdose or serious injury, those who have had a drug overdose associated with a suicide attempt, and those who have caused significant family turmoil should be considered for referral to a substance abuse treatment program (see Chapter 5).

Children, and especially adolescents, usually resist consultation with a psychiatrist or psychologist, and referral to a treatment center almost always is met with anger and opposition. The patient's family is not always convinced of the need for intervention and often shares with the patient a denial that a problem exists and even a rejection of conventional values about drug use. Many adolescents (and sometimes their families) adopt an arrogant or abusive attitude toward the physician who recommends formal treatment. The physician must avoid being critical or judgmental and not take on an adversarial role. Although coercion is indicated in life-threatening situations, it should be reserved for patients and families who have not responded to more positive approaches.

Primary care physicians should become familiar with the treatment programs available in their communities and develop a relationship with at least one such facility so that smooth referrals can be made on a regular basis. It is important that treatment programs recognize the patient's cultural strengths, values, and experiences while encouraging behavioral and attitudinal changes.[24] After referral, the primary care physician should monitor the patients' progress and maintain contact with the adolescent and family. Follow-up not only provides the opportunity to continue to learn about substance abuse treatment programs but also gives the distinct message to the family that the primary care physician cares about the patient and family, despite disapproval of the adolescent's drug practices and behaviors.

Family Support

Primary care physicians recognize their responsibility to the family. At least 3 issues must be faced with respect to the family: (1) confidentiality, (2) the family "problem," and (3) prevention and intervention.

Confidentiality

To obtain a reliable drug history, the primary care physician must assure the adolescent patient of qualified confidentiality (see Chapter 7).[20] This confidentiality must be respected unless the adolescent's immediate health and welfare are at stake or the adolescent's life or that of another person is at risk. One could argue that any alcohol or drug use by an adolescent automatically carries the threat of serious harm or even death. Each physician must make that judgment on the basis of the age of the patient, the amount and nature of the drug use, the particular family involved, and other available information. The adolescent who is in the later stages of drug abuse and is dependent on drugs is obviously in immediate danger, and confidentiality is no longer an issue. Clearly, the patient suffering serious negative consequences of substance abuse has relinquished the right to confidentiality and should no longer be provided confidential care. Confidentiality is also less applicable for the child and cognitively or judgmentally immature preadolescent or early adolescent, even when there is little substance abuse.

Drug Use as a Family Problem

Children and adolescents of the 1960s and 1970s are now parents. A reasonable question asked by modern parents is: "How do I tell my children to 'say no to drugs' when in the 1960s, I said, 'yes'?" This should be asked in the context of the knowledge they gleaned from their experiences and the desire to avoid such problems for their children. Although parents may no longer be using drugs, permissive attitudes about substance abuse may persist and be discerned by children. It is possible, even likely, that the adolescent who is using alcohol or drugs is part of a family whose members also use such substances. This possibility may be explored with the adolescent, with the parents, or with the family as a whole. It must be done in a nonjudgmental, open, sincere, and compassionate manner. Parents with a drinking problem often will do nothing about it until they see the same problem in their offspring. To help their children, they may be willing to reveal their secrets and seek help for themselves.

Prevention and Intervention

Parents are obligated to discuss the use of alcohol, tobacco, and other drugs with their children. Children and adolescents should have no doubts about where their parents stand on the issue. Unfortunately, many parents condone and even encourage the use of legal (for them) drugs, such as alcohol, tobacco, and prescription or over-the-counter drugs. Some, surprisingly, also condone the use of what they consider harmless illicit drugs, such as marijuana. Their attitudes about drug use cannot be kept secret from their children, but more importantly, their behavior—drinking, smoking, and drug use and abuse—is obvious to their offspring. Like it or not, parents teach by example; children rarely do what parents tell them to do but almost always do what their parents do.

Early in the relationship with the family, primary care physicians can begin to counsel parents about the effects of parental attitudes and behavior on children. There is a risk that parents will interpret the physician's attempts to open such a discussion as prying or meddling in their private affairs. This risk of misunderstanding and unpleasantness should not deter the physician from embarking on this important line of questioning and counseling. On the contrary, many parents welcome the physician's moral support when trying to make changes in their own lives and when attempting to broach this difficult area of discussion with their children. This support is needed especially by parents who have a dependency problem themselves, by those already alienated from their children, and by single parents, including noncustodial parents.

Parents too often delay seeking help for disruptive behaviors associated with substance abuse until the problem has escalated to a critical level. They firmly try to keep the problem within the family, hoping it will improve or go away. By the time the physician is confronted with the problem, the child and family may already be suffering the devastating effects of substance abuse on family life. Often, the child is failing in school, disobeys parents, has dropped out of usual activities, breaks curfews, and in general, creates total chaos at home. Parents fear that they have lost control, are concerned for their child's safety and well-being and about the example being set for their other children, and are sure that their child will leave home if they use more punitive measures. They are wary about sharing their concerns with teachers for fear that this sensitive information will not be kept confidential, and they worry that their disclosures will adversely affect their child's standing at school. They fear involving juvenile authorities and are terrified that their child may be taken from them. They fear for their child's future and even fear the child's death. Above all, they fear that they are losing their child's love, that their anger will make matters worse, and that they will lose their child forever. Finally, they delay seeking help from their family physician because of fear, denial, and also embarrassment, because they believe they have failed as parents. There should be no doubt that the primary care physician has a critical role in the support and guidance of parents and other family members through this trying period of their lives.

When the child or adolescent must be referred to a drug treatment program, the parents will need additional encouragement and support. Frequent contact by phone and in person may be necessary. Fears about sending the adolescent to a residential treatment program may need to be allayed if, in fact, such fears are not well founded. It is best to focus on what drug use has done to the adolescent and how it has affected his or her behavior rather than to try to explain why the problem has developed and how it has evolved. By temporarily focusing on the "here and now" and the child's need for help, the primary care physician can help overcome the denial of 1 or both parents. This early focus on what drugs have done to the child often will give parents the courage to follow through with the referral and will help relieve the guilt that is almost always experienced. In all cases, the physician should not withdraw from the situation but rather should continue to help the family see clearly what is needed and help them follow through on recommendations. Withdrawal from the clinical situation, unfortunately, often is perceived by the parents as abandonment by the physician.

Education

Primary care physicians devote a major part of their daily activities to educating patients and families. Education is a vital component of providing medical care. Like other areas of medical care, the physician has an important role in educating patients and families about the hazards of alcohol, tobacco, and other drugs of abuse. This role may be fulfilled in many ways. In addition to 1-on-1 encounters with patients and families, the primary care physician can schedule group sessions for children, adolescents, and parents and other family members. Group encounters are an efficient way to accomplish anticipatory guidance and to educate a large number of people at one time. The use of posters in the waiting area and examining room not only provides important health messages but also tells the patient and parents that substance abuse is a topic the physician is willing to discuss. Brochures are helpful but should be personalized if possible and always viewed by the physician before distribution to patients. The primary care physician also has a role in the community as a health educator and advisor about drug and alcohol use. The physician often is viewed as an authority in matters related to substance abuse, and the physician's opinion is highly regarded by members of the community.

Community Action

Beyond the traditional role of physicians in providing direct care to young people and their families is the opportunity to participate in school and community health initiatives. Although such activities may be less personal than a physician-patient relationship, they offer the opportunity to influence the well-being of a large number of children, adolescents, and their families. Moreover, physicians involved in these programs gain from the sharing of perspectives among educators, clergy, government officials, the judiciary system, concerned parents, and other health professionals. Pooled knowledge and shared perspectives most often result in a more worthwhile initiative and increased benefits to the young people served. In a complex area such as substance abuse in which education and ethics, legislation and law enforcement, and family values and actions are as important as or more important than medical concerns, community-based health intervention is improved greatly through physician involvement.

Advocacy Roles and Opportunities

Although physicians have many opportunities to assume advocacy roles within their communities, such participation generally has remained at a relatively low level. A first step toward involvement is the identification of individuals or groups, such as the following, already addressing issues of substance abuse. Many such nonprofessional self-help and advocacy groups have achieved national prominence (Appendix 1).

Medical societies

Most national and regional medical and specialty societies have substance abuse committees or youth and adolescent committees. Whether dedicated specifically to substance abuse or to a broader range of health problems, these groups may provide a variety of opportunities for involvement. Included within their activities may be education programs for physicians or the public, consultation with other community agencies, local legislative action, and opportunities to influence the policies and practices of the national parent organization. Such committees would welcome the participation of interested physicians (Appendix 2).

Local schools

Perhaps the widest range of opportunities for physician involvement exists in participation in school-related activities. Local school boards often welcome assistance with the formulation of drug abuse policies and curricula. Meetings of the school board provide a forum for expressing concern and offering direction. Beyond such informal opportunities, it is not uncommon for physicians to be appointed to school committees addressing drug abuse curricula or policy issues. State law may mandate physician representation on such committees.

Local parent-teacher organizations have by and large maintained an active posture about issues related to adolescent substance abuse. Their activities have included educational programs for parents and students and initiatives designed to prevent or delay drug use or to minimize the consequences of such use.

Local governments

Most localities have health advisory boards or have created committees or umbrella agencies to address issues of substance abuse. The statute that created these agencies often requires physician membership. The structure, functions, and names of such agencies may differ. Some agencies are purely advisory; however, many control the expenditure of governmental funds or receive funding with which to initiate programs and projects.

Citizen-parent action groups

Particular to the area of adolescent drug abuse prevention efforts has been the emergence of a multitude of community-based initiatives. Independent of professional or governmental affiliation, such groups usually comprise and are led by concerned parents. These local groups are often part of a national network, but a variety of independent initiatives may be found in any locality.

Conclusion

Despite many not having the time, knowledge, or skills to treat the more seriously drug-involved adolescent, primary care physicians can have a critical role in addressing issues of substance abuse among adolescents. Through anticipatory guidance, the emergence of drug abuse problems may be prevented or minimized. Most often, the primary care physician is the only health care professional who is in a position to recognize problems of drug abuse as they evolve and is the clinician most likely to be called to treat the acute consequences of drug use. The longitudinal relationship with the child or adolescent and the family is an asset not only in the referral process but also for offering support throughout the process of evaluation and treatment. Finally, as an educator and a facilitator of community action, the primary care physician has the opportunity to exert influence on issues of drug abuse beyond the confines of the practice setting or the individual physician-patient relationship.

References

1. American Academy of Pediatrics. *Periodic Survey of Fellows No. 19: Substance Abuse Among Colleagues and Patients: Pediatricians' Views, Patient Identification, and Educational Needs.* Elk Grove Village, IL: American Academy of Pediatrics; 1993
2. Comerci GD. Office assessment of substance abuse and addiction. *Adolesc Med.* 1993;4:277-293
3. Fleming M, Barry K, Davis A, et al. Medical education about substance abuse: changes in curriculum and faculty between 1976 and 1992. *Acad Med.* 1994;69:362-369
4. Adger H, McDonald EM, DeAngellis C. Substance abuse education in pediatrics. *Pediatrics.* 1990;86:555-560
5. Bergmann MA, Smith MB, Hoffmann NG. Adolescent treatment: implications for assessment, practice guidelines, and outcome management. *Pediatr Clin North Am.* 1995;42:453-472
6. American Academy of Pediatrics, Committee on Substance Abuse. Tobacco, alcohol, and other drugs: the role of the pediatrician in prevention and management of substance abuse. *Pediatrics.* 1998;101:125-128
7. Green M, ed. *Bright Futures: Guidelines for Health Supervision of Infants, Children, and Adolescents.* Arlington, VA: National Center for Education in Maternal and Child Health; 1994

8. American Medical Association. *AMA Guidelines for Adolescent Preventive Services (GAPS)*. Elster AB, Kuznets NJ, eds. Baltimore, MD: Williams & Wilkins; 1994

9. Comerci GD, Schwebel R. Substance abuse: an overview. *Adolesc Med.* 2000;11:79-101

10. Johnston LD, O'Malley PM, Bachman JG. *National Survey Results on Drug Use From the Monitoring the Future Study, 1975-1997. Volume I: Secondary School Students.* Rockville, MD: National Institute on Drug Abuse; 1998. NIH Publication No. 98-4345

11. O'Malley PM, Johnston LD, Bachman JG. Adolescent substance use: epidemiology and implications for public policy. *Pediatr Clin North Am.* 1995;42:241-260

12. Comerci GD. Office assessment and brief intervention with the adolescent suspected of substance abuse. In: Graham AW, Schultz TK, eds. *Principles of Addiction Medicine.* 2nd ed. Washington, DC: American Society of Addiction Medicine; 1998:1145-1151

13. Cohen E, MacKenzie RG, Yates GL. HEADSS, a psychosocial risk assessment instrument: implications for designing effective intervention programs for runaway youth. *J Adolesc Health.* 1991;12:539-544

14. Bell DL, Ragin DF, Cohall A. Cross-cultural issues in prevention, health promotion, and risk reduction in adolescence. *Adolesc Med.* 1999;10:57-69

15. American Academy of Pediatrics, Committee on Substance Abuse. Testing for drugs of abuse in children and adolescents. *Pediatrics.* 1996;98:305-307

16. American Academy of Pediatrics, Committee on Bioethics. Informed consent, parental permission and assent in pediatric practice. *Pediatrics.* 1995;95:314-317

17. *Vernonia School District 47 J v Acton,* 94-590 Sct (9th Circ 1995)

18. Substance Abuse and Mental Health Services Administration, Office of Applied Studies. *Preliminary Results from the 1997 National Household Survey on Drug Abuse.* Rockville, MD: US Department of Health and Human Services; 1998

19. Werner MJ. *Adolescent Substance Abuse Risk Factors and Prevention Strategies.* Washington, DC: Maternal and Child Health Bureau and National Center for Education in Maternal and Child Health, US Dept of Health and Human Services; 1991

20. American Academy of Pediatrics. Confidentiality in adolescent health care. *AAP News.* April 1989. Available at: http://www.aap.org/policy/104.html. Accessed April 27, 2001

21. American Society of Addiction Medicine. *Patient Placement Criteria for the Treatment of Psychoactive Substance Use Disorders.* Washington, DC: American Society of Addiction Medicine; 1991

22. Armentano ME. Assessment, diagnosis, and treatment of the dually diagnosed adolescent. *Pediatr Clin North Am.* 1995;42:479-490

23. American Academy of Pediatrics, Committee on Substance Abuse. Drug-exposed infants. *Pediatrics.* 1995;96:364-367

24. Substance Abuse and Mental Health Services Administration, Center for Substance Abuse Treatment. *Cultural Issues in Substance Abuse Treatment.* Rockville, MD: US Department of Health and Human Services; 1999. DHHS Publication No. SMA 99-3278

Chapter 3

Evaluation by Interview and Questionnaire

Trina Menden Anglin, MD, PhD, FAAP*

Evaluation by Interview and Questionnaire

The clinical interview remains the standard of practice in the primary care setting for assessing adolescent patients' use of substances. However, many structured questionnaires and interview instruments have been developed or adapted for adolescents in clinical settings and show promise as objective and efficient tools for documenting the nature and extent of adolescent patients' involvement with drugs and alcohol. The field of addiction medicine is moving toward the use of formal assessment instruments to standardize patient diagnoses among health care professionals, determine severity of patients' addiction, and match treatment to need.[1] This chapter presents balanced descriptions of interviewing strategies for clinical screening and for more detailed evaluation of adolescent substance use as well as the clinical use of structured questionnaires and interviews for screening and assessment; discusses recommended content; develops a scheme by which the health care professional can synthesize data and formulate a conclusion about an adolescent's probable depth of involvement with substances; and provides guidance for discussing substance use problems with adolescents and their parents and conducting brief motivational interventions.

---

*This chapter is based on the article, "Interviewing Guidelines for the Clinical Evaluation of Adolescent Substance Abuse," from *Pediatric Clinics of North America* 1987;34:381-398. Permission to adapt and update this article for publication as a chapter in this book has been granted by WB Saunders Company, Philadelphia, PA. The opinions expressed in this chapter are the author's and do not necessarily represent the views or policies of the Health Resources and Services Administration, US Department of Health and Human Services.

Context of Evaluation

Given the high prevalence of tobacco, alcohol, and illicit drug use by contemporary adolescents, it is recommended that all adolescents be screened for substance use and abuse as part of every visit for clinical preventive services.[2-4] (The US Preventive Services Task Force recommended that all adolescents be screened for problem drinking using a routine interview or standardized questionnaire but was less forceful in its recommendation regarding routine clinical screening for drug abuse.[5] It stated that there is insufficient evidence to recommend for or against routine screening for drug abuse using standardized questionnaires. On the basis of the high prevalence of drug use and the serious nature of the consequences of drug abuse and dependence, the Task Force recommended, however, that questions about drug use be included as part of the medical history. In addition, the Task Force recommended that all adolescents be counseled to avoid underage drinking and illicit drug use.) Clinical preventive services encounters include examinations for school and camp, preparticipation sports evaluations, preemployment examinations, and for females, assessment for contraception. All adolescents, including those well-known to the health care professional since childhood, deserve periodic reassessment of their psychosocial development and functioning (see Chapter 2).

Screening for substance use and abuse should be placed in the context of assessing an adolescent's general health status and psychosocial well-being. Certain populations of adolescents may have heightened vulnerability to substance use and abuse. For example, adolescents who are gay, lesbian, or bisexual are at higher risk of substance use as part of a set of responses to such serious stressors as social isolation, stigmatization, and hate crimes.[6] Adolescents with chronic diseases, such as diabetes mellitus, cystic fibrosis, and sickle cell disease, have significant risks of using tobacco, alcohol, and marijuana even though their use rates are somewhat lower than those of their healthy peers.[7] It is not clear whether adolescents with serious visual or hearing impairment have different risk levels for substance abuse compared with the general

population of adolescents.[8] Adolescents at risk of human immunodeficiency virus infection are at high risk of substance abuse
problems.[9] In addition, adolescents who have a substance abuse
disorder are also more likely to suffer from other psychiatric
disorders, including such problems as conduct disorder, attention-
deficit/hyperactivity disorder, major depressive disorder, bipolar
disorder, anxiety disorder, and bulimia (see Chapter 11).[10-12]
Finally, adolescents and young adults with major disabilities
incurred from trauma, such as spinal cord injury and traumatic
brain injury, are at high risk of substance abuse; intoxication may
have contributed to causing the injury.[8] Clinical circumstances for
which adolescents should be carefully screened for use and abuse
of substances are listed in Table 3.1.

Although it can be fairly simple to identify adolescents with
serious substance use disorders, it can be challenging to identify
adolescents whose problems are subtle or who have not experienced significant adverse consequences. Early identification of
youth with substance use problems should help to target timely
and appropriate intervention.[13] One objective of this chapter is to
enhance the health care professional's ability to detect adolescents
who are having substance use problems before serious impairment
develops.

---

table 3.1 **Clinical Circumstances and Problems Meriting
Evaluation for Substance Use and Abuse**

- Physical symptoms outlined in Chapter 2
- Mental health symptoms and problems outlined in Chapter 11
- Evaluation for deteriorating school performance
- Evaluation for behavioral problems (eg, school truancy, fighting, running away,
  property destruction, stealing, lying, attending all-night parties)
- Entry into mental health care
- Intake into juvenile justice system
- Trauma (eg, vehicle, boat, falls, near drowning, burns, sexual assault)
- Emergency department visit (eg, for intoxication or suicide attempt)
- Any use by children younger than 11 years

Interviewing Process

General Interviewing Techniques

Assessing adolescents for substance use and abuse should be based on the principles of the general adolescent health interview. Although the health care professional's immediate goal is to collect accurate information, the interview also promotes the understanding of each adolescent as an individual, building of the adolescent's and family's trust, and enhancement of the adolescent's and family's compliance with any plans for further evaluation, treatment, and behavioral change. The development of a therapeutic alliance, or rapport, between health care professional and adolescent is essential to the task of gathering accurate and comprehensive information. The health care professional's style and behavior during the clinical encounter is a very important factor influencing the success of the visit.[14] Even health care professionals who incorporate a structured questionnaire into their evaluation protocol of adolescent patients' health status need to use the principles of interviewing.

Every interview has a structure. It includes an introduction or beginning; this important opening phase sets the stage for the remainder of the encounter, helps to establish rapport, and influences how successfully the health care professional can complete the visit's agenda. The middle of the interview defines the history; it is largely concerned with data gathering. The end or conclusion of the interview, which usually follows the physical examination, provides closure for the visit and looks toward the future; it includes a summation of the visit's content and process, health counseling, opportunities for discussion, and formulation of plans for further evaluation and management.[15]

Table 3.2 suggests general interviewing techniques. Consideration of the following points will help the interview's process flow smoothly. Think of the interview as a directed, patient-centered conversation rather than as an interrogation. Do not barrage the adolescent with questions. As much as possible, questions should be phrased open-endedly, which encourages the adolescent to respond in sentences or phrases. Do not ask questions that provide negative expectations of response (for example, "You don't drink and drive, do you?"). The adolescent's answers, comments, and questions should dominate the interview time. A health care professional experienced in interviewing adolescents can flexibly guide the interview tempo and topic sequence.

At the beginning of the visit, let the adolescent and parents know what to expect. Establish the procedure of the visit to help prepare them for the procedure of interviewing and examining the adolescent alone, interviewing the parents privately, and interviewing the family as a small group. The sequence of these steps may vary on the basis of familial dynamics and the health care professional's usual practice.

Occasionally, worried parents may use pretense in scheduling an appointment for evaluation of an adolescent's substance use. For example, the patient may believe that the appointment's purpose is for evaluation of recurrent knee symptoms and is unaware that the parents had privately requested the health care professional

table 3.2 **Suggesting Interviewing Techniques**

- Interview the adolescent privately.

- Discuss the parameters of confidentiality.

- Avoid parental subterfuge.

- Ask open-ended questions. Do not ask questions that provide negative expectations of response that can be construed as "setups" or that can heighten a patient's defensiveness.

- Do not barrage the adolescent with questions.

- Do not lecture or moralize.

- Be sensitive to the adolescent's responsiveness to your style and to specific questions. Determine what types of information the adolescent would like to learn or verify, and then provide it.

- If the adolescent has no questions, offer information that is developmentally appropriate using the technique of generalization.

Adapted with permission from *Current Pediatric Diagnosis and Treatment.* Hay WW Jr, Groothius JR, Hayward AR, Levin MJ, eds. 13th ed. Stamford, CT: Appleton & Lange; 1997:161

to address the more sensitive issue of the adolescent's heavy drinking every weekend. The health care professional should avoid involvement in such subterfuge and ask the parents to share their concerns with the adolescent before the visit. It is important for the health care professional to be honest with the parents and the adolescent; the health care professional needs to disclose gently the parents' concerns to the adolescent and inform the parents of the need to discuss their concerns with the adolescent. The health care professional can often bring about more effective and constructive communication between parents and adolescent as part of the resolution of this clinical circumstance (see Chapter 2).

Demonstrate respect by encouraging the adolescent to tell his or her side of the story and by allowing the adolescent to have a sense of control over the process of the visit. For example, if a cooperative adolescent demonstrates discomfort with a particular topic, the health care professional can briefly empathize with the adolescent's feelings and state, "We can return to this topic a little later." Another technique is to allow the adolescent to choose to have private time with the health care professional first or have the parents go first. Pay attention to the adolescent's verbal and nonverbal messages. How comfortable is the patient with a topic? Is interview fatigue developing? The health care professional can enhance the accuracy of data collection by discussing positive, not just problematic, issues; by discussing less sensitive topics first; and by creating a context for sensitive question sets. For example, the health care professional could preface a series of questions about alcohol use with the statement, "It is medically important to know about your drinking, because alcohol can sometimes injure the lining of the stomach and cause pain similar to yours." To confirm that the health care professional's understanding recognizes the adolescent's and the parents' perspectives, it is wise to restate and summarize key responses.

Confidentiality of Information Disclosed by the Adolescent
It is important to discuss the parameters of confidentiality with adolescents and their parents. Health care professionals may want

to view their relationships with adolescent patients and their parents as all being members of the same team with the mutual goal of guiding the adolescent toward a healthy adulthood. Adolescents often spontaneously give their consent for the health care professional to share information with their parents, which demonstrates maturity and trust. However, confidentiality of patient care and protection of a patient's privacy are maxims of adolescent health care for the following reasons: adolescents are more willing to share sensitive information more accurately if they know it will remain confidential, adolescents can be encouraged to seek care for sensitive issues that can jeopardize their own health or the health of others, adolescents can be shielded from the discrimination or humiliation that could result from nonconfidential disclosure, and honoring adolescents' confidentiality and privacy supports the development of their autonomy as they move toward adulthood.[16]

Health care professionals generally honor adolescent patients' requests for confidentiality unless there is concern that the adolescent is engaging in life-jeopardizing or serious health-compromising behavior. Substance use can clearly endanger an adolescent's health and safety. Most health care professionals would agree that parents need to be included in the process if an adolescent is experiencing serious behavioral dysfunction from substance use or if referral to a treatment program is necessary. However, state laws vary regarding need for parental consent for treatment. Statutes of almost all states permit minors to consent to outpatient counseling for drug and alcohol abuse, but more than half of states have placed various limitations on minors' ability to consent, which include age restrictions and mandated physician notification of parents (see Chapter 7).[16] In practice, the need for financial reimbursement for treatment services often necessitates parental involvement.

It is always the health care professional's decision whether parents should be informed of their adolescent's harmful involvement with substances and at what point the parents should be informed. However, once this decision is made, the health care professional should involve the adolescent in deciding how the parents will be informed. One approach is to have the adolescent patient decide to tell his or her parents or to have the health care professional tell them and decide whether the other party will remain in the room during the discussion with the parents. Self-disclosure guided by the health care professional may help an adolescent retain self-respect and may also strengthen familial bonds. Regardless of whether the adolescent or health care professional serves as primary spokesperson to the parents, the visit should conclude with a family discussion to ensure that the parents and the adolescent have a full understanding of the situation and hear the same messages together and to determine what the next steps should be.

Although this chapter appears to discuss the evaluation of a substance-abusing adolescent as being able to take place during a single visit, formal assessment often requires more than 1 planned encounter. However, screening for involvement with alcohol and drugs should take place during 1 visit. Even though defined visit time may be devoted to a formal assessment, in reality, the evaluation of substance use by an adolescent is an evolving process that should be addressed throughout a patient's tenure with a health care professional. A variety of time management approaches may be used for formal assessment. Some health care professionals routinely schedule separate appointments for the parents and the adolescent and use a third appointment for a group meeting to summarize the findings and plan next stages. It may take a health care professional more than 1 encounter to develop a sufficiently strong relationship with a patient to be able to obtain meaningful information. Substance-abusing adolescents commonly have many problems that need to be addressed and that may compete for clinical priority with (or even override the clinical priority of) comprehensive assessment of the substance abuse (eg, new diagnosis of pregnancy, serious acute physical trauma, sexual assault, running away from home, attempted suicide). The time and effort spent in addressing these other issues may help forge a therapeutic alliance between adolescent and health care professional so that a more formal assessment of substance use is conducted in an atmosphere of trust and respect and may enhance investment in the adolescent's well-being.

Many health care professionals' practices have time constraints that permit them to screen adolescent patients for substance use problems but not to perform more detailed assessments. These health care professionals need time-efficient strategies to screen their adolescent patients for substance use and abuse. This chapter also considers instruments that can help quickly to determine that an adolescent potentially has a substance abuse problem and deserves referral for comprehensive assessment.

Strategies for Interviewing Adolescents for Substance Abuse

Most adolescents who seek health and medical care, including those who abuse drugs and alcohol, are pleasant and cooperative. However, substance-abusing adolescents often attempt to conceal the extent of their involvement, especially if interviewed in the presence of their parents.[17] It is unlikely that they will spontaneously introduce the topic of alcohol and drug use, because they do not perceive it as problem that needs to be addressed.[14] They may use different defenses if they feel that their use is threatened. These behaviors are not directed personally at the health care professional. It is important to recognize and outwardly acknowledge these behaviors as protective strategies before returning the interview to its course. Frightened or anxious adolescents may appear silent and noncommunicative. Angry adolescents have commonly been brought to the health care professional against their will and may behave defiantly. The health care professional can often diffuse this behavior by validating the patient's feelings and describing them in a friendly but firm way. For example: "You seem quite upset and unhappy about coming here today. I can understand your not wanting to come." The health care professional can positively acknowledge the patient's keeping the appointment in recognition of its importance and can state that the primary goal of the visit is to help the patient and health care professional to achieve an accurate and thorough understanding of the nature of the patient's involvement with drugs and alcohol; it is not to coerce the patient into doing anything against his or her will. Angry adolescents may also use profanity or vulgar language to express themselves or to attempt to disconcert the interviewer. Calmly accepting the language by acknowledging its use is an appropriate response.

Adolescents who abuse substances may also attempt to divert attention from themselves. One tactic is to disclose another family member's problem behavior, such as physical abuse or drinking. This information is obviously valuable for the clinical evaluation. However, for the time being, it should remain tangential to the interviewer's focus. It is appropriate to acknowledge receiving the information by saying, "I can understanding your being concerned about that. Let's talk about it a little later. Right now, however, I need to ask you . . ."

Adolescents who abuse substances may minimize their involvement or distort factual information, and their parents may perceive them as liars. These behaviors are strategies that help the adolescent maintain the pattern of use. Adolescents may appear glib, verbally facile, charming, and obsequious. Such behavior may conceal a disdain for authority and indicate a belief that it is possible to deceive or manipulate adults and get away with substance abuse and even illegal behaviors; these adolescents may have a comorbid conduct disorder.

It is important to let the adolescent know that attempts to mislead or even delude the health care professional will not succeed. During an initial assessment, however, direct confrontation is usually counterproductive. For example, if the adolescent presents obviously inconsistent information, the health care professional might say, "That doesn't make sense. Earlier you said that . . . Now you are telling me . . . It just doesn't add up." Attempts to mislead the interviewer should be entered into the assessment record.

Occasionally, an adolescent might arrive for a health care visit in an obviously intoxicated state. It is not usually possible to obtain contextual information or to complete an assessment in this circumstance. However, the intoxicated state certainly provides documentation of a problem.

Psychosocial Assessment

A general psychosocial assessment of an adolescent provides the framework for addressing substance use. It helps determine what roles psychoactive substance use may play in the adolescent's life. Information should be gathered that will help determine whether an adolescent is at risk of abusing substances, is making satisfactory developmental progress, or has experienced any negative consequences from substance abuse. Table 3.3 outlines key areas of exploration.

Substance abuse interferes with an adolescent's developmental progress.[18] It interferes with reality testing and learning how to make sound decisions. It can exaggerate the egocentric worldview of adolescents, and on the basis of the psychoactive properties of the substances used, can make the adolescent alternate between sensations of grandeur and loss of control. Adolescents who abuse substances lose opportunities for developmental growth; fail to address their academic, environmental, and vocational responsibilities; and are not able to define work and play roles. They may isolate themselves within a subgroup that is internally cohesive but negativistic toward and incongruent with wider cultural values. Although adolescents who abuse substances may feel liberated from societal constraints, they may become more dependent on their families and society as they fail to make psychoemotional developmental progress toward responsible adulthood.

Assessment of adolescent substance abuse can be difficult for the following reasons[19]:

- Compared with adults, adolescents have a relatively short life history of substance use and have not always experienced m any negative consequences that can be directly related to it. However, they may have other problems in association with substance abuse, such as depression, anxiety, school failure, juvenile delinquency, or a history of physical or sexual abuse, that complicate the evaluation process and require simultaneous attention.

---

table 3.3 Substantive Areas of Psychosocial Assessment

- Home and family relationships (constellation, shared activities, respect for parents, organization of family's daily life, isolation, conflict, breaking of family rules, running away)

- Family history (use by parents, siblings, and relatives)

- School (performance and classroom placement, attendance, behavior, ability to concentrate and remember, involvement in sports and extracurricular activities)

- Peers (developmental appropriateness, shared activities, fighting, substance use, involvement in gang activities and gang membership, legal involvement, motor vehicle crashes and traffic citations)

- Sexual behavior (romantic involvement, use by boyfriend or girlfriend, risk of pregnancy or fatherhood and sexually transmitted diseases, number of partners, prostitution, trading sex for drugs)

- Leisure activities (fun, relaxation, preferred music and video genres, community organizations and service)

- Employment (position, schedule, disposition of earnings)

- Role of religion and faith (religiosity of parents and of adolescent, any unique beliefs associated with their religion's tenets, involvement with youth faith group activities)

- Physical health (general health and somatic concerns, symptoms of withdrawal, toxic reactions to specific drugs or alcohol, overdoses, blackouts, history of trauma and injuries, bulimic binging and purging)

- History of victimization by abuse (physical, sexual)

- Motor vehicle history (driving record, crashes and near-misses, traffic citations, boating mishaps)

- Access to weapons (family, peers, firearm ownership)

- Police and court involvement (probation status, history of illegal activities, incarceration, pattern of charges and offenses)

- Mental health (depression and moods, alienation, anxiety, hallucinations, suicidal ideation and attempts, anger, impulsivity, history of intervention and hospitalization)

- Aspirations and goals for the future (hopes and plans for beyond high school)

- Self-perception (self-liking and satisfaction with current life)

Adapted with permission from *Current Pediatric Diagnosis and Treatment.* Hay WW Jr, Groothius JR, Hayward AR, Levin MJ, eds. 13th ed. Stamford, CT: Appleton & Lange; 1997:162

- There is normative acceptance of excessive levels of alcohol and drug use among groups of substance-abusing young people, so an adolescent who consumes similar quantities will not consider the behavior abnormal or deviant.
- The psychologic, familial, and social dysfunction that commonly accompanies a substance abuse problem may have existed previously or may have been exacerbated by it. Other family members, including the parents, may themselves have substance abuse or other mental health problems and may not cooperate fully with the evaluation process or accept its conclusions.
- Most adolescents' cognitive skills are not yet fully developed. Self-definition and effective problem solving skills may be limited by an adolescent's cognitive immaturity.

Levels of Assessment for Substance Abuse

The assessment process for substance abuse can be divided into 3 levels of completeness and detail.[20] The first level is the *clinical screening*. Its goal is to help health care professionals identify patients that deserve comprehensive assessment. Clinical screening cannot establish a diagnosis or determine treatment needs. However, a screening test or procedure should be able to differentiate patients with and without a specified disease process. An initial screening test should be highly sensitive to detect patients with the disease and ideally should also be highly specific to limit the number of individuals with false-positive results who would require further assessment. It should be simple and quick and have a high rate of acceptability to patients and health care professionals.[21,22] Clinical screening for substance use and abuse should occur in the following circumstances: adolescent visits for clinical preventive services, follow-up visits for problems known to be associated with substance abuse (eg, trauma), and whenever it is important to obtain a general psychosocial profile (see Table 3.1). The second level of assessment for substance abuse is the *mid-range evaluation*. An ideal tool for this level should have a high sensitivity for detecting problems in multiple areas of functioning as it identifies the patterns of behavioral, psychologic, and physiologic conditions associated with substance abuse. It should help the health care professional to gain an in-depth understanding of the patient's problems. In addition, it should provide sufficient quality information to make accurate decisions about the scope and intensity of intervention needed.[23]

Both of these levels of assessment can be conducted by a health care professional in an office-based practice. All health care professionals who provide health and medical care to adolescents should become proficient in the clinical screening of their patients for substance use problems. Health care professionals who lack the time or who feel unprepared to conduct more comprehensive evaluations may decide to refer adolescent patients whom they suspect to have substance abuse problems for further assessment. Health care professionals who specialize in the health and medical care of adolescents and those who are particularly interested in behavioral issues should be able to perform comprehensive mid-range, or second level, assessments. The in-depth interview described in the following section is an example of a mid-range evaluation, as are 2 validated instruments, the Personal Experience Inventory (PEI)[24] and the Teen Addiction Severity Index (TASI),[25,26] which are both described later in this chapter.

The third level of assessment represents the *specialized evaluation.* It is usually conducted by a team as part of the formal intake process into a substance abuse treatment program and is not easily accomplished in its entirety by a single primary care health care professional.

Detailed Substance Use History by Interview

Sequence of Interview Process
The health care professional should discuss more general lifestyle questions before inquiring about use of substances. There are 2 important reasons for this sequence. The first is that the adolescent needs time to develop or renew a relationship with the health

care professional before being asked to discuss a sensitive subject. The second reason is that the health care professional will be able to use general psychosocial information as a database to help determine how at risk an adolescent may be for substance abuse. This information will help to determine how deeply the health care professional should probe.

One strategy that can provide order to the interview process and improve the quality of information gathered is to start with the least threatening and then move on to more sensitive topics. Use of tobacco products, including cigarettes and smokeless tobacco, is so common among adolescents in the United States that it can almost be considered normative behavior even though purchase of tobacco by minors is illegal. Questions about use of tobacco are currently considered a mildly sensitive area. Learning about use of alcohol is the next step on the continuum. Again, drinking by adolescents can almost be considered normative behavior, but the sensitivity is somewhat intensified, because the sale of alcoholic beverages to minors carries clear legal sanctions. Inquiry about marijuana is the next step. Use of this substance is considered more sensitive than use of alcohol, because marijuana is a federally illicit substance for individuals of all ages. Furthermore, adolescents' parents are far less likely to use marijuana than they are to drink alcoholic beverages. This gulf increases adult social (and therefore, societal) disapproval. The fact that, compared with alcohol use, a significantly smaller proportion of adolescents use marijuana is consistent with its decreased social acceptability and contributes to its greater sensitivity as a topic of discussion. Finally, the health care professional should ask about the use of other illicit drugs, reviewing major techniques of use (eg, taking pills, smoking, sniffing or huffing, snorting, injecting), as well as classes of drugs. In summary, this organization of the interview provides a natural order of progression, moving from the socially accepted, to the socially tolerated, to the socially disapproved, to the overtly illegal.

Initial Exploration

People who abuse substances tend to minimize their involvement with them. They commonly do not perceive or experience this behavior as problematic.[27,28] On the other hand, substance users can provide a valid history if they trust and respect the health care professional. In particular, most adolescents whose lifestyles do not revolve around substance use will provide sufficient information about their use of alcohol and drugs to allow the health care professional to complete an accurate evaluation. It is critical, however, for the health care professional to establish an appropriate atmosphere for the interview and to convey trustworthiness and sincerity. The purpose of initial exploratory inquiries is to help establish the tone for this section of the interview. During this process, the health care professional may be tested by the adolescent. If the interviewer appears to register disapproval, dismay, or condescension in reaction to initial disclosure statements, it is doubtful that the adolescent will provide accurate information about substance use. The health care professional will have failed the adolescent's test and will not be deemed trustworthy or credible. In addition, the health care professional can measure the adolescent's willingness to offer information during this exploratory phase.

Exploratory issues are phenomenologic; they address the adolescent's perceptions of how widely drugs and alcohol are accepted by and used by other adolescents. Specifically, the health care professional can inquire about the adolescent's perceptions about peer attitudes toward use of tobacco, alcohol, and drugs and can then narrow the frame of reference to the adolescent's own friends. The health care professional can next inquire about actual behavior. For example: "How large a group of students at your school are into drinking or doing drugs? If someone wanted to buy marijuana, crack, ecstasy, or uppers, how easy would it be? What happens at parties, social occasions, and clubs you have heard about or have personally attended?" This approach is less threatening, because it does not ask for information about personal involvement, yet it provides valuable information about levels of risk.

Elements of a Formal Substance Use History

The goal of this set of questions is to determine the quality and depth of the relationship the adolescent has with substances. Minimal time is needed to discuss these issues with an adolescent patient who is functioning well and who admits to little or no use of alcohol and drugs. These questions are very useful, however, when the health care professional needs to explore an adolescent's use of substances more intensively. Table 3.4 summarizes the elements of a substance use history.

The pediatric health care professional needs to be familiar with and should use colloquial street names of drugs popular in the geographic area, especially if the adolescent has limited English language skills or is developmentally unsophisticated. The health care

---

table 3.4 **Elements of a Substance Use History**

- First use: age, circumstances, feeling effects

- Past substance use patterns

- Current motivation to use (perceived benefits of use)

- Current feeling effects of use (include both pleasant and negative experiences)

- Current patterns of use (substances used, frequency, binging behavior, circumstances of use)

- Current frequency of intoxication or becoming "high"

- Tolerance (how much alcohol does it take to get high now? What about 6 months ago? A year ago?)

- Substance of choice

- Personal limits to categories of substances willing to try

- How substance is obtained

- Financial resources

- Dealing activities

- Perceptions of significant others about use (family members, peers, boyfriend or girlfriend)

Adapted with permission from *Current Pediatric Diagnosis and Treatment.* Hay WW Jr, Groothius JR, Hayward AR, Levin MJ, eds. 13th ed. Stamford, CT: Appleton & Lange; 1997:163

professional may need to ask the adolescent for assistance in grounding an unfamiliar name in a particular class of drugs.

It is less threatening to establish a historical perspective when asking an adolescent to discuss personal use of alcohol and drugs. Before addressing current use patterns, find out about the adolescent's first experiences with alcohol and with marijuana. For example: "Tell me about the first time you ever had anything to drink. What was it like? When was the first time that you ever got really high?" With these questions, the health care professional is trying to help the adolescent disclose accurate information and determine whether the adolescent is preoccupied with the experience of getting high from psychoactive substances. Although the health care professional cannot ask specific questions that directly address the latter goal, he or she can commonly document this preoccupation through the adolescent's enthusiastic descriptions of what it feels like to be high.

The pediatric health care professional should gradually move the questions forward to the present time. For example: "About how much are you drinking now compared with last fall when school started?" By identifying patterns of use, the health care professional will learn how often the adolescent uses particular substances and how much is consumed at a time. For example: "How many times did you get high in the last month?" (A 30-day time frame has proven quite useful. It is short enough to allow accurate recall but is sufficiently long to determine recent patterns of use.)

Forced multiple-choice answers are a useful strategy for adolescents who find it difficult to answer spontaneously. For example, the health care professional could provide choices as follows: "Do you use about once every month, Saturday nights only, or 3 times a week? When was the last time you got high? Are you using drugs or alcohol at school, on school nights, or only on weekends?"

It may be less threatening to determine approximate quantities of substances consumed by using the concept of tolerance rather than asking for this information directly. Increasing tolerance for specific agents is associated with increasing use. Tolerance can be addressed historically by determining how much it takes to get a little high and how much to get really high. Have the adolescent compare these amounts with what was necessary to get high 3 months, 6 months, and a year ago. However, the relevance of the concept of tolerance to the definition of substance use disorders in adolescents in not clear. Tolerance is a complex construct to measure.[29]

The health care professional should learn about the circumstances of use. Does the adolescent use substances only during parties or also when alone? Has the adolescent ever used at school? What does the adolescent gain from the experience of becoming high? Examples of possible questions that can explore this experience include the following: "What is it like to be high? Has anything really good ever happened while you've been high? What does getting high do for you?" The appetitive effects of substances serve as important motivators for individuals to continue their use once they experience pleasurable sensations.[27,28]

Another important area concerns the benefits substance use may offer the adolescent. Does intoxication relieve negative pressures and enhance the ability to relax? Adolescents who have learned to use substances for anxiety relief may be at special risk of developing more serious problems. In addition, they have not been able to learn healthy mechanisms for coping with stress or for addressing troublesome issues. A possible exploratory question is: "How do you make yourself feel better when you're really upset or nervous about something? Does drinking (or using drugs) help?"

The concept outlined above—that adolescents who use substances perceive benefits from their use—has been elaborated into a brief screening instrument. This instrument is discussed later in Perceived benefits scales (see p 72).[30,31] The 5 items that compose the empirically validated scale can be incorporated into the clinical interview by asking the adolescent how much drugs and alcohol help make it easier to relax, be friendly, be with friends who drink or do drugs, forget problems, and feel good about oneself. When used in this manner, these questions are meant to enrich clinical information and to help youngsters gain insight into their relationships with substances.

Learning how an adolescent obtains drugs and alcohol may not be possible unless a trusting relationship has developed with the health care professional. To obtain supplies, adolescents who have become substance dependent commonly resort to deviant and illegal behaviors, such as stealing, dealing, prostitution, and exchanging sex for drugs. An adolescent engaging in such activities obviously has a very serious problem (however, some sophisticated adolescent dealers may not use so that they may retain a sharp business acumen). There is an excellent chance, however, that such an adolescent will exhibit problem behavior in other areas. Even though an adolescent may vociferously deny stealing from parents, it may be this very behavior that finally forces parents to seek help. Some exploratory questions include: "How much do you spend a week on drugs? (Try to be as specific as possible, naming drugs that you know the adolescent favors.) Have you ever needed to borrow money or take something that didn't belong to you so you could get a supply? Have you ever traded sex for drugs? Have you ever gotten into trouble with the law trying to get drugs? How much do you deal?"

It is often enlightening to learn who is concerned about an adolescent's use of alcohol and drugs. The concerns of family members, friends, and romantic partners who worry that an adolescent may be using alcohol or drugs excessively are usually well placed. Heightened media coverage of drug use, however, may overly sensitize cautious parents about an adolescent's experimentation. An adolescent who abuses substances may be able to admit that a parent is anxious about the use even while minimizing or belittling the concern. It is unusual, however, for a substance-abusing adolescent to admit spontaneously that the involvement is dysfunctional even when use has caused significant problems.

Adverse Consequences

Even though adolescents who are abusing alcohol and drugs may not recognize adverse consequences associated with the abuse, health care professionals can play an important role by pointing out to the family and the adolescent that use has caused problems. The impact of associating a negative consequence with use of substances is more powerful if it occurs close to the time that the consequence occurred. For example, during recovery from the adverse effects of an overdose or acute intoxication, the adolescent and family may be more receptive to intervention. The need for an emergency department visit or hospitalization for substance-associated trauma, cardiovascular or neurologic event, behavioral aberration, or mental status impairment is a medical consequence that a health care professional should target. Such episodes can be helpful in convincing a family that a substance abuse problem exists; when people are frightened, they feel vulnerable and can be more open to offers of help. As discussed later in this chapter, such events may serve as a turning point by which addicted adolescents are able to make a causal connection between use of substances and their serious life problems.[27,28]

The health care professional should seek other common consequences associated with the use of substances by focused interview questions. Table 3.5 outlines areas that should be explored. Many of them are embedded in the psychosocial history, and positive responses to them (eg, motor vehicle trauma, fighting, multiple sexual partners), even during an earlier section of a general interview, may prompt the health care professional to consider the need for a careful assessment of an adolescent's substance use.

Brief Clinical Screening by Interview

When limited time is available, health care professionals can incorporate direct questions about use of substances into the psychosocial history (Table 3.3). These questions should be asked

table 3.5 **Exploration for Adverse Consequences of Substance Abuse***

Medical and physical

Somatic symptoms

Disturbed sleep

Blackouts

Trauma and unintentional injury

Visits to emergency department for intoxication or overdose

Psychologic

Labile mood

Anger control

Low frustration tolerance

Impulsivity and poor self-control

Depression

Anxiety

Interpersonal

Conflict with family

Loss of friends

Loss of a romantic relationship

Fighting

Impulsive sexual behavior

School, community, and safety

Motor vehicle or boat crashes and near-misses

Destruction of property

Theft

School absenteeism

Poor school performance or failure

Poor job performance or job absenteeism

Disciplinary action (arrest for driving under the influence, other legal involvement,
    school suspension, dropped from sports team)

*These common examples of consequences of substance use are embedded in the psychosocial
history.

Adapted with permission from *Current Pediatric Diagnosis and Treatment.* Hay WW Jr, Groothius JR,
Hayward AR, Levin MJ, eds. 13th ed. Stamford, CT: Appleton & Lange; 1997:165

only after less sensitive topics (eg, home, school, peer relationships, employment, community involvement, leisure activities)
have been explored. It is possible that asking these questions
abruptly and without consideration of the patient's comfort level
with the interview may increase the risk of responses that minimize use. The health care professional should frame screening
questions about substance use on the basis of information that is
readily available, such as a patient's age. For example, it would
be appropriate to ask a young adolescent about experimental use
("Have you ever . . ."), but it may be permissible to assume that
some older adolescents have already tried alcohol at least once.
Examples of questions include: "Have you ever tried drinking
beer? What about wine coolers? Have you ever tried drinking hard
liquor?" Screening questions for older adolescents and second-
level questions for younger adolescents who disclose any use of
alcohol could include: "About how often do you drink alcohol?
About when was the last time you drank any alcohol? What
is your favorite alcoholic beverage? About how much do you
drink at parties or when you go out to clubs?"

Further information about alcohol use (eg, age when first started to drink, quantities needed to feel a little high and very drunk,
and description of how it feels to be high) can be obtained in a
conversational manner from patients who give positive responses.

Screening questions about marijuana use should follow. The
health care professional should then inquire about any experiences
with other drugs that have lower prevalence of use.

Formal clinical screening instruments (outlined in the next
section) are contrasting approaches that attempt to determine
whether an adolescent patient is at risk of a substance use problem or disorder by asking indirect questions. It is possible to
blend these 2 approaches so that adolescents who respond affir-
matively to the indirect questions of a formal screening instrument can be asked about their patterns of use. Use of these 2
approaches together may strengthen the health care professional's
ability to discern which adolescent patients need comprehensive
assessments.

The health care professional can reinforce the behavior of adolescent patients who do not use substances by finding out why use has not occurred and helping them to affirm decisions not to use.

Formal Assessment Instruments

Health care professionals may prefer to use formal clinical screening instruments, which include interview and written self-report questionnaire formats and provide a highly structured and time-efficient approach to screening. More detailed instruments can also yield severity scores. Some formal instruments have been empirically validated and standardized. There are several significant advantages to using a standardized instrument: its psychometric properties are known; questions are internally consistent with each other; if a patient were to be given the same instrument at a later point in time, answers would remain the same unless changes had occurred in the use pattern of substances; the instrument measures what it was intended to measure; the instrument is able to differentiate individuals at high risk of substance abuse from those at low risk; and normative scores have been obtained that represent results that individuals from different populations or with differing levels of substance use tend to receive. In summary, some standardized instruments can provide an accurate, objective, and reliable way to identify adolescents with substance use problems, document the extent of engagement and severity of the addiction, and help determine the level of treatment care needed.[32] In addition, formal questionnaires and interview schedules help provide a structure and focus to the assessment interview. Because patients' answers are recorded before the interview or are short answers, they enhance the health care professional's opportunity to engage the patient during their review.[14]

The use of questionnaires for obtaining sensitive information from adolescents is still controversial partly because of concern about adolescents minimizing the extent of involvement with substances.[22,33] It is possible that formal screening instruments, especially those that use indirect methods to detect harmful involvement with substances, may have difficulty in detecting adolescents with milder problems. These instruments address adverse consequences of use and may miss adolescents who have not yet experienced any harmful consequences. In addition, not all published screening instruments have been validated.

Innovative, interactive computer-assisted technology for identification of sensitive health issues, including substance abuse, has been found to be preferred by adolescents and to yield a higher rate of positive responses to screening questions, compared with personal interview and written questionnaire.[34,35] Used interactively, computers appear to increase the interpersonal ambience of assessment for adolescents.[36] At this time, however, resource constraints have limited the use of such technology in most primary care clinical settings.

In contrast to standardized formal instruments, the detailed clinical interview, as outlined in earlier sections, is descriptive, open ended, and interactive. If conducted skillfully, it can offer a contextual richness that is missing from more structured approaches. However, the completeness and accuracy of information is dependent on the skill of the interviewer, and the interpretation of nonstandardized interviews is subjective. In 1990, the Institute of Medicine recommended that treatment for alcohol problems begin with a comprehensive assessment that maximizes objectivity and is a positive experience for the patient.[36] Because no single tool is foolproof and able to meet the needs of all patients, the Institute of Medicine recommended that a mixture of approaches be used, including face-to-face interviews, self-administered testing, and computerized testing.[36]

The most common reason given by adolescents who disclosed that they had not answered a health care professional's questions regarding use of alcohol and drugs honestly was that a parent had been present during the interview.[17] In clinical settings, a written questionnaire cannot be administered in the absence of interaction between the patient and health care professional. In addition, it is helpful if the instrument also considers general psychosocial functioning. Interview and questionnaire approaches to the process of assessment can help the health care professional achieve the following goals: to describe the adolescent's problems clearly; to identify the pattern of behavioral, psychologic, and physiologic conditions associated with substance use; and to determine whether referral to an appropriate professional facility for further evaluation and intervention is indicated.

Screening instruments should be highly sensitive so that they can identify adolescent patients at risk of substance abuse. To cover a range of substances, they should also have a wide scope. Screening instruments are not meant to be diagnostic or very specific; their purpose is to identify adolescents who need further assessment of a potential substance abuse problem.[32] However, a successful screening instrument needs to achieve a reasonable balance between sensitivity and specificity. Additional considerations include cost, ease of administration, and how well it is accepted by patients.[21]

Eleven instruments that are available to health care professionals have been selected for discussion. They represent the assessment levels of clinical screening and mid-range evaluation. Most of these screening instruments, especially those that are more complex, have been at least partly validated. Two are part of a larger tiered systems approach to evaluation. Instruments designed for specialized assessment are beyond this chapter's purview. Questions are provided for brief screening instruments that are in the public domain.

Clinical Screening Instruments

CRAFFT mnemonic tool

The CRAFFT was developed as a 9-item brief screening test designed specifically for adolescents.[37] Its questions were adapted from 3 independent instruments, each of which is briefly discussed later, including the RAFFT,[38] the Drug and Alcohol Problem Quickscreen (DAP),[39] and the Problem-Oriented Screening Instrument for Teenagers (POSIT).[40] The CRAFFT was validated using a sample of 99 adolescent outpatients arriving for general health care; the Personal Involvement with Chemicals Scale from the PEI,[24] which is also discussed below, served as the criterion standard. The CRAFFT demonstrated 82% correlation with its standard. A linear regression analysis found that 6 items from the CRAFFT explained 68% of the variance and also demonstrated an internal consistency of 0.68. On the basis of the final 6-item model, if a patient had a score of at least 2, then the CRAFFT was able to identify 92% of adolescents with an intensive need for treatment with 82% specificity, a calculated positive predictive value of 67%, and a negative predictive value of 97%.[37] The following 6 questions compose the final CRAFFT model:

- Have you ever ridden in a **C**ar driven by someone (including yourself) who was high or had been using alcohol or drugs?
- Do you ever use alcohol or drugs to **R**elax, feel better about yourself, or fit in?
- Do you ever use alcohol or drugs while you are by yourself (**A**lone)?
- Do you ever **F**orget things you did while using alcohol or drugs?
- Do your **F**amily or **F**riends ever tell you that you should cut down on your drinking or drug use?
- Have you ever gotten into **T**rouble while you were using alcohol or drugs?

RAFFT mnemonic tool

The RAFFT was developed by Project Adept at Brown University in 1989 as a clinically useful component of adolescent patient interviews.[38] Its goal is to determine quickly whether an adolescent's use of alcohol and drugs is harmful. It addresses the following 5 areas through single questions: perceived benefits, social pattern of use, peer use, genetics and family use, and psychosocial consequences. Although it is clinically endorsed by practitioners and by trainees, it has not been formally evaluated; its validity is unknown. In addition, no scoring system has been developed for it, so the health care professional must rely on best judgment. The questions are framed dichotomously and assume use. Questions include:

- Do you drink or use drugs to **R**elax, feel better about yourself, or fit in?
- Do you ever drink alcohol or use drugs while you are by yourself, **A**lone?
- Do you or any of your closest **F**riends drink or use drugs?
- Does a close **F**amily member have a problem with alcohol or drug use?
- Have you ever gotten into **T**rouble from drinking or drug use (eg, skipping school, bad grades, trouble with the law or parents)?

Adolescent CAGE

The third screening interview is the adolescent CAGE.[13] This instrument is based on the adult CAGE, a 4-question mnemonic interview originally developed for screening adult male patients for alcohol abuse, which has adequate sensitivity and specificity in different medical settings for adult patients.[41-43] The following questions address the pattern and consequences of use:

- Have you ever felt the need to **C**ut down on drinking or drug use?
- Have you ever felt **A**nnoyed by criticism about your drinking or drug use?
- Have you ever felt **G**uilty about your drinking or drug use? Have you ever felt **G**uilty about something you said or did while you were drinking or using drugs?
- Have you ever taken a morning **E**ye-opener?

These questions can also be easily adapted to inquire about family members. For example, the health care professional could ask: "Do you think your father needs to cut down on his alcohol use? Does his drinking ever worry or bother you?"

The adolescent CAGE was adapted for use as a flexible but structured clinical tool in 1992 (the adult CAGE was developed in 1968 and was first validated in 1974[41]). Two to 3 affirmative answers create a high index of suspicion for substance abuse, and 4 affirmative answers are considered pathognomonic. The mnemonic tool helps the health care professional remember the content areas. Although the adolescent CAGE has been highly endorsed by health care professionals as a clinical and teaching tool, it has only been formally validated among college students for alcohol use. By itself, the adolescent CAGE appears to be most useful in identifying male students with more severe alcohol problems. Despite its clinical usefulness in adult patients, the CAGE has had variable success in accurately identifying university students with alcohol problems.[44-47] It may be particularly insensitive to detecting drinking problems among female college students.[46-48]

The adolescent CAGE probably cannot stand by itself as an adequate screening instrument for substance abuse or for alcohol abuse as a single problem. However, in combination with another instrument, the perceived benefits of drinking scale (this 5-question instrument is discussed later),[30,31] and inquiries about tobacco use, the drinking behavior of the student's best friend, and age of first drinking (especially younger than 15 years), a significant proportion of college students (including females) could be correctly identified regarding problematic alcohol use. Any 2 affirmative responses to this 12-question set is considered a positive result that warrants further evaluation.[45,48] This version of the adolescent CAGE has not been validated on younger adolescents.

However, the CAGE-AA (CAGE **A**dapted for **A**dolescents), a further modification of the original instrument, has been studied in adolescents 15 to 18 years of age in an outpatient medical setting.[49] The questions have been reworded, especially the fourth question, and include the following:

- Have you ever tried to **C**ut down on your drinking or using drugs?
- Have you ever been **A**nnoyed with someone because they criticized your drinking or using drugs?
- Do you feel bad or **G**uilty about your drinking or drug use?
- Do you ever use alcohol or drugs **E**arly in the day?

The internal reliability of the CAGE-AA is generally acceptable (α 0.60), except with 2 major populations: male (α 0.42) and Hispanic (α 0.43) adolescents.[49]

Perceived benefits scales

The perceived benefits of drinking scale and the perceived benefits of drug use scale were developed to be quickly and easily administered screening instruments that could serve as proxy measures of adolescents' substance abuse.[30,31] The authors reasoned that a phenomenologic approach could yield valuable information regarding substance use without needing to elicit information about an adolescent's specific patterns of substance use or negative consequences resulting from alcohol and drug use. Such information can be difficult to obtain accurately during an initial interview because the adolescent may not trust the interviewer or may deny heavy use patterns or the occurrences of negative consequences. The questions from these scales were briefly presented as a strategy to supplement and help enrich other clinical information in the section ***Elements of a Formal Substance Use History*** (see p 59). This section discusses the clinical use of the perceived benefits scales when used as formal instruments to screen for adolescent substance abuse. The alcohol and drug scales each contain the following 5 parallel questions:

- Drinking (or using drugs) helps me relax.
- Drinking (or using drugs) helps me be friendly.
- Drinking (or using drugs) helps me be with friends who drink or use drugs.
- Drinking (or using drugs) helps me forget my problems.
- Drinking (or using drugs) helps me feel good about myself.

Adolescents' answers are dichotomized; that is, replies are given in a "yes" or "no" format. Each separate item receives a score of 1 if an adolescent endorses it. The authors recommend that a cutoff score of 3 be used for each scale so that scores of 3 or higher would suggest an abuse problem. Using this cutoff score in a classroom setting yielded a mean accuracy rate of 77% for the perceived benefit of drinking scale and 80% for the perceived benefit of drug use scale. In addition, the perceived benefits of drinking scale has demonstrated capability of identifying female college students (but not male students) with moderate drinking problems.[30,31] The perceived benefits scales can serve as a useful adjunct to interviewing youngsters who are already known to have some life experience with substance use. They probably function best as a supplementary assessment tool for adolescents who are known to use alcohol or illicit drugs.

Personal Experience Screening Questionnaire
A fifth clinical screening instrument, the Personal Experience Screening Questionnaire (PESQ), is a validated, shortened (38-item) version[50] of the PEI, a second-level assessment tool, which is discussed later.[24] The PESQ covers 3 areas (problem severity, psychosocial risk, and drug use history) and can be completed in 10 to 15 minutes. Its purpose is to determine whether an adolescent patient merits more complete evaluation. The problem severity scale correlates 0.94 with the main problem severity scale of its parent instrument and is estimated to have an accuracy rate of 88% in predicting need for further assessment.[50] Given its brevity, this instrument is practical for use in a busy primary care setting. In contrast to the other clinical screening instruments, its psychometric properties have been very well established. It is available for a fee from Western Psychological Services, 12031 Wilshire Boulevard, Los Angeles, CA 90025-1251; 800/648-8857 or 310/478-2061.

Simple Screening Instrument for Alcohol and Other Drug Abuse
The Simple Screening Instrument for Alcohol and Other Drug Abuse (SSI-AOD) was developed by a consensus panel for the Substance Abuse and Mental Health Services Administration of the US Department of Health and Human Services for screening diverse individuals in a variety of settings.[32] The SSI-AOD includes the following 5 content domains: consumption pattern of alcohol and drugs; preoccupation with matters pertaining to substance use and loss of control over use of substances; adverse physical, psychologic, and social consequences; self-recognition of a problem; and physiologic effects as evidenced by tolerance and withdrawal. This instrument was not designed for any particular age group, and the sources for its items include previously

validated instruments targeted at adults and adolescents. The 16 questions composing the SSI-AOD, which are in the public domain, are available in interview and self-administered format at http://www.health.org/govpubs/bkd143/11m.htm. Each question is answered in a dichotomous "yes" or "no" fashion. The following is a summary of the questions:

During the last 6 months:

1. Have you used alcohol or other drugs? (Multiple examples of drugs are listed.)
2. Have you felt that you use too much alcohol or other drugs?
3. Have you tried to cut down or quit drinking or using alcohol or other drugs?
4. Have you gone to anyone for help because of your drinking or drug use? (Several examples are listed.)
5. Have you had any health problems? For example, have you:
   - Had blackouts or other periods of memory loss?
   - Injured your head after drinking or using drugs?
   - Had convulsions or delirium tremens (DTs)?
   - Had hepatitis or liver problems?
   - Felt sick, shaky, or depressed when you stopped drinking or using drugs?
   - Felt "coke bugs" or a crawling feeling under the skin after you stopped using drugs?
   - Been injured after drinking or using drugs?
   - Used needles to shoot drugs?
6. Has drinking or other drug use caused problems between you and your family or friends?
7. Has your drinking or other drug use caused problems at school or work?
8. Have you been arrested or had other legal problems? (Several examples of legal problems are listed.)
9. Have you lost your temper or gotten into arguments or fights while drinking or using other drugs?
10. Are you needing to drink or use drugs more and more to get the effect you want?

11. Do you spend a lot of time thinking about or trying to get alcohol or other drugs?
12. When drinking or using drugs, are you more likely to do something you wouldn't normally do, such as break rules, break the law, sell things that are important to you, or have unprotected sex with someone?
13. Do you feel bad or guilty about your drinking or drug use?

Within your lifetime:
14. Have you ever had a drinking or other drug problem?
15. Have any of your family members ever had a drinking or drug problem?
16. Do you feel that you have a drinking or drug problem now?

Each item with a positive or "yes" response receives a score of 1, and each item with a negative or "no" response receives a score of 0; items 1 and 15 provide background information but are not included in the scoring. Preliminary scoring guidelines suggest that a score of 0 to 1 indicates little or no risk of abuse of alcohol or other drugs, a score of 2 to 3 indicates minimal risk, and a score of 4 or greater indicates a moderate to high risk and need for further assessment. However, there is no published empirical evaluation of this scoring protocol, and it is possible that patients with low scores may not be providing accurate information. In addition, the scoring protocol does not consider adolescents separately from adults. This instrument was developed by a consensus panel, and little formal work has been done to validate it. However, its questions are drawn from several other instruments that have been validated, largely with adults. The items of the SSI-AOD demonstrate good internal consistency (α 0.83) for adolescents.[49]

Adolescent Substance Abuse Subtle Screening Inventory
The Adolescent Substance Abuse Subtle Screening Inventory (SASSI), an empirically validated screening tool, was first made commercially available in 1988. The adolescent version, which

contains about 60 questions and requires about 15 minutes to complete, is between 80% and 90% accurate in identifying adolescents with substance abuse problems.[51] The SASSI is composed of 6 scales, which are meant to be used to generate hypotheses regarding individuals' adjustment and treatment needs, including: face valid alcohol, face valid other drug, obvious attributes (willingness to admit symptoms), subtle attributes (relatively little insight into the basis for problems), correctional (risk of legal problems), and defensiveness (unconscious denial or deliberate concealment of problems) scales. It also contains a random answering pattern scale designed to detect nonmeaningful response sets, and its multiple scales are meant to be used in combination to develop individual profiles. When the psychometric properties of an updated version of this instrument, the SASSI-2, were assessed on college students, its reliability and validity were found comparable to instruments in the public domain oriented toward adults.[52] In addition, even though the SASSI was designed to minimize intentional faking, on instruction, students were able to purposefully minimize and exaggerate their use of alcohol without the instruments being able to detect such misrepresentation.[52] The SASSI is copyrighted by the SASSI Institute and can be ordered for a fee at http://www.sassi.com.

Tiered Systems Approaches to Evaluation

Two additional clinical screening instruments, the Drug Use Screening Inventory (DUSI)[53,54] and the POSIT,[40,54] are embedded in a tiered systems approach for screening, diagnostic evaluation, and comprehensive assessment. These instruments are longer and more complex than the clinical screening instruments presented earlier and address problems in several psychosocial arenas in addition to substance abuse. Health care professionals may use either of these screening instruments independently without proceeding through the entire evaluation system. Both instruments have been validated.

Drug Use Screening Inventory

The DUSI is the initial component of a 3-stage integrated assessment and treatment planning protocol for adolescents suspected of abusing substances.[53,54] It was developed by an expert consensus panel and uses a decision tree format so that the assessment activities of each successive stage are based on the results of the previous stage.

The initial stage is the screening assessment, which consists of 2 written questionnaires, the Personal History Form to document the adolescent's background, and the DUSI. The purpose of the DUSI is to identify the psychosocial, psychiatric, and medical problems that are commonly associated with substance abuse in adolescents. The DUSI (revised) contains 159 questions, most of which have dichotomous responses, and measure problems in the following 10 domains: substance use, behavior patterns, health status, psychiatric disorder, social competence, family system, school adjustment, work, peer relationships, and leisure or recreation. It also checks for validity of reporting by use of a "lie scale." It is scored in 3 ways: the absolute problem density for each of the 10 domains, the relative problem severity for each domain in relation to the overall number of problems by domain, and the summary problem index, which measures the absolute severity of problems relative to the universe of problems regardless of domain. Scoring can be performed manually, by a computer scoring service, or by personal computer software. The DUSI is aimed at a fifth grade reading level and takes subjects 20 to 30 minutes to complete.

The second stage is the diagnostic evaluation, which uses specific instruments to explore each screened problematic domain more comprehensively. For example, to evaluate the first domain, it uses the Chemical Dependency Assessment Scale, which must be computer scored. The Achenbach Child Behavior Checklist is used to evaluate the second domain, behavior patterns. Health status is determined by a comprehensive medical history and physical examination. Some recommend performing a structured psychiatric interview and a comprehensive self-report instrument (Symptom Checklist-90) to assess an adolescent for possible psychiatric disorders. Other previously validated indices are used to measure the remaining domains. A diagnostic formulation is then developed for each adolescent, usually by members of a treatment team. Finally, an adolescent's treatment plan is built to address specific problems diagnosed during the second stage of assessment.

This thoughtful conceptualization of a semistandardized strategy for assessing adolescent substance abuse clearly requires a multidisciplinary effort that surpasses the capability of an individual primary care health care professional. However, a busy health care professional may want to use the DUSI as a structured screening instrument. It has 2 limitations. First, because most answers are dichotomized ("yes" or "no" format), it may be difficult for an adolescent to endorse either answer entirely. Second, the DUSI may not be appropriate for all adolescents (eg, those who have severe psychiatric disturbances or pronounced patterns of socially deviant behavior), and certain populations may give unique cultural interpretations to the meanings of certain items. The DUSI is under copyright and is available for a fee from The Gordian Group, PO Box 1587, Hartsville, SC 29550; 843/383-2201; http://www.dusi.com. Clinical support for use of the DUSI is available from Ralph Tarter, PhD, at 412/624-1070.

Adolescent Assessment/Referral System

The National Institute on Drug Abuse published the *Adolescent Assessment/Referral System (AARS) Manual* in 1991.[40,54] It was designed to help health care professionals screen and evaluate individual adolescents suspected of using alcohol or drugs. The AARS targets multiple functional areas of evaluation to help health care professionals match appropriate treatment resources to the needs of individual adolescents. A major purpose is to provide a standardized approach to assessment so individuals who are not experts in the field of substance abuse can determine which adolescents need more extensive evaluation. The structure of the AARS conforms to a "behavioral assessment funnel" described by Donovan[20] with the following components: initial screening, comprehensive assessment, establishment of diagnoses, and development of treatment plan based on local resources.[40]

Initial screening is accomplished by the completion of 2 written questionnaires by individual adolescents. The first is the POSIT, which is available in English and Spanish and has a sixth grade reading level. The POSIT is the best known component of the AARS. It was designed by a consensus panel of expert clinician researchers and consists of 139 questions with dichotomized ("yes" or "no") responses. In practice, about 25 minutes are needed for adolescents to complete it. POSIT screens 10 functional areas for problems: substance use and abuse, physical health status, mental health status, family relationships, peer relations, educational status, vocational status, social skills, leisure and recreation, and aggressive behavior and delinquency. Each relevant question adds 1 point to the risk score for a functional area. It is scored using a template; each functional area has been assigned a cutoff score that indicates an individual adolescent may be experiencing a problem in that area and probably needs further assessment. Certain items are "red flags" that by themselves indicate an adolescent is at high risk of a problem and deserves further assessment in that functional area.

To allow complete detection of problems, POSIT cutoff scores were assigned to be very sensitive. However, such sensitivity may falsely identify adolescents who have no problems. It may be possible to estimate the severity of substance abuse problems by the level of the score. Other possible issues that POSIT presents include its dichotomization, which may make it more difficult for adolescents to endorse high- and low-risk answers, and the reading level needed to understand certain questions. (However, POSIT has been successfully used as an interview for adolescents with poor reading skills.) Research is ongoing on the cultural relevance of the POSIT's Spanish language version. Finally, POSIT cannot be scored without its template.

Validation of the POSIT on a large sample of adolescents undergoing evaluation for substance abuse found a sensitivity of 0.84 and a specificity of 0.41 for the substance use and abuse scale.[55] In addition, there was adequate convergence of findings when the POSIT was compared with the PEI, for which psychometric properties have been well studied. (The PEI[24] is discussed later.) The POSIT's substance use and abuse scale contains 17 items; when using a positive score cutoff of 2, its diagnosis classification accuracy was found to be 84%, its sensitivity was 95%, and its specificity was 79%.[56] A shortened version of this scale with 11 items had test characteristics similar to those of the complete scale.[56] The 11 questions, which are meant to be answered by "yes" or "no," (positive cutoff score is 2) include the following (each question's original number is indicated for reference purposes):

- Do you ever feel you are addicted to drugs? (17)
- Have you started using more and more drugs or alcohol to get the effect you want? (18)
- Does your alcohol or drug use ever make you do something you would not normally do, like breaking rules, missing curfew, breaking the law, or having sex with someone? (19)
- Do you forget things you did while drinking or using drugs? (20)
- Do your family or friends ever tell you that you should cut down on your drinking or drug use? (21)
- Do you have a constant desire for alcohol or drugs? (22)
- Do you ever feel you can't control your alcohol or drug use? (23)
- Do you have serious arguments with friends or family members because of your drinking or drug use? (24)
- Do you miss out on activities because you spend too much money on drugs or alcohol? (25)
- Does alcohol or drug use cause your moods to change quickly, like from happy to sad or vice versa? (26)
- Have you accidentally hurt yourself or someone else while high on alcohol or drugs? (27)

Two supplementary instruments that are based on the POSIT have been developed. The first is the Problem-Oriented Screening Instrument for Parents (POSIP), which uses a subset of 73 questions to ask parents about their adolescent children's substance use and behaviors. It is meant to provide collateral information. The second instrument, the POSIT Follow-up Questionnaire, is meant to monitor adolescents' involvement in psychoactive substances using a 6-month retrospective time frame. Its 86 items were also derived from the original POSIT questionnaire.

The second component of the AARS's initial screening of adolescents suspected of having possible substance use or abuse problems is the Client Personal History Questionnaire.[40] This companion questionnaire elicits demographic information as well as information about religion, living status, school performance, employment status, membership in a street gang, health status and behavior, familial socioeconomic status, adolescent and familial involvement with the justice system, substance use by family members, treatment by a mental health professional, and special education needs. The Client Personal History Questionnaire also helps to determine the adolescent's exposure to 40 stressful life events, to profile the current level of stress in the adolescent's life and environment. This questionnaire asks the adolescent to share very sensitive information in a written format; if it is used as part of an intake process in the absence of skilled interviewing, it is possible that the adolescent would feel too threatened to disclose some information accurately.

If the POSIT has indicated that a possible problem exists in any of the 10 functional domains, the AARS recommends 2 specific tools to provide further definition to the problem. Together, these 19 instruments (in general, 2 choices are recommended for each domain) compose the Comprehensive Assessment Battery (CAB). These instruments represent the more complex level of more thorough but targeted assessment of areas identified as problematic by the POSIT. The tools composing the CAB were recommended by national experts; most have been psychometrically validated on adolescents and have been successfully used in clinical settings. The expert panel attempted to recommend instruments that are readily available and can be administered and scored with a minimum of training. However, because many of these tests are time consuming and carry monetary costs, the health care professional should exercise judgment in their application. In addition, it is not clear how health care professionals should choose between the 2 recommended instruments for each domain. Examples of instruments include the PEI (which is discussed later) to assess substance abuse; the Diagnostic Interview Schedule for Children (DISC) to assess mental health status; and the Youth Self Report (YSR) of the Child Behavior Checklist to assess aggressive behavior and delinquency. A complete list of the CAB instruments and their purchase information are contained in the *AARS Manual.*

In summary, the AARS provides an integrated approach to help health care professionals evaluate adolescents for possible substance abuse. The POSIT appears to have acceptable content validity and clinical utility. However, it is likely that busy health care professionals would refer adolescents for further evaluation if they were concerned about the results of the POSIT rather than attempting the second level of assessment themselves. Health care professionals should also remember that in clinical settings, structured questionnaires should not be administered in the absence of individual interaction with the health care professional. The AARS is in the public domain and is available from the Substance Abuse and Mental Health Services Administration's National Clearinghouse for Alcohol and Drug Information; 800/729-6686 (stock No. BKD-59). A brief description of it is also available at http://www.nida.nih.gov:80/ICAW/ICAWTeens/html and at http://www.nida.nih.gov:80/TXInit/TXInit8a.html.

Instruments for Mid-range Evaluation

Two instruments, the PEI,[24] which represents a trio of tools, and the TASI,[25,26] have been validated for use in clinical settings to assess adolescents' use of substances and place the use in a psychosocial context.

Personal Experience Inventory

The PEI is a 260-item, written, structured questionnaire geared for a sixth grade reading level.[24,54] Its goal is to provide detailed diagnostic and treatment information. It has been extensively validated for construct validity and reliability. It is divided into 2 components: substance use problem severity scales and psychosocial and environmental risk factors and influences. It contains a total of 18 indices, reviews drug use history, and screens for 6 clinical problems associated with substance abuse, including physical and sexual abuse. It also contains 3 validity scales that allow the scorer to determine whether the adolescent is answering questions accurately. Validation of the PEI includes normative data by gender on adolescents 12 to 15 years of age and 16 to 18 years of age.[57,58]

The Adolescent Diagnostic Interview (ADI) was designed to be able to supplement the PEI or to be used as an independent assessment for substance abuse. This interview follows a structured format and addresses the symptoms of psychoactive substance use disorders covered by the *Diagnostic and Statistical Manual of Mental Disorders, Fourth Edition Text Revision (DSM-IV-TR).*[59] It also screens for other mental health disorders and measures psychosocial stressors and level of functioning.

Personal Experience Inventory-Parent Version

The Personal Experience Inventory-Parent Version (PEI-PV), a standardized, clinically oriented self-report questionnaire, has been developed specifically to target parents as part of the assessment of an adolescent's use of drugs and alcohol.[60] As a companion to the adolescent-oriented PEI,[24,54] the parent version's questions are congruent with it. The PEI-PV consists of 18 scales that are categorized into 3 domains: problem severity scales, personal adjustment scales, and environment scales. The last category, which includes scales on sibling drug use, family history, family drug use, family estrangement, parental support, and parental control, measures core parenting practices thought to be related to adolescent substance use. Significant convergence between parents' and adolescents' responses was obtained for 11 of the 15 scales that were directly correlated. Parents tended to underreport their adolescent children's involvement with substances and problems resulting from the use.[60]

Teen Addiction Severity Index

The TASI[25,26] was modified from an adult instrument, the Adult Severity Index. It is a semistructured interview that takes about 30 minutes to administer the 126 questions. The TASI includes 7 domains: psychoactive substance use, school status, employment and support status, family relationships and functioning, legal status, peer and social relationships, and psychiatric status. It provides a severity rating for each domain. It can also provide helpful collateral information if it is administered to parents. Each domain consists of a 5-point scale that subjectively measures the severity of the problem and need for treatment. It has been partially validated on adolescents admitted to an inpatient dual diagnosis program, and except for the family relationships subscale, has demonstrated good interrater reliability. It was able to discriminate between patients with and without psychoactive substance use disorders. In addition, scores on selected subscales have been found to correlate with well-validated criterion measures. Although the TASI has not been validated in an outpatient medical setting, it may provide a structured format for health care professionals who want to conduct a more complete assessment than a brief screen but who do not feel confident in their substance abuse interviewing skills or who want to use a standardized approach. In addition, because it is designed to measure severity of addiction, the TASI is useful for monitoring post-treatment or aftercare status. The TASI is not in the public domain. However, it is available on request from its developers.[25,26]

Synthesizing Clinical Information

The health care professional must synthesize available information to be able to judge its historical accuracy and determine the severity of an adolescent's substance abuse. The accuracy of an adolescent's substance use history should be judged by indirect measures. The health care professional can compare the adolescent's individual historical use of substances with empirical information that supports the "stage theory."[61] It has been demonstrated that most adolescents follow a specific sequence of substance use. They rarely begin with an illicit drug; the usual sequence is beer or wine, followed by tobacco or hard liquor, and then marijuana. Escalation of alcohol consumption may occur after initiation of marijuana use. The use of these substances precedes involvement with other illicit drugs, such as cocaine. For example, if there is evidence that an adolescent has used amphetamines but denies having used other substances, this information is not consistent with empirically described patterns. Even though an adolescent may have a substance of choice, other drugs previously used on a regular basis are not usually abandoned. There is more likely to be an addition rather than a substitution. However, adolescents may avoid categories of substances that have caused unpleasant or frightening effects in the past.

Dimensions of adolescent substance use can be categorized by a transitional framework. The first stage, *initiation,* represents experimental use, or the transition from a nonuser to a user. The second stage is *continuation* of a certain class of substances; this stage may represent substance abuse for some adolescents. *Maintenance and progression within a class of substances* is usually dependent on the practices of an adolescent's peer group. However, individual adolescents may start using more concentrated forms of a substance. Examples include drinking distilled liquor rather than beer and injecting cocaine rather than snorting. The fourth stage of the continuation is *progression across drug classes.* It represents polysubstance abuse and dependence. Adolescents may also have *regression, cessation, and relapse cycles.*[11]

Formal Diagnostic Classification Systems

A continuum of severity exists for substance abuse; it is not a dichotomous phenomenon. Two commonly accepted classification and definitional systems are used to frame clinical diagnoses. Although their working definitions are widely accepted for adults, the nosology of substance use disorders is problematic for the adolescent population. Adult criteria may not always apply to adolescents; adolescents may have differing patterns of use, a different developmental course, and somewhat different adverse consequences of use.[62] For example, even though substance abuse and substance dependence are separated by major classification systems, an epidemiologic study found that this framework is not supported empirically for the adolescent population and that it may be more meaningful to combine selected criteria to determine problem severity.[63] However, no empirically derived, developmentally based set of definitional criteria exist for diagnosing adolescents with substance use disorders. One study of diagnostic assignments made using *DSM-IV-TR*[59] criteria determined that these criteria are probably "defensible" for adolescents but recommended the need to tailor substance use disorder criteria for adolescents.[29] With these caveats, the 2 major existing diagnostic classification systems are described, and the linkages between the *DSM-IV* criteria and *International Classification of Diseases, Ninth Edition, Clinical Modification (ICD-9-CM)*[64] codes are discussed.

The first system, *The Classification of Child and Adolescent Mental Diagnoses in Primary Care: Diagnostic and Statistical Manual for Primary Care (DSM-PC), Child and Adolescent Version,*[65] considers the developmental differences among children, adolescents, and adults. It recognizes that many adolescents use alcohol and marijuana on an experimental basis and considers this behavior a developmental variation ("substance use variation"). The *DSM-PC* also recognizes the diagnosis of a "substance use problem," which it defines as the repeated use of alcohol or an illicit substance that has not become a behavioral pattern and has not significantly impaired psychosocial functioning. Adolescents who use substances in the context of emotional or behavioral difficulties are also considered to have a substance use problem.[65] The *DSM-PC* uses the general term "substance abuse disorder" for more serious problems; it includes substance abuse and substance dependence. These latter diagnostic categories are consistent with the classification system contained in the *DSM-IV-TR,*[59] which is discussed later. The developmentally oriented system of the *DSM-PC,* which is geared primarily for pediatric health care professionals, is easily available for purchase but is not in wide general use.

In contrast, the *DSM-IV-TR*[59] does not recognize the use of the terms "developmental variation" and "substance use problem." The main diagnostic category of the *DSM-IV-TR* is "substance use disorders," which includes substance abuse and substance dependence. (Substance-induced disorders are beyond the purview of this chapter.) The *DSM-IV-TR* defines substance abuse as a "maladaptive pattern of substance use leading to clinically significant impairment of distress" as manifested by 1 or more of the following criteria:

- Recurrent substance use resulting in a failure to fulfill major role obligations at work, school, or home (eg, substance-related absences or suspensions from school, being fired from a job)
- Recurrent substance use in circumstances that are physically hazardous (eg, driving an automobile; skiing; swimming; rock climbing; riding a bicycle, scooter, or skateboard; or operating machinery while impaired by a substance's effects)
- Recurrent substance-related legal problems (eg, arrest for driving under the influence, disorderly conduct, or vandalism while impaired by a substance's effects)
- Continued substance use despite having persistent or recurrent social or interpersonal problems caused or exacerbated by the effects of the substance (eg, physical fights or unpleasant arguments, damaging furniture or punching holes in the wall, sexual behavior that is later regretted)

Substance dependence is the most serious type of substance use disorder. In addition to the criteria outlined for substance abuse, individuals who are substance dependent must manifest at least 3 of the following 7 criteria:

- Tolerance: increased amounts of the substance are needed to achieve the desired effect or intoxication or if the same amount of the substance is used over time, it produces a lesser effect
- Withdrawal: adverse physiologic and cognitive changes that may cause maladaptive behaviors when blood or tissue levels of a substance decrease in an individual who had used it heavily over a prolonged time period
- Taking the substance in larger amounts or over a longer time period than intended
- Having a persistent desire or a history of unsuccessful efforts to regulate or control substance use
- Spending a great deal of time and effort in activities necessary to obtain or use the substance or to recover from its effects
- Reducing or giving up important school- or work-related and social or recreational activities because of the substance use (eg, not participating in family activities to use or to spend time with substance using friends)
- Continued use of the substance in the face of knowing that it has caused a significant physical or psychologic problem.[59]

Major *ICD-9-CM* coding categories are compatible with *DSM-IV-TR* categories for substance use disorders, although differences exist at finer levels.[64] Relevant *ICD-9-CM* codes include alcohol dependence syndrome (303 with a fourth or fifth digit specifier needed); drug dependence (304 with a fourth or fifth digit specifier needed); nondependent abuse of drugs (305 with a fourth or fifth digit modifier needed). Nondependent alcohol abuse is coded as 305.0 (fourth digit specifier), cannabis abuse is coded as 305.2, and unspecified drug abuse is coded as 305.9. Fifth digit subclas-sification systems for dependence syndromes and nondependent abuse of drugs and alcohol include 0 (unspecified), 1 (continuous), 2 (episodic), and 3 (in remission).[64]

Stage Change Models of Addiction: Moving Toward Intervention

The stage change model of the natural history of addiction provides a developmental framework for understanding the emergence of an addiction and looks ahead toward the evolution of recovery. Stages of change theories are based on empirical observations. The transtheoretical model of change was originally elaborated by Prochaska and DiClemente and others about 2 decades ago as they used previously developed behavioral theories to explain the process of successful cessation of smoking behavior.[66-68] They identified 5 dynamic stages or sets of steps and tasks that individuals go through as they attempt to change their behavior.

The *precontemplation stage* represents lack of awareness of the nature and extent of a problem or an unwillingness to change the behavior. The *contemplation stage* involves serious thinking about change and includes a decision-making evaluation and relative weighing of the problem behavior and the change. The *preparation* or *determination stage* represents resolution of the decision-making process and making a commitment to a change plan in a defined time span, often measured as 1 month. During the *action stage,* the patient implements a change plan, changes the behavior, and learns to cope with the changes and the loss of the problem behavior. Patients who successfully maintain their behavior change for at least 3 to 6 months move into the *maintenance stage,* and they learn how to integrate the behavior change into their lifestyle.[69,70]

The 10 processes of change (eg, consciousness raising, self-liberation, helping relationship) compose the second component of the transtheoretical model of change; they facilitate movement through the stages of change. The third component of the transtheoretical model is made up of the 5 levels of change, which emphasize that individuals can be in different stages of change with respect to such problem areas as symptoms, interpersonal and intrapersonal problems, and systems and family problems. The second and third components of the model are not as widely known as the 5 stages of change.[69]

Stage change theory can be applied psychologically to clarify and guide treatment approaches across the life span of an addictive process.[27,28] The psychologically applied model provides a conceptual explanation of why some patients with substance abuse problems are more ready to accept help than others and provides the foundation for intervention in the primary care setting. It consists of 6 applied stages of change. The first stage is the initial use of substances or *initiation* into this behavior and the *emergence of addiction.* During the second stage of *positive consequences,* the individual has positive experiences that are direct, such as psychologic reinforcement, and indirect, such as enhanced social esteem, which fuel the addictive process. *Adverse consequences* emerge during the third stage; nonaddicted individuals would recognize and heed them and would alter their behavior toward moderation in use or abstinence, but the addicted individual is initially unaware of the adverse consequences and is unable to use this information for behavioral feedback. During this stage, which is termed *precontemplation* in the transtheoretical model, individuals who are addicted are not able to see that the adverse effects of their substance use are the cause of their suffering; they tend to blame their problems on others. Simultaneously, however, they continue to receive some positive consequences from using substances.[27,28]

Addicted individuals who recover eventually have a turning point, which allows them insight into the causal connection between their addictive behaviors and adverse life consequences. Often, the turning point is marked by a life crisis, which helps addicted individuals realize that the substance use must cease if they are to regain control. This fourth stage, which the transtheoretical model terms *contemplation,* is marked by ambivalence—the addicted individual simultaneously wants and does not want to quit. There is desire to shed the adverse experiences but reluctance to leave the positive experiences associated with use of substances. Individuals who move forward toward quitting eventually accept personal responsibility for their behavior and self-control rather than delegating it to others. The fourth stage is called *acceptance of responsibility* and serves as the true turning point toward *active quitting,* the fifth stage of the applied model, which is synonymous with the transtheoretical model's *action stage of change.* During this time, affected individuals make energetic organizational changes to their lives to quit. Finally, most addicted individuals who have quit can relapse, so individuals must work continuously to *maintain the change* and prevent relapse.[27,28]

The health care professional can determine the severity of an adolescent's substance abuse by determining what stage the pattern of use represents and by analyzing this information in the context of the adolescent's general psychosocial functioning. The following framework has been recommended for assessing severity of involvement: consideration of symptoms; functioning at home, at school, and in the community; burden of suffering; and risk and protective factors. The health care professional should also consider the adolescent's developmental stage; a preadolescent's or young adolescent's involvement in any substance use should always be treated as a problem unless it can be determined to be an isolated episode of experimentation. Finally, the health care professional should be alert to the possibility that a substance-abusing adolescent has a comorbid mental health problem, such as a depressive disorder, anxiety disorder, or conduct disorder.[23]

Counseling Strategies for Adolescents Involved With Substance Abuse

Most health care professionals will not—and probably should not—assume the responsibility of treating adolescents with substance abuse or substance dependence disorders. However, they can use counseling strategies to ensure effective communication and referral. Health care professionals' interviewing skills and negotiating style are critical to patient compliance with recommendations for further assessment and treatment and, ultimately, outcome.[71,72]

Many substance-abusing adolescents and even their families have not previously considered substance use to be a source of concern, even though it is objectively associated with adverse consequences. These adolescents and their families may be less able to accept the recommendation that treatment would be helpful. How the pediatric health care professional interacts with the adolescent and family is critical for engaging them in addressing the substance abuse problem and its treatment. As discussed previously, a stages of change model helps to make sense of the developmental progression of the addictive process as well as recovery from it.[27,28] Using the stages of change model,[68,69,73] these individuals may be placed in the *precontemplation stage,* which describes the substance use pattern before any active consideration of change. The health care professional may need to modify the counseling goal for these adolescents and their families and may need to accept success in calling their attention to the substance abuse as a problem behavior. Over time, the health care professional's ongoing interest and investment in the patient and the patient's recognition of the causal role of substance use on adverse experiences may help the patient to proceed to the *contemplation stage.* Although individuals in this stage are clearly considering addressing the substance abuse problem, they also experience motivational conflict and ambivalence and may need their perceived self-efficacy bolstered. The health care professional's goal for adolescents and their families who are at this second stage is to move them forward to the *determination* or *preparation substage* of contemplation and finally to an *action stage,* in which they make active attempts to change. A successful counseling outcome for adolescents and their families at the action stage would be acceptance of the screening evaluation and follow-up with a recommendation for full assessment and therapeutic intervention.

Counseling strategies that the pediatric health care professional can use to help adolescents and their families accept that a substance abuse problem exists, want to make behavioral changes, and accept referral for further assessment or treatment are summarized in Table 3.6. They are based on the concept of brief clinical intervention and motivational interviewing[74,75] and include the following elements: providing empathic and objective data, meeting patient expectations, dealing with the ambivalence of

table 3.6 Motivational Counseling Strategies Based on Principles
of Brief Intervention

Counseling Steps and Sample Approaches	Brief Intervention Principle
Summarize information from interview and any collateral sources.	Direct feedback after assessment
Clarify problem behaviors related to substance use and make links between use of substances and adverse consequences experienced by the adolescent. Use the adolescent's description of problems.	
Provide accurate normative information about the percentages of adolescents who use similar substances.	
Express concern for the adolescent's health and well-being.	
Ask the adolescent to express his or her understanding of the substance use and why the health care professional is concerned.	Enhancement of motivation to change through building of discrepancy
Elicit self-motivational statements from the patient.	Addressing ambivalence about changing substance use behaviors
Help patient to identify good and bad feelings or things related to using substances.	
Point out important facts about risks and adverse consequences associated with substance use.	
Ask patient what might occur if the substance use continues.	
Ask patient to identify important reasons to change substance use behaviors.	
Provide clear advice to decrease or stop use of substances or to obtain further assessment or treatment.	Negotiation and goal setting
Offer a short menu of options from which the patient can choose regarding next steps (patient can help design the treatment program).	
With the adolescent, set a short-term goal (eg, trial of abstinence over the next 2 weeks).	

the patient and family, assessing the patient's readiness for change, assessing barriers and strengths, reinterpreting past experiences in the context of current consequences, negotiating a follow-up plan, and offering hope for the future.[71]

The health care professional can use strategies developed for brief interventions for adult patients with alcoholism to help facilitate successful referral to a substance abuse treatment program (see Chapter 5). Multiple studies across a wide range of age groups (including adolescents and young adults), settings, and cultures have demonstrated the clinical effectiveness of brief interventions, which represent a time-limited, patient-centered counseling strategy that focuses on changing patient behavior and enhancing patient compliance with treatment.[72,76-78] In addition to helping health care professionals refer patients for specialized treatment, brief intervention has been shown to help patients with alcohol problems decrease their use of alcohol. Brief intervention focuses on increasing patients' readiness to change their behavior and emphasizes harm reduction.

First, the health care professional should allow the adolescent to describe perceptions of the substance use and the problems it may be causing. Regardless of the adolescent's perceptions, the health care professional should then summarize the information gathered during the assessment.[76] This approach demonstrates respect for the adolescent and allows the health care professional to make adjustments in communication style to respond most effectively to the adolescent's concerns.[74,75] It also may help adolescents who are in the precontemplation stage to kindle doubts about the wisdom of using substances. In addition to preparing the adolescent and family for future steps, summarization ensures that the health care professional understands the historical information and can communicate the problem accurately. A descriptive summary provides a clear statement of the problem behaviors to the adolescent and family. It is helpful to outline adverse experiences and dysfunctional behavior in the context of substance use and to use the patient's own descriptions of problems. The following example illustrates this process:

"I know that many adolescents smoke marijuana sometimes. However, since this school year started, you have been using marijuana more often than you did last year, and several things have happened that have aroused my concern. First, you haven't been feeling well—you are tired all the time and have been coughing. Second, school isn't going well for you— you've already been suspended twice for fighting, you've dropped out of band and quit soccer, and your grades are down. Third, you were really shaken up last week by that traffic accident when your friend was driving after drinking. And fourth, you have been feeling very sad, and other people see you as being angry all the time. I am very worried about you."

After communicating concern, the next step is to provide clear information without moralizing or lecturing.[76] For example: "When a person becomes really involved with drinking or doing drugs, without realizing it or even wanting it to happen, the alcohol and drugs can take over a person's life. This is what I believe is happening to you."

It is helpful for the health care professional to again ask for input from the adolescent patient. The health care professional could ask the patient why he or she is worried about the substance use and what possible health and safety consequences it poses. For example: "I know that it is difficult to hear this. What do you think about what I have been saying? As your doctor, why am I so worried about you?" The health care professional needs to listen to the patient actively and reflectively.

Next, the health care professional needs to provide clear advice.[76] For example: "I believe that the best thing for you is to stop smoking marijuana and drinking alcohol." At this point, the adolescent may again need a chance to respond. Do not expect your assessment to be automatically accepted by the adolescent or the family, even if the adolescent is experiencing serious dysfunction or has had multiple adverse consequences. It is possible that the patient is not ready to acknowledge the seriousness of the substance use and is unwilling to proceed with further assessment or intervention. As the health care professional, you need to recognize that the patient is in the precontemplation stage, agree to disagree about the substance abuse, and continue to provide caring health and medical care to the patient on a regular basis. Each visit provides an additional opportunity to assess the patient's involvement with substances and readiness to change.[75]

It is also important to recognize the intense ambivalence that commonly accompanies a patient's recognition that a problem exists (contemplation stage).[27,28,74,75] Assisting a patient to become actively aware of the internal conflict can help to mobilize and resolve it so that further progress may be made. Your goal is to tip the balance toward determination to change. For example: "It sounds like you are torn between wanting to continue and wanting to stop. Let's examine what you like about using and what it means to you, as well as what you don't like about it. If we write your thoughts down in 2 columns, you'll be able to examine each set of reasons later."

If the patient is ready to work on changing the substance use behaviors (preparation or determination stage), it is important to involve the adolescent in planning steps for more complete evaluation or for treatment.[76] This strategy enhances the patient's commitment to changing behaviors. For example: "These are our options: we can work together over the next month to see whether you can stop using alcohol and marijuana and then make a decision about what might work best, or you can see another doctor who specializes in working with people who have substance abuse problems."

The health care professional needs to accomplish 2 agendas simultaneously: to help the patient achieve personal responsibility for change and to support the patient's self-efficacy for change.[71,74-76,78] For example: "I would like us to work together to help you to make these important changes, but it is up to you to make them happen. Even though it seems difficult, I know that you can do it if you try. What other things have you worked on to change in your life?" It is also necessary to help the patient to identify potential barriers and challenging situations and to prepare for them by developing specific strategies to avoid or overcome them. For example: "What might get in the way of your being able to stop drinking and using marijuana for the next month?"

If you decide that an adolescent needs to be referred for further evaluation or intervention, clarify your role as you facilitate the referral process. Try not to allow the adolescent and family to perceive the referral as rejection by you. Two techniques you can use to avoid this issue are commitment to continued appropriate involvement with the adolescent and personalization of the referral process. For example: "I believe that it would really help you to feel better if you and your family learned more about substance abuse and enrolled in a treatment program for adolescents who have problems with drugs and alcohol. I would like you to meet a friend of mine who knows a lot about adolescents, families, and the problems that drugs and alcohol can cause. I don't have the background to give you really expert help for this problem. I will continue to be here for you as your doctor, but you also need counseling help."

Many adolescent patients benefit from reading and self-help exercises. There are several sources of high-quality literature on substance abuse for adolescents and their parents, and there are also interesting Web sites. Some adolescents may find it helpful to record their thoughts as well as their activities in a journal. Others may want to express themselves through artwork. Bibliotherapy has been found to be part of successful brief intervention programs for adults.[76]

It is very important to provide clear instructions for follow-up care. Patients should end the visit with a definite return appointment.[76] It is helpful to provide concrete assistance in facilitating referral to a treatment agency. The health care professional should be familiar with community and school-based resources and the treatment philosophies of various programs, the services they provide, and their fee schedules. Families who belong to health care plans will need to determine what benefits their plans provide.

Establish personal contact with program staff members. Adolescents and families often feel overwhelmed and powerless when they are confronted with serious problems. Your status as their health care professional will help provide the stimulus they need to complete the referral successfully. You may want the patient or family to telephone the counseling professional or treatment agency from your office. Ask the family to call you after their first appointment. Let them know that you will have the agency or counselor contact you if the adolescent misses the first appointment. This strategy enhances the probability of successful referral. Additional ways to increase a return visit rate include a handwritten note mailed to the patient's home, an interim telephone call, or an e-mail message. These strategies all demonstrate concern and caring by the health care professional.[74]

Conclusion

Health care professionals have the skills to assess their adolescent patients' use of alcohol and drugs. They can include questions that help define the extent of patient use of alcohol and drugs as part of their comprehensive interview; they can use formal questionnaires or interview schedules; or they can incorporate previously validated instruments into their overall psychosocial assessments. At a minimum, health care professionals need to identify patients who require more detailed assessment of their use of substances. Health care professionals who have the interest and adequate time are able to evaluate adolescent patients in more depth and formulate diagnoses relevant to substance abuse. Pediatric health care professionals should be able to provide brief interventions on the basis of a motivational interviewing and health counseling style to adolescent patients and their families, to decrease or eliminate the adolescent's use of substances and enhance the effectiveness of referral, when needed, for further evaluation and treatment.

References

1. Gastfriend DR, Baker SL, Najavits LM, Reif S. Assessment instruments. In: Graham AW, TK Schultz, eds. *Principles of Addiction Medicine.* 2nd ed. Chevy Chase, MD: American Society of Addiction Medicine; 1998:273-278

2. American Medical Association. *Guidelines for Adolescent Preventive Services (GAPS): Recommendations and Rationale.* Elster AB, Kuznets NJ, eds. Baltimore, MD: Williams & Wilkins, 1994:117-130

3. Green M, Palfrey J, eds. *Bright Futures. Guidelines for Health Supervision of Infants, Children and Adolescents.* 2nd ed. Arlington, VA: National Center for Education in Maternal and Child Health; 2000: 231-298

4. American Academy of Pediatrics, Committee on Psychosocial Aspects of Child and Family Health. *Guidelines for Health Supervision III.* Elk Grove Village, IL: American Academy of Pediatrics; 1997:147-192

5. US Preventive Services Task Force. *Guide to Clinical Preventive Services.* 2nd ed. Baltimore, MD: Williams & Wilkins; 1996:567-593

6. Stronski HSM, Remafedi G. Adolescent homosexuality. *Adv Pediatr.* 1998;45:107-144

7. Valencia LS, Cromer BA. Sexual activity and other high-risk behaviors in adolescents with chronic illness: a review. *J Pediatr Adolesc Gynecol.* 2000;13:53-64

8. Heinemann AW. Persons with disabilities. In: Lowinson JH, Raiz P, Millman RB, Langrod JG, eds. *Substance Abuse: A Comprehensive Textbook.* 3rd ed. Baltimore, MD: Williams & Wilkins; 1997:716-725

9. Huba GJ, Melchior LA, Trevithick L, et al. Predicting substance abuse among youth with, or at high risk for, HIV. *Psychol Addict Behav.* 2000;14:197-205

10. Crowley TJ, Riggs P. Adolescent substance use disorder with conduct disorder and comorbid conditions. In: Rahdert E, Czechowicz D, eds. *Adolescent Drug Abuse: Clinical Assessment and Therapeutic Interventions.* Rockville, MD: National Institute on Drug Abuse, US Department of Health and Human Services; 1995:49-111

11. Kaminer Y. *Adolescent Substance Abuse. A Comprehensive Guide to Theory and Practice.* New York, NY: Plenum Medical Book Co; 1994

12. Armentano ME. Adolescent substance abuse and psychiatric comorbidity. In: Graham AW, Schultz TK, eds. *Principles of Addiction Medicine.* 2nd ed. Chevy Chase, MD: American Society of Addiction Medicine; 1998:1161-1167

13. Werner MJ, Adger H. Early identification, screening, and brief intervention for adolescent alcohol use. *Arch Pediatr Adolesc Med.* 1995;149:1241-1248

14. Washton AM. Clinical assessment of psychoactive substance use. In: Washton AM, ed. *Psychotherapy and Substance Abuse: A Practitioner's Handbook.* New York, NY: The Guilford Press; 1995:23-43

15. Othmer E, Othmer SC. *The Clinical Interview Using DSM-IV. Vol 1: Fundamentals.* Washington, DC: American Psychiatric Press; 1994: 271-314

16. English A. Health care for the adolescent alone: a legal landscape. In: Blustein J, Levine C, Dubler NN, eds. *The Adolescent Alone: Decision Making in Health Care in the United States.* New York, NY: Cambridge University Press; 1999:78-99

17. Friedman LS, Johnson B, Brett AS. Evaluation of substance abusing adolescents by primary care physicians. *J Adolesc Health Care.* 1990;11:227-230

18. Hird S, Khuri E, Dusenbury L, Millman RB. Adolescents. In: Lowinson JH, Ruiz P, Millman RB, Langrod JG, eds. *Substance Abuse. A Comprehensive Textbook.* 3rd ed. Baltimore, MD: Williams & Wilkins; 1997:683-692

19. Bright GM, Hawley DL, Siegel PP. Ambulatory management of adolescent alcohol and drug abuse. *Semin Adolesc Med.* 1985;1:279-282

20. Donovan DM. Assessment of addictive behaviors: implications of an emerging biopsychosocial model. In: Donovan DM, Marlatt GA, eds. *Assessment of Addictive Behaviors.* New York, NY: The Guilford Press; 1988:3-48

21. Sullivan E, Fleming M. *A Guide to Substance Abuse Services for Primary Care Clinicians.* Rockville, MD: Substance Abuse and Mental Health Services Administration, US Department of Health and Human Services; 1997:1-50. DHHS Publication No. SMA 97-3139

22. Winters KC, Stinchfield RD. Current issues and future needs in the assessment of adolescent drug abuse. In: Rahdert E, Czechowicz D, eds. *Adolescent Drug Abuse: Clinical Assessment and Therapeutic Interventions.* Rockville, MD: National Institute on Drug Abuse, US Department of Health and Human Services; 1995:146-170

23. McLellan T, Dembo R. Screening and assessment of alcohol and other drug-abusing adolescents. Rockville, MD: Substance Abuse and Mental Health Services Administration, US Department of Health and Human Services; 1994. DHHS Publication No. SMA 95-3058

24. Winters KC, Henley GA. *Personal Experience Inventory Test and Manual.* Los Angeles, CA: Western Psychological Services; 1989

25. Kaminer Y, Bukstein O, Tarter RE. The teen-addiction severity index: rationale and reliability. Int J Addict. 1991;26:219-226

26. Kaminer Y, Wagner E, Plummer B, Seifer R. Validation of the teen addiction severity index (T-ASI): preliminary findings. *Am J Addict.* 1993;2:250-254

27. Shaffer HJ, Robbins M. Psychotherapy for addictive behavior: a stage-change approach to meaning making. In: Washton AM, ed. *Psychotherapy and Substance Abuse. A Practitioner's Handbook.* New York, NY: The Guilford Press; 1995:103-123

28. Shaffer HJ. Psychology of stage change. In: Lowinson JH, Ruiz P, Millman RB, Langrod, JG, eds. *Substance Abuse. A Comprehensive Textbook.* 3rd ed. Baltimore, MD: Williams & Wilkins; 1997:100-106

29. Winters KC, Latimer W, Stinchfield RD. The *DSM-IV* criteria for adolescent alcohol and cannabis use disorders. *J Stud Alcohol.* 1999;60:337-344

30. Petchers MK, Singer MI. Perceived-benefit of drinking scale: approach to screening for adolescent alcohol abuse. *J Pediatr.* 1987;110:977-981

31. Petchers MK, Singer MI, Angelotta JH, Chow J. Realization and expansion of an adolescent substance abuse screening measure. *J Dev Behav Pediatr.* 1988;9:25-29

32. Winters KC, Zenilman J. *Simple Screening Instruments for Outreach for Alcohol and Other Drug Abuse and Infectious Diseases.* Rockville, MD: US Department of Health and Human Services; 1994:3-18. DHHS Publication No. SMA 94-2094

33. Comerci GD. Office assessment and brief intervention with the adolescent suspected of substance abuse. In: Graham AW, Schultz TK, eds. *Principles of Addiction Medicine.* 2nd ed. Chevy Chase, MD: American Society of Addiction Medicine; 1998:1145-1151

34. Paperny DM, Aono JH, Lehman RM, Hammar SL, Risser J. Computer-assisted detection and intervention in adolescent high-risk health behaviors. *J Pediatr.* 1990;116:456-462

35. Millstein SG, Irwin, CE. Acceptability of computer-acquired sexual histories in adolescent girls. *J Pediatr.* 1987;103:815-819

36. Institute of Medicine. *Broadening the Base of Treatment for Alcohol Problems.* Washington, DC: National Academy Press; 1990:242-278

37. Knight JR, Shrier LA, Bravender TD, Farrell M, Bilt JV, Shaffer HJ. A new brief screen for adolescent substance abuse. *Arch Pediatr Adolesc Med.* 1999;153:591-596

38. Dube CE, ed. *The Project ADEPT Curriculum for Primary Care Physician Training.* Providence, RI: Brown University; 1989

39. Schwartz RH, Wirtz PW. Potential substance abuse. Detection among adolescent patients using the drug and alcohol (DAP) Quick Screen: a 30-item questionnaire. *Clin Pediatr.* 1990;29:38-43

40. Rahdert ER, ed. *The Adolescent Assessment/Referral System Manual.* Rockville, MD: Alcohol, Drug Abuse and Mental Health Administration, US Department of Health and Human Services; 1991. DHHS Publication No. AM 91-1735

41. Ewing JA. Detecting alcoholism: the CAGE questionnaire. *JAMA.* 1984;252:1905-1907

42. Bush B, Shaw S, Cleary P, Delbanco TL, Aronson MD. Screening for alcohol abuse using the CAGE questionnaire. *Am J Med.* 1987;82:231-235

43. Liskow B, Campbell J, Nickel EJ, Powell BJ. Validity of the CAGE questionnaire in screening for alcohol dependence in a walk-in (triage) clinic. *J Stud Alcohol.* 1995;56:277-281

44. Ross HE, Tisdall GW. Identification of alcohol disorders at a university mental health center using the CAGE. *J Alcohol Drug Educ.* 1994;39:119-126

45. Werner MJ, Walker LS, Greene JW. Screening for problem drinking among college freshmen. *J Adolesc Health.* 1994;15:303-310

46. O'Hare T, Tran TV. Predicting problem drinking in college students: Gender differences and the CAGE questionnaire. *Addict Behav.* 1997;22:13-21

47. Heck EJ, Williams MD. Using the CAGE to screen for drinking-related problems in college students. *J Stud Alcohol.* 1995;56:282-286

48. Werner MJ, Walker LS, Greene JW. Longitudinal evaluation of a screening measure for problem drinking among female college freshmen. *Arch Pediatr Adolesc Med.* 1994;148:1131-1337

49. Knight JR, Goodman E, Pulerwitz T, DuRant RH. Reliabilities of short substance abuse screening tests among adolescent medical patients. *Pediatrics.* 2000;105:948-953

50. Winters KC. Development of an adolescent alcohol and other drug abuse screening scale: personal experience screening questionnaire. *Addictive Behav.* 1992;17:479-490

51. Risberg RA, Stevens GJ, Graybill DF. Validating the adolescent form of the substance abuse subtle screening inventory. *J Child Adolesc Subst Abuse.* 1995;4:25-41

52. Myerholtz L, Rosenberg H. Screening college students for alcohol problems: psychometric assessment of the SASSI-2. *J Stud Alcohol.* 1998;59:439-446

53. Tarter RE. Evaluation and treatment of adolescent substance abuse: a decision tree method. *Am J Drug Alcohol Abuse.* 1990;16:1-46

54. Friedman AS, Granick S. *Assessing Drug Abuse among Adolescents and Adults: Standardized Instruments.* Rockville, MD: National Institute on Drug Abuse, US Department of Health and Human Services; 1994. NIH Publication No. 94-3757

55. McLaney MA, Del Boca F, Babor T. A validation study of the problem-oriented screening instrument for teenagers (POSIT). *J Ment Health.* 1994;3:363-376

56. Latimer WW, Winters KC, Stinchfield RD. Screening for drug abuse among adolescents in clinical and correctional settings using the problem-oriented screening instrument for teenagers. *Am J Drug Alcohol Abuse.* 1997;23:79-98

57. Winters KC, Stinchfield RD, Henly GA, Schwartz RH. Validity of adolescent self-report of alcohol and other drug involvement. *Int J Addict.* 1990-91;25:1379-1395

58. Winters KC, Stinchfield RD, Henly GA. Further validation of new scales measuring adolescent alcohol and other drug abuse. *J Stud Alcohol.* 1993;54:534-541

59. American Psychiatric Association. *Diagnostic and Statistical Manual of Mental Disorders, Fourth Edition Text Revision (DSM-IV-TR).* Washington, DC: American Psychiatric Association; 2000:175-191

60. Winters KC, Anderson N, Bengston P, Stinchfield RD, Latimer WW. Development of a parent questionnaire for use in assessing adolescent drug abuse. *J Psychoactive Drugs.* 2000;32:3-13

61. Kandel D, Yamaguchi K. From beer to crack: developmental patterns of drug involvement. *Am J Public Health.* 1993;83:851-855

62. Bukstein O, Kaminer Y. The nosology of adolescent substance abuse. *Am J Addict.* 1994;3:1-13

63. Harrison PA, Fulkerson JA, Beebe TJ. DSM-IV substance use disorder criteria for adolescents: a critical examination based on a statewide school survey. *Am J Psychiatry.* 1998;155:486-492

64. *International Classification of Diseases, 9th Revision, Clinical Modification (ICD-9-CM).* 5th ed. Vol. 1. Los Angeles, CA: Practice Management Information Corporation; 2000:215-217

65. Wolraich ML, Felice ME, Drotar D, eds. *The Classification of Child and Adolescent Mental Diagnoses in Primary Care. Diagnostic and Statistical Manual for Primary Care (DSM-PC), Child and Adolescent Version.* Elk Grove Village, IL: American Academy of Pediatrics; 1996:133-141

66. Prochaska JO, DiClemente CC. Stages and processes of self-change of smoking: toward an integrative model of change. *J Consult Clin Psychol.* 1983;51:390-395

67. Prochaska JO, DiClemente CC, Velifer WF, Fava J. Measuring processes of change: applications to the cessation of smoking. *J Consult Clin Psychol.* 1988;56:520-528

68. DiClemente CC, Prochaska JO, Fairhurst SK, Velicer WF, Velasquez MM, Rossi JS. The process of smoking cessation: an analysis of precontemplation, contemplation, and preparation stages of change. *J Consult Clin Psychol.* 1991;59:295-304

69. DiClemente CC, Prochaska JO. Toward a comprehensive, transtheoreti cal model of change. In: Miller WR, Heather N, eds. *Treating Addictive Behaviors.* 2nd ed. New York, NY: Plenum Press; 1998:3-24

70. Prochaska JO. Enhancing motivation to change. In: Graham AW, Schultz TK, eds. *Principles of Addiction Medicine.* 2nd ed. Chevy Chase, MD: American Society of Addiction Medicine; 1998:595-607

71. Graham AW, Fleming MS. Brief interventions. In: Graham AW, TK Schultz, eds. *Principles of Addiction Medicine,* 2nd ed. Chevy Chase, MD: American Society of Addiction Medicine; 1998:615-630

72. Bien TH, Miller WR, Tonigan JS. Brief interventions for alcohol problems: a review. *Addiction.* 1993;88:315-336

73. Werner MJ. Principles of brief intervention for adolescent alcohol, tobacco, and other drug use. *Pediatr Clin North Am.* 1995;42:335-349

74. Miller WR. Enhancing motivation for change. In: Miller WR, Heather N, eds. *Treating Addictive Behaviors.* 2nd ed. New York, NY: Plenum Press; 1998:121-132

75. Rollnick S, Morgan M. Motivational interviewing: increasing readiness to change. In: Washton, AM, ed. *Psychotherapy and Substance Abuse: A Practitioner's Handbook.* New York, NY: The Guilford Press; 1995:179-191

76. Fleming MF, Manwell LB. Brief intervention in primary care settings. A primary treatment method for at-risk, problem, and dependent drinkers. *Alcohol Res Health.* 1999;23:128-137

77. Fleming MF, Mundt MP, French MT, Manwell LB, Stauffacher EA, Barry KL. Benefit-cost analysis of brief physician advice with problem drinkers in primary care settings. *Med Care.* 2000;38:7-18

78. Fleming MF, Barry KL, Manwell LB, Johnson K, London R. Brief physician advice for problem drinkers. A randomized controlled trial in community-based primary care practices. *JAMA.* 1997;13:1039-1045

Chapter 4

Scientific Issues in Drug Testing and Use of the Laboratory

Walter Rosenfeld, MD, FAAP, and William E. Wingert, PhD

Although controversy persists about legal and ethical issues involved in drug testing and the application of testing to individuals and groups[1] (see Chapters 2 and 7), the methods for testing continue to improve. In view of these controversies and advancements, the health care professional should have an understanding of the issues and technologies that apply to drug testing so as to provide optimal patient care.

Scientific Issues in Drug Testing

As the result of several factors, the technology for testing for drugs of abuse in urine has improved recently. Typically, the testing process involves 2 steps: screening by immunoassay and confirmation by gas chromatography/mass spectrometry (GC/MS). Forensic laboratories, which are accredited by the federal Substance Abuse and Mental Health Services Administration (SAMHSA), the College of American Pathologists, or a number of state agencies, are required to use immunoassay methods.

Manufacturers continue to develop initial screening assays that are more sensitive and reliable and that can be automated. However, immunoassays are not specific for a single drug or drug metabolite. Manufacturers provide laboratories with a list showing the cross-reactivity of an immunoassay with other compounds. These lists cannot be considered totally inclusive, because cross-reactivity is possible with a substance not studied. Therefore, whenever accuracy is required for forensic purposes, the screening result should be confirmed by using GC/MS. Methods of GC/MS continue to improve, and laboratories have developed procedures to confirm positive results from newer immunoassays and to meet the standards of the accrediting agencies and the expectations of their clients.

Screening tests ideally should be designed for maximum sensitivity (few false-negative results). Otherwise, a false-negative result would terminate the testing process. "Screen-only" testing without confirmation is less expensive, but the potential for a false-positive result from the screen is high when the prevalence of drug use is low in the population being tested. Therefore, screen-only testing should be avoided except in the management of known substance abusers when frequent testing is required and cost issues are critical.

Confirmation by GC/MS yields a highly accurate result with maximum specificity (few false-positive results). GC/MS using selected ion monitoring for the targeted drug has become the laboratory gold standard. This method of confirmation is not suitable for large-scale screening, because it is expensive. Together, the combination of immunoassay (high sensitivity) and GC/MS (high specificity) provides the most accurate diagnostic information. A number of questions must be addressed when designing a drug-testing program. These questions include the following:

1. *How wide a variety of drugs is being assayed?*

   This may vary from a single drug when a particular substance is being monitored to a broad variety when there is no apparent drug of choice. Typically, the laboratory tests for a limited menu of drugs (Table 4.1), and the numbers and types of specific drugs assayed vary among laboratories. Pediatricians should also be familiar with what drugs are included in a particular screening panel before ordering a test. A small but important number of other abused substances, such as lysergic acid diethylamide (LSD), ketamine hydrochloride, and anabolic steroids, also may be of interest but may not detected by a screening immunoassay. Tests for these substances should be specifically ordered in addition to or in place of the usual screening panel.

2. *Should the immunoassay result be confirmed?*

   The necessity of confirmation testing to complement the immunoassay screen depends on the population being tested. Typically, in a general population undergoing urine drug testing, 5% of the

table 4.1 Duration of Detectability and Common Cutoffs for Selected Drugs in Urine by Immunoassay and GC/MS[2]

Drug	Approximate Detection Time in Urine*	Immunoassay Cutoff (ng/mL)	GC/MS Cutoff (ng/mL)
Amphetamines	3-4 d	1000	Amphetamine, 500; methamphetamine, 500
Cocaine	2-3 d	300	150
Cannabinoids	Varies with use: casual use, 2-3 d; long-term use, up to 1 mo	20/50/100	10/15
Opiates	2-3 d	300/2000	300/2000
Phencyclidine	8-10 d	25	25
Methadone	10-14 d	300	100
Propoxyphene	3-6 d	300	300
Barbiturates	Short-acting, 3-7 d; intermediate-acting, up to 2.5 wk	200	200
Benzodiazepines	Up to 2 wk	300	300
Methaqualone	4-6 d	300	300

*Detection times are considered to be independent of actual cutoffs used. Chronic users' detection time may be up to 1 mo.

results are positive. An almost ideal immunoassay with 99% specificity and 99% sensitivity used to screen a population with a 5% prevalence of use will yield a predictive value of 83.9%. That is, if 10 000 persons are screened and 500 (5%) are using a particular drug, 495 of the 500 would have positive test results (99% sensitivity), and 95 of the 9500 nonusers would have positive test results (1% false-positive results, or 99% specificity). The predictive value would be 495 of 590, or 83.9%. Clearly, a test that has almost 16% false-positive results is unacceptable when the results may affect a person's education, employment, or reputation. In such cases, the GC/MS confirmation must follow. On the other hand, if the population being tested has an 80% prevalence of use (eg, a group entering drug rehabilitation), the predictive value for the screening assay would be 99.7% (7920 true-positive results and only 20 false-positive results). Under these circumstances, a confirmation test may be unnecessary. As a general rule, however, positive screening results should always be confirmed by GC/MS.

3. *How broad a screen should be performed?*
The test menu of most forensic urine testing laboratories consists of approximately 10 tests, which can be screened by immunoassay and confirmed by GC/MS. The cost varies little whether few, several, or all drugs are being tested. Drug availability and use patterns depend somewhat on geography, and the physician may be able to limit the extent of testing through knowledge of the drugs most commonly used in a particular locale. Compared with broad screening batteries, testing strategies that focus on only 1 drug and, therefore, are less expensive are used in the periodic evaluation of subjects enrolled in drug treatment programs. Under these circumstances, the adolescent's drug of choice usually is known, and repeated testing for multiple drugs would be unproductive and unnecessarily expensive.

4. *What is the sensitivity of the screening procedure?*
Immunoassays are extremely sensitive screening procedures (Table 4.1). Manufacturers have adjusted the sensitivity of the immunoassays so that there is optimal response at the cutoff

concentration used to determine whether the test result is positive or negative. Because most drugs can only be detected in urine for a short time, it is advantageous to use the lowest cutoff available, which will then lead to confirmation by GC/MS.[3] A much discussed concern with low cutoffs for immunoassays for marijuana has been that positive results might be attributable to passive inhalation of second-hand smoke. However, numerous studies have demonstrated that it is unlikely that someone could unknowingly or passively be exposed to a sufficient amount of marijuana smoke to have a positive test result.[4-7]

5. **What is the specificity of the confirmatory procedure?**
Confirmatory procedures are often costly because of the extensive labor and expensive instrumentation required. However, when results may affect a person's education, sports participation, employment, or rights, the results must meet forensic standards so as to withstand the scrutiny of litigation and avoid unjustly injuring the person. The 3 key elements that must be met include establishment of the identity of the compound by a dependable analytical method with high specificity (such as GC/MS), accurate quantification of the drug (by GC/MS), and chain of custody documentation of the specimen and aliquots.[8]

6. **Is there a well-documented chain of custody?**
When circumstances may lead to litigation or punishment, the chain of custody must not be overlooked, because it is challenged more often in legal procedures than are the analytical results. The person responsible for the collection must follow an established written protocol. Guidelines for such protocols have been well established.[8,9] Often, the collection of a specimen is not observed directly, because such observation violates social taboos about individual rights to privacy. Some laboratories use a urine collection protocol developed by the SAMHSA[10] that does not involve direct observation. Patients are required to empty their pockets before giving a specimen, are sent into a collection room where the water has been turned off and blue dye added to standing water to prevent dilution or adulteration,

and a temperature is taken of the collected specimen immediately after it is obtained. However, for the adolescent who has already agreed to produce a urine specimen for drug testing, it is appropriate and logical to explain that this needs to be done under direct observation. Failure to observe the collection of the specimen allows for adulteration and interferes with the establishment of a chain of custody. Ideally, the collector seals the specimen in the presence of the donor, completes the chain of custody documentation, and arranges for the specimen to be forwarded to the laboratory. The chain of custody is continued once the laboratory receives the specimen and breaks the seal as a precursor to testing. Any transfers of the specimen bottle must be documented properly. Specimens are handled and stored in a secure location separate from the testing area. Aliquots of the specimen for testing must have a chain of custody equivalent to that for the original specimen. Specimens for which test results are positive are commonly stored frozen for 1 year and indefinitely if the results are being challenged in court or if the client requests longer storage.

7. *Should urine be the specimen of choice?*

Many body tissues and fluids other than urine can be used for drug testing.[11,12] Included in this list of tissues and fluids are hair, nails, saliva, and sweat (Table 4.2). Hair, in particular, has evoked much interest as an alternative to urine.[13,14] However, urine remains the most widely used specimen for the following reasons:

a. The collection of urine is noninvasive.
b. Adequate volumes for testing are collected easily.
c. Because of the concentrating function of the kidney, drugs or their metabolites are present in sufficiently high concentrations.
d. Because of the usual absence of protein and cellular components, urine is a relatively clean substance for analysis.
e. Drugs and metabolites usually are stable in frozen urine, permitting long-term storage of samples for which test results are positive.

A disadvantage of using urine for testing is that often the specimen is not collected under direct observation, allowing the opportunity for tampering by substitution of a "clean" urine specimen or by the addition of an adulterant that may interfere with testing

table 4.2 Detection Times and Apparent Advantages and Disadvantages of Unconventional Samples

Sample	Detection Time	Advantages	Disadvantages
Hair	Months	• Long-term measure of drug use • Easily obtainable • Ability to obtain similar sample for reanalysis • Low potential for manipulations of samples to alter test outcome	• New technology • Recent drug use not readily detected • Potential environmental contamination • Potential ethnic bias • Limited number of laboratories that offer hair testing services
Nail	Months	• Long-term measure of drug use	• New technology • Not readily obtainable • Recent drug use not detected • Potential environmental contamination
Saliva	12-24 h	• Easily obtainable • Parent drug present • Saliva concentration correlates to free drug concentration in plasma	• New technology • Short-term measure of drug use • Potential oral drug contamination
Sweat	1-4 wk	• Cumulative measure of drug use • Easily obtainable • Parent drug present • Monitor drug use for a period of weeks with drug patch	• New technology • Potential environmental contamination • High intersubject variability

Adapted with permission from Cone EJ. *New Developments in Biological Measures of Drug Prevalence: The Validity of Self-reported Drug Use: Improving the Accuracy of Survey Estimates.* Bethesda, MD: National Institute on Drug Abuse; 1994.

procedures.[15-17] The potential for adulteration has assumed greater importance as substances that interfere with testing, such as potassium nitrite,[18,19] glutaraldehyde,[20] and others, have become available commercially and advertised widely for their ability to sabotage urine testing. As laboratories develop methods to detect these adulterants, new ones undoubtedly will appear.

A partial means of detecting possible adulteration or manipulation of the urine specimen is to check the specific gravity. A urine-specific gravity less than 1.010 is deemed too dilute for drug testing by the United States Olympic Committee and the National Collegiate Athletic Association.[21]

Even an accurate drug testing procedure differentiates only between the persons who have used a drug recently and those who have not. The time after exposure during which test results will be positive is relatively short (Table 4.1). The results of a single urine test do not indicate the pattern of drug use, the method of administration, the frequency of use, or the amount used. No interpretation can be made about whether the person is dependent or addicted or whether the person is physically or mentally impaired by the drug.[22] These limitations hold true for urinary ethanol concentrations, which often do not correlate well with blood alcohol concentrations.[23] The assignment of impairment must rely on overt behavioral signs, tests of cognitive function, or more extensive psychosocial assessments designed for this purpose.[24,25]

Urine drug testing always should be performed in a laboratory that is accredited by an established regulatory body, such as SAMHSA, the College of American Pathologists, or a designated state agency, and that engages in regular proficiency testing. Accreditation by these agencies requires that the laboratory director be a physician or a doctoral-level scientist with extensive experience and background in forensic toxicology and related disciplines. An important criterion for selecting a laboratory is the ready availability of the director or other qualified personnel for necessary consultation or clarification.

Screening Techniques

Color or Spot Tests

These tests are used to test for the presence of specific drugs that are not detected readily by other techniques used for broad-spectrum analysis. Spot tests are used to detect drugs such as salicylates,[26] ethchlorvynol,[27] and ethanol.[28] The tests are performed by adding urine to a reagent that produces a specific color change if the suspected drug is present. Usually, the tests are performed manually, and the color change is observed visually. If a semiquantitative result is desired, the color may be measured spectrophotometrically. Advantages of spot testing include the low cost of the reagents and the immediate availability of results. Disadvantages include production of a similar color change by other substances so that the reaction is not totally specific. Also, the sensitivity is low, and a high concentration of the drug may be necessary to produce the color change.

Thin-Layer Chromatography

Thin-layer chromatography (TLC) was one of the earliest methods used to screen for drugs of abuse.[29,30] The sensitivity of TLC is not as good as immunoassays, and it is labor intensive, requiring an extraction and concentration step before application to the thin layer plate. The identification of a drug by migration distance and characteristic color can be subjective. Nevertheless, TLC performed by an experienced analyst remains an excellent tool for the identification of a broad spectrum of drugs.

Immunoassays

Protocols for workplace drug testing require the use of an immunoassay for initial screening. Six major types of immunoassays are in use, and they are discussed in descending order by volume of tests performed. All immunoassays share common features, including an antibody that has the required specificity and sensitivity, a mechanism for reaction of the antibody with the analyte (drug) to produce a product that can be measured, and a detection system that can measure this product (eg, color, fluorescence, radioactivity).

Enzyme-Multiplied Immunoassay Technique

Enzyme-multiplied immunoassay technique (EMIT [Behring, San Jose, CA]) is the most commonly used technology in urine drug testing. The assay is based on the competition between drug in the urine and drug labeled with an enzyme (glucose-6-phosphate dehydrogenase [G6PD]) for antibody binding sites. The enzyme activity decreases on binding to the antibody so that the resulting absorbance change is directly proportional to the amount of drug in the urine. The reaction occurs in 1 phase (homogeneous assay), which permits adaptation on many high-volume clinical analyzers.

Kinetic Interaction of Microparticles in Solution

Kinetic interaction of microparticles in solution (KIMS [Abuscreen Online {Roche Diagnostic Systems, Branchburg, NJ}]) is a more recent technology now in common use in urine drug testing. In KIMS, there is competitive binding of latex particle-labeled drugs with the analyte (drug of abuse, if present) for a limited amount of available antibody. In the absence of a drug of abuse in the urine, the antibody cross-links to sufficient particle-labeled molecules to result in agglutination. The degree of agglutination produces a change in absorbance that is measurable and inversely proportional to the amount of abused drug in the specimen. Similar to EMIT, KIMS is a homogeneous immunoassay and has been adapted for use on a number of clinical analyzers.

Cloned-Enzyme Donor Immunoassay

Cloned-enzyme donor immunoassay (CEDIA [Microgenics, Concord, CA]) is a newer immunoassay based on a genetically engineered enzyme (β-galactosidase). The amount of drug in the urine determines the amount of active enzyme produced from an inactive precursor. The active enzyme then is responsible for hydrolysis of a chromophore to produce a measurable absorbance change.

Radioimmunoassay

Radioimmunoassay (RIA) is one of the first and most sensitive techniques for urine drug testing.[31] RIA uses competition between radioactive-labeled drug and free unlabeled drug for a limited amount of antibody. Because the required separation step adds to the complexity of the technique, RIA has not been adapted for use on clinical analyzers as have EMIT, KIMS, and CEDIA.

Fluorescence Polarization Immunoassay

Fluorescence polarization immunoassay (FPIA) also is based on competitive binding between labeled antigen and unlabeled antigen. The label is a compound that fluoresces. The assay is based on the amount of polarized fluorescent light detected when the fluorescent-labeled drug is excited with plane polarized light. FPIA is used primarily for measurement of drugs and other low–molecular-weight compounds. FPIA procedures have been automated and have good sensitivity.

Enzyme-Linked Immunosorbent Assay

Another emerging method is enzyme-linked immunosorbent assay (ELISA). Testing by ELISA involves antibodies to specific drugs that are bound to a microtiter plate. ELISA is particularly useful in screening for drugs and metabolites that are not detected by the previously described methods. ELISA methods have been adapted for use with specimens other than urine.[32,33]

Immunoassays have advantages and disadvantages. Among the disadvantages is the fact that immunoassays cannot stand alone when used for forensic purposes, because they are not totally specific. Cross-reactivity may occur with other drugs or with other substances that cannot be identified. This cross-reactivity is of particular concern when testing for amphetamines and opiates. A number of sympathomimetic amines, including pseudoephedrine, ephedrine, and phenylpropanolamine hydrochloride, are available without a prescription and are not typically drugs of abuse. Similarly, opioids, such as hydrocodone, hydromorphone hydrochloride, oxycodone hydrochloride, and oxymorphone hydrochloride, all of which may be prescribed legitimately, cross-react with the opiate immunoassay but will not be confirmed by GC/MS specific for morphine or codeine. Manufacturers supply testing laboratories with a list that shows the cross-reactivity of the immunoassay with drugs. The cross-reactivity differs among types of immunoassays and even within the same immunoassay when a different antibody is used. Yet another disadvantage is that immunoassays are at best semiquantitative over a limited concentration range and should be regarded primarily as qualitative tests only.

Among the advantages of immunoassays is the fact that they are available for almost all drugs commonly abused by adolescents (Table 4.1). Immunoassays that have been adapted for clinical analyzers can be processed rapidly and interfaced to a computer system for reporting. Although immunoassays are not totally specific, broad cross-reactivity may be an advantage when screening for a class of drug, such as benzodiazepines, or when assessing for an unknown drug in a specimen from an emergency room.

Confirmation Techniques

Gas Chromatography

Gas chromatography is a commonly used technique for the detection of drugs in body fluids.[34-36] The substance being analyzed is extracted from the urine into an organic solvent and placed in a capillary column. Compounds are separated by their differing retention times on the capillary column. The capillary columns in use have the capacity to differentiate among many compounds. Compounds with similar structures may be extremely difficult to separate by gas chromatography, and therefore, an additional step using a detector to definitively identify a unique compound is needed. The sensitivity is excellent when combined with a suitable detector for the drug being analyzed. A variety of detectors are available, including flame ionization, nitrogen-phosphorus, electron capture, and mass spectrometry. The performance of gas chromatography requires a highly trained analyst and expensive equipment. It is also time consuming, as only 1 sample can be analyzed at a time.

Gas Chromatography/Mass Spectrometry

GC/MS combines the high resolving power of gas chromatography with the molecular identifying capacity of mass spectrometry.

GC/MS represents the gold standard for the confirmation of the presence of drugs in the urine.[37] After separation of compounds by gas chromatography, the mass spectrometer breaks the compound eluting from the gas chromatography column into ion fragments. These ion fragments are unique to particular drugs, and thus, mass spectrometry provides an identifying fingerprint of a detected substance. The time-consuming process of extracting the drug from the urine, the cost of the equipment to perform GC/MS, and the technical expertise necessary to perform the test contribute to the reality that this technique, however accurate, should be used for confirmatory rather than screening purposes.

High-Performance Liquid Chromatography

High-performance liquid chromatography (HPLC) is another established chromatographic technique available to separate and analyze a large variety of compounds.[38] It is particularly useful for the confirmation of drugs that cannot be analyzed by gas chromatography because they are not volatile or they decompose when exposed to the high heat of gas chromatography. As with gas chromatography, a detector must be used to identify a particular substance of abuse definitively.

A variety of other methods continue to emerge as confirmatory tests for drugs of abuse. HPLC with diode array detector has evolved with the development of the diode array/ultraviolet-visible spectral detector, which allows for the computerized comparison of the light spectrum of an unknown substance with a library of known spectra, yielding a high degree of specificity.[39] As with GC/MS, the time necessary for sample preparation, the technical expertise necessary to perform the analysis, and the cost of the equipment prohibit the use of HPLC with diode array detector as a screening tool. Liquid chromatography/mass spectrometry is useful for the analysis of a variety of compounds that are too fragile for accurate analysis by GC/MS.[40] Liquid chromatography/mass spectrometry combines liquid chromatography with tandem mass spectrometry; it is a sophisticated method with great specificity and sensitivity and is useful for the analysis for compounds present in very low levels, such as LSD.[41]

Conclusion

In addition to legal and ethical considerations, physicians should be aware of the strengths and limitations of drug testing methods. Standards for testing body fluids for drugs of abuse are well established, and many laboratories are accredited by state agencies or national groups, such as SAMHSA or the College of American Pathologists. Forensic drug testing requires that the initial screening immunoassay, which lacks specificity, be followed by a highly specific confirmatory method that unequivocally establishes the identity of the suspect compound. Currently, GC/MS is the widely accepted confirmatory method, although new technologies continue to emerge.

Health care professionals should be cognizant of the objectives of any drug testing program in which they participate. They should be comfortable with the criteria for selecting persons to be tested, the validity of the procedures used to collect specimens, and the adequacy of the laboratory methods for screening and confirmation. Furthermore, because health care professionals are often placed in the role of interpreting and responding to the results of drug testing, they should be aware that even a positive result does not provide information about the extent of abuse or any attendant physical or mental impairment.

References

1. American Academy of Pediatrics, Committee on Substance Abuse. Testing for drugs of abuse in children and adolescents. *Pediatrics.* 1996;98:305-307
2. Moffat AC, Jackson JV, Moss MS, Widdop B, eds. *Clarke's Isolation and Identification of Drugs.* 2nd ed. New York, NY: Rittenhous; 1986
3. Wingert WE. Lowering cutoffs from initial and confirmation testing for cocaine and marijuana: large scale study of effects on rates of drug positive results. *Clin Chem.* 1997;43:101-103
4. Cone EJ, Johnson RE. Contact highs and urinary cannabinoid excretion after passive exposure to marijuana smoke. *Clin Pharmacol Ther.* 1986;40:247-255
5. Cone EJ, Johnson RE, Darwin WD, Yousefnejad D, Paul BD, Mitchell J. Passive inhalation of marijuana smoke: urinalysis and room air levels of delta-9 tetrahydrocannabinol. *J Anal Toxicol.* 1987;11:89-96

6. Mule SJ, Lomax P, Gross SJ. Active and realistic passive marijuana exposure tested by three immunoassays and GC-MS in urine. *J Anal Toxicol.* 1988;12:113-116

7. Perez-Reyes M, DiGuiseppi S, Mason AP, Davis KH. Passive inhalation of marijuana smoke and urinary excretion of cannabinoids. *Clin Pharmacol Ther.* 1983;34:36-41

8. Mandatory guidelines for federal workplace drug testing programs, 53 *Federal Register* 1170 (1988)

9. Center for Substance Abuse Prevention. *Urine Specimen Collection Handbook for Federal Workplace Drug Testing Programs.* Rockville, MD: Substance Abuse and Mental Health Services Administration, US Department of Health and Human Services; 1996. DHHS Publication No. SMA 96-3114

10. Vogl W. *Urine Specimen Collection Handbook for Federal Workplace Drug Testing Programs.* DHHS Publication No. SMA 96-3114. Rockville, MD: Substance Abuse and Mental Health Services Administration, US Department of Health and Human Services; 1996

11. US Department of Health and Human Services, Substance Abuse and Mental Health Services Administration, Drug Testing Advisory Board. Report from the Scientific Meeting on Drug Testing of Alternative Technologies; April 28-30, 1997; Rockville, MD. Available at: http://www.health.org/workpl.htm. Accessed March 8, 2001

12. Baumgartner WA, Hill VA, Blahd WH. Hair analysis for drugs of abuse. *J Forensic Sci.* 1989;34:1433-1453

13. Baumgartner WA, Hill V. Hair analysis for organic analytes: methodology, reliability issues, and field studies. In: Kintz P, ed. *Drug Testing in Hair.* Boca Raton, FL: CRC Press Inc; 1996:223-266

14. Inoue T, Seta S, Goldberger BA. Analysis of drugs in unconventional samples. In: Liu RH, Goldberger BA, eds. *Handbook of Workplace Drug Testing.* Washington, DC: American Association for Clinical Chemistry Press; 1995:131-158

15. Cody JT. Adulteration of urine specimens. In: Liu RH, Goldberger BA, eds. *Handbook of Workplace Drug Testing.* Washington, DC: American Association for Clinical Chemistry Press; 1995:181-208

16. Liu RH. Comparison of common immunoassay kits for effective application in workplace drug urinalysis. *Forensic Sci Rev.* 1964;6:19

17. Baiker C, Serrano L, Lindner B. Hypochlorite adulteration of urine causing decreased concentration of delta 9-THC-COOH by GC/MS. *J Anal Toxicol.* 1994;18:101-103

18. El Sohly MA, Feng S, Kopycki WJ, et al. A procedure to overcome interferences caused by adulterant "Klear" in the GC-MS analysis of 11-nor-delta9-THC-9-COOH [letter]. *J Anal Toxicol.* 1997;21:240

19. Urry FM, Komaromy-Hiller G, Staly B, et al. Nitrite adulteration of workplace urine drug-testing specimens, I: sources and associated concentrations of nitrite in urine and distinction between natural sources and adulteration. *J Anal Toxicol.* 1998;22:89-95

20. Goldberger BA, Caplan YH. Effect of glutaraldehyde (Urinaid) by immunoassay. *Clin Chem.* 1994;40:1605-1606

21. Davis A, Sample B. Drug testing procedures for athletes. In: Fuentes RJ, Rosenberg JM, Davis A, eds. *Athletic Drug Reference '95.* Durham, NC: Glaxo Inc; 1995:141-159

22. Kapur BM. Drug-testing methods and clinical interpretations of test results. *Bull Narc.* 1993;45:115-154

23. Baselt RC. Disposition of alcohol in man. In: Garriott JC, ed. *Medicolegal Aspects of Alcohol.* 3rd ed. Tucson, AZ: Lawyers & Judges Publishing Co Inc; 1996:65-83

24. Westrich LM, Rosenthal RN. Physical examination of substance abusers: how to gather evidence of concealed problems. *Postgrad Med.* 1995;97:111-123

25. Fuller PG, Cavanaugh RM. Basic assessment and screening for substance abuse in the pediatrician's office. *Pediatr Clin North Am.* 1995;42:295-315

26. Trinder P. Rapid determination of salicylate in biological fluids. *Biochem J.* 1954;57:301-303

27. Frings CS, Cohen PS. Rapid colorimetric method for the quantification of ethchlorvynol (Placidyl) in serum and urine. *Am J Clin Pathol.* 1970;54:833-836

28. Kozelka FL, Hine CH. Method for the determination of ethyl alcohol for medicolegal purposes. *Ind Engl Analyt Chem Educ.* 1941;15:905

29. Sunshine I. Use of thin-layer chromatography in the diagnosis of poisoning. *Am J Clin Pathol.* 1963;40:576-582

30. Sunshine I, Fike WW, Landesman H. Identification of therapeutically significant organic bases by thin-layer chromatography. *J Forensic Sci.* 1977;11:428-439

31. Liu RH. Evaluation of commercial immunoassay kits for effective workplace drug testing. In: Liu RH, Goldberger BA, eds. *Handbook of Workplace Drug Testing.* Washington, DC: American Association for Clinical Chemistry Press; 1995:67-130

32. Speihler V, Faye J, Fogerson R, Schoendorfer D, Niedbala RS. Enzyme immunoassay validation for qualitative detection of cocaine in sweat. *Clin Chem.* 1996;42:34-38

33. Cassells NP, Craston DH, Hand CW, Baldwin D. Development and validation of a non-isotopic immunoassay for the detection of LSD in human urine. *J Anal Toxicol.* 1996;20:409-415

34. Mule SJ. Routine identification of drugs of abuse in human urine, I: application of fluorometry, thin-layer and gas-liquid chromatography. *J Chromatogr.* 1971;55:255-266

35. Costello CE, Hertz HS, Sakai T, Biemann K. Routine use of a flexible gas chromatograph–mass spectrometer–computer system to identify drugs and their metabolites in body fluids of overdose victims. *Clin Chem.* 1974;20:255-265

36. Ullucci PA, Cadoret R, Stasiowski PD, Martin HF. A gas chromatographic mass spectrometric drug screening procedure in current use. *Clin Chem.* 1976;22:1197

37. Mandatory guidelines for federal workplace drug testing programs: revised mandatory guidelines, 59 *Federal Register* 29908-29931 (1994)

38. Wallace JE, Hamilton HE. Analytical principles. In: Cravey RH, Baselt RC, eds. *Introduction to Forensic Toxicology*. Davis, CA: Biomedical Publications; 1981:87-109

39. Elliott SP, Hale KA. Applications of a HPLC-DAD drug screening system on retention indices and UV spectra. *J Anal Toxicol.* 1998;22:279-289

40. Hoja H, Marquet P, Verneuil B, Lofti H, Penicaut B, Lachatre G. Applications of liquid chromatography-gas spectrometry in analytical toxicology: a review. *J Anal Toxicol.* 1997;21:116-126

41. de Kanel J, Vickery WE, Waldner BA, Monahan RM, Diamond FX. Automated extraction of lysergic acid diethylamide (LSD) and N-demethyl-LSD from blood, serum, plasma, and urine samples using the Zymark RapidTrace with LC/MS/MS confirmation. *J Forensic Sci.* 1998;32:622-625

Chapter 5

The Role of the Primary Care Physician in the Referral Process

Paul G. Fuller, Jr, MD, FAAP

The primary care physician is faced daily with the direct or indirect consequences of substance abuse affecting patients and their families. The spectrum ranges from the effects of environmental tobacco smoke on the infant or physical or sexual abuse of the young child to severe emotional, educational, physical, or legal consequences for adolescents and frequent violent drug-related deaths. This chapter focuses on guidelines for referral of the adolescent who is known or suspected to be abusing or addicted to mood-altering drugs. This is a difficult and uncertain area of clinical practice for the average health care professional who commonly has not had sufficient education or experience to acquire a sense of competence or expertise for managing these patients.

To approach such adolescents, the primary care physician first must identify risk factors for substance abuse and then recognize signs and symptoms that may be consequences of substance abuse rather than of primary medical, behavioral, or psychiatric conditions. These signs and symptoms include frequent injuries, chronic respiratory complaints, sexually transmitted diseases, pregnancy, family problems, truancy or school suspension, and depression or suicide attempts. The patient's denial system and that of teachers, parents, physicians, and friends often delays or makes diagnosis difficult, especially because the diagnosis of substance abuse disorders is made predominantly on the basis of a thorough history, which may not be presented truthfully.

During the last decade, the pediatric and adolescent medical literature has grown substantially as clinicians and researchers have reported their observations and work in the field of adolescent substance abuse. Prevention techniques are being subjected to scientific scrutiny as efforts to curb the desire to use mood-altering chemicals become more urgent in the face of increased use. The stages of adolescent substance abuse leading to dependency were defined more than a decade ago (Table 5.1).[1] Since then, the AAP has published many related policy statements and

table 5.1 Stages of Adolescent Substance Abuse

Stage	Description
1	Potential for abuse
	• Decreased impulse control
	• Need for immediate gratification
	• Available drugs, alcohol, inhalants
	• Need for peer acceptance
2	Experimentation: learning the euphoria
	• Use of inhalants, tobacco, marijuana, and alcohol with friends
	• Few, if any, consequences
	• Use may increase to weekends regularly
	• Little change in behavior
3	Regular use: seeking the euphoria
	• Use of other drugs, eg, stimulants, LSD, sedatives
	• Behavioral changes and some consequences
	• Increased frequency of use; use alone
	• Buying or stealing drugs
4	Regular use: preoccupation with the "high"
	• Daily use of drugs
	• Loss of control
	• Multiple consequences and risk-taking
	• Estrangement from family and "straight" friends
5	Burnout: use of drugs to feel normal
	• Poly substance use/cross-addiction
	• Guilt, withdrawal, shame, remorse, depression
	• Physical and mental deterioration
	• Increased risk-taking, self-destructive, suicidal

Reprinted with permission from Comerci GD. Recognizing the five stages of substance abuse. *Contemp Pediatr.* 1985;2:57-68.

has defined the role of the pediatrician in the management of substance abuse.[2] The treatment community continues to study therapeutic approaches, relapse prevention strategies, and outcomes. The challenge for the primary care physician remains, however, to determine the severity of the adolescent's drug involvement and then make a decision about continued office follow-up or referral for treatment. Risk factor assessment and evaluation by interview are addressed in earlier chapters and form the basis on which further management can be accomplished.

When to Follow Up and When to Refer

The early stages of substance abuse in adolescents are often the most difficult to evaluate. Although early experimentation with mood-altering chemicals, including nicotine, is normative, it is important that it not be condoned or permitted by adults in the adolescent's life or medical professionals caring for the adolescent. The first and only use of certain gateway drugs, such as inhalants or alcohol, occasionally has resulted in tragic consequences, including unintentional injuries and death. Often the early user is naive about the effects of a substance and uninitiated in its use and lacks tolerance for the effects of the drug.

For the new experimenter (stage 2) with or without an adverse consequence, education and close follow-up are indicated. The primary care physician can have an important role in the education process at this stage of use for the patient and the family. For the adolescent with an adverse consequence (eg, acute intoxication, an injury, school suspension), an evaluation by an experienced adolescent drug counselor or physician might be an appropriate intervention and would underscore the significance of the behavior. Follow-up office visits should address current use. Families should be advised to set firm rules about their adolescent's involvement with nicotine and other drugs, and consequences for use should be clearly defined with unequivocal understanding of expectations and compliance. Enabling behavior by parents, teachers, other adults, and health care professionals must be recognized and avoided. The primary care physician can become part of a chain of adults who emphasize the nonuse message by providing clear and consistent information to parents and their adolescents while maintaining a trusting and caring relationship. A nonjudgmental health risk-based approach is paramount. An adversarial relationship must be avoided if continued discussion of substance abuse and other high-risk behaviors is the goal.

The decision to refer more drug-involved adolescents (stages 3 through 5) is straightforward if the symptoms and signs are recognized as being caused by substance abuse or dependence. Where to refer the identified adolescent in need of treatment is often more complicated. For admission to a reimbursable level of care, most treatment programs require an abuse or dependence diagnosis according to *Diagnostic and Statistical Manual of Mental Disorders, Fourth Edition*[3] *(DSM-IV)* criteria, although in some communities, treatment programs with education and prevention services are available for adolescents with substance abuse problems who are identified early. Although most primary care physicians do not have a working knowledge of *DSM-IV* diagnoses, an understanding of "substance abuse" and "substance dependence" criteria can be helpful in determining whom or where to refer (Tables 5.2 and 5.3).[3] Unless the primary care physician has additional knowledge or training in addiction medicine, it is highly recommended that any adolescent meeting *DSM-IV* criteria for abuse or dependence be referred at least for an evaluation and treatment recommendation by a professional experienced in adolescent chemical dependency. If the patient or family is unwilling to proceed with this phase of intervention, an adversarial relationship might ensue as the primary care physician makes referral recommendations that are clearly indicated but not accepted by the patient or family. It is important to stand firm on what is best for the adolescent and family but remain available and supportive.

---

table 5.2 *DSM-IV* **Criteria for Substance Abuse**

A. A maladaptive pattern of substance use leading to clinically significant impairment or distress, as manifested by one (or more) of the following, occurring within a 12-month period:

   (1) recurrent substance use resulting in a failure to fulfill major role obligations at work, school, or home (eg, repeated absences or poor work performance related to substance use; substance-related absences, suspension, or expulsion from school; neglect of children or household)

   (2) recurrent substance use in situations in which it is physically hazardous (eg, driving an automobile or operating a machine when impaired by substance use)

   (3) recurrent substance-related legal problems (eg, arrests for substance-related disorderly conduct)

   (4) continued substance use despite having persistent or recurrent social or interpersonal problems caused or exacerbated by the effects of the substance (eg, arguments with spouse about consequences of intoxication, physical fights)

B. The symptoms have never met the criteria for Substance Dependence for this class of substance.

Reprinted with permission from American Psychiatric Association. *Diagnostic and Statistical Manual of Mental Disorders, Fourth Edition (DSM-IV)*. Washington, DC: American Psychiatric Association; 1994:183-183.

Where to Refer

In the field of addiction medicine, the concept of "patient-treatment matching" has become increasingly important for determining appropriate clinical (and economic) levels of care for the patient with a diagnosis of substance abuse or dependence.[4] Patient-treatment matching is based on a comprehensive biopsychosocial assessment of the patient and considers current and past drug use, previous treatment, health consequences, psychiatric comorbid conditions, family and social issues, vocational-educational effects, legal history, motivation for treatment, and support systems available.

table 5.3 *DSM-IV* **Criteria for Substance Dependence**

A maladaptive pattern of substance use, leading to clinically significant impairment or distress, as manifested by three (or more) of the following, occurring at any time in the same 12-month period:

1. Tolerance, as defined by either of the following:
   a. A need for markedly increased amounts of the substance to achieve intoxication or desired effect.
   b. Markedly diminished effect with continued use of the same amount of the substance.

2. Withdrawal, as manifested by either of the following:
   a. The characteristic withdrawal syndrome for the substance.
   b. The same (or a closely related) substance is taken to relieve or avoid withdrawal symptoms.

3. The substance is often taken in larger amounts or over a longer period than was intended.

4. There is a persistent desire or unsuccessful efforts to cut down or control substance use.

5. A great deal of time is spent in activities necessary to obtain the substance (eg, visiting multiple doctors or driving long distances), use the substance (eg, chain-smoking), or recover from its effects.

6. Important social, occupational, or recreational activities are given up or reduced because of substance use.

7. The substance use is continued despite knowledge of having a persistent or recurrent physical or psychological problem that is likely to have been caused or exacerbated by the substance (eg, current cocaine use despite recognition of cocaine-induced depression or continued drinking despite recognition that an ulcer was made worse by alcohol consumption).

Reprinted with permission from American Psychiatric Association. *Diagnostic and Statistical Manual of Mental Disorders, Fourth Edition (DSM-IV)*. Washington, DC: American Psychiatric Association; 1994:181.

Managed care dictates treatment options for chemical dependency and mental health as rigorously as for medical and surgical
treatments. The primary care physician routinely is required to
approve referrals for substance abuse and mental health treatment.
Firm guidelines are being established that dictate level of care and
length of treatment. Inpatient treatment is no longer the norm for
the initial referral. More commonly, the patient first must have
unsuccessful results from outpatient treatment.

The American Society of Addiction Medicine (ASAM) has
published *ASAM Patient Placement Criteria for the Treatment
of Substance-Related Disorders, Second Edition-Revised* that
defines levels of adult and adolescent treatment.[5] Adolescent
levels include early intervention, outpatient treatment, intensive
outpatient treatment, partial hospitalization, clinically managed
low-intensity residential treatment, clinically managed medium-
intensity residential treatment, medically monitored high-intensity
residential/inpatient treatment, and medically managed intensive
inpatient treatment. Placement is determined on the basis of 6
multidimensional criteria: (1) acute intoxication or withdrawal
potential; (2) previous medical conditions and complications;
(3) emotional and behavioral conditions and complications;
(4) treatment acceptance or resistance; (5) relapse and continued
use potential; and (6) recovery environment (Table 5.4). The
ASAM criteria also include parameters for continued stay
and discharge from various levels of treatment.

A more comprehensive and detailed description of the continuum of adolescent treatment options based on multiple client
assessment criteria has been published by the Center for Substance
Abuse Treatment.[6] These treatment levels include more intensive
outpatient options as well as long-term residential psychosocial
care (therapeutic communities), halfway houses, and group home
living arrangements for seriously involved adolescents.

If the primary care physician chooses to use these criteria, at
least a basic understanding of the principles of substance abuse

table 5.4 Crosswalk of the Adolescent Placement Criteria Levels 0.5 through IV

Levels of Care

CRITERIA DIMENSIONS	LEVEL 0.5 Early Intervention	LEVEL I Outpatient Treatment	LEVEL II.1 Intensive Outpatient Treatment	LEVEL II.5 Partial Hospitalization	LEVEL III.1 Clinically Managed Low-Intensity Residential Treatment	LEVEL III.5 Clinically Managed Medium-Intensity Residential Treatment	LEVEL III.7 Medically Monitored High-Intensity Residential Inpatient Treatment	LEVEL IV Medically Managed Intensive Inpatient Treatment
DIMENSION 1: Acute Intoxication and/or Withdrawal Potential	The adolescent is not at risk of withdrawal.	The adolescent is not at risk of withdrawal.	The adolescent is experiencing minimal withdrawal or is at risk of withdrawal.	The adolescent is experiencing mild withdrawal or is at risk of withdrawal.	The adolescent's state of withdrawal (or risk of withdrawal) is being managed concurrently at another level of care.	The adolescent is experiencing mild to moderate withdrawal (or is at risk of withdrawal), but does not need pharmacological management or frequent medical or nursing monitoring.	The adolescent is experiencing mild to moderate withdrawal (or is at risk of withdrawal), but this is manageable at Level III.7-D.	The adolescent is experiencing severe withdrawal (or is at risk of withdrawal) and requires intensive active medical management.
DIMENSION 2: Biomedical Conditions and Complications	None or very stable.	None or very stable.	None or stable, or distracting from treatment at a less intensive level of care. Such problems are manageable at Level II.1.	None or stable, or distracting from treatment at a less intensive level of care. Such problems are manageable at Level II.5.	None or stable.	None or stable; the adolescent is receiving concurrent medical monitoring as needed.	The adolescent requires medical monitoring, but not intensive treatment.	The adolescent requires 24-hour medical and nursing care.

table 5.4 Crosswalk of the Adolescent Placement Criteria Levels 0.5 through IV, cont.

Levels of Care

CRITERIA DIMENSIONS	LEVEL 0.5 Early Intervention	LEVEL I Outpatient Treatment	LEVEL II.1 Intensive Outpatient Treatment	LEVEL II.5 Partial Hospitalization	LEVEL III.1 Clinically Managed Low-Intensity Residential Treatment	LEVEL III.5 Clinically Managed Medium-Intensity Residential Treatment	LEVEL III.7 Medically Monitored High-Intensity Residential Inpatient Treatment	LEVEL IV Medically Managed Intensive Inpatient Treatment
DIMENSION 3: Emotional, Behavioral, or Cognitive Conditions and Complications	The adolescent evidences no or very stable problems in Dimension 3. These are being addressed through concurrent mental health services and do not interfere with addiction treatment at this level of care.	The adolescent's status in Dimension 3 is characterized by all of the following:	The adolescent's status in Dimension 3 features one or more of the following:	The adolescent's status in Dimension 3 features one or more of the following:	The adolescent's status in Dimension 3 features one or more of the following:	The adolescent's status in Dimension 3 features one or more of the following:	The adolescent's status in Dimension 3 features one or more of the following:	The adolescent's status in Dimension 3 features one or more of the following:
(a) *Dangerousness/Lethality*		(a) The adolescent is not at risk of harm.	(a) The adolescent is at low risk of harm, and he or she is safe between sessions.	(a) The adolescent is at low risk of harm, but he or she is safe overnight.	(a) The adolescent needs a stable living environment for safety.	(a) The adolescent is at moderate but stable risk of harm and thus needs medium-intensity 24-hour monitoring or treatment for safety.	(a) The adolescent is at moderate risk of harm and needs high-intensity 24-hour monitoring or treatment, or secure containment, for safety.	(a) The adolescent is at severe risk of harm.

table 5.4 Crosswalk of the Adolescent Placement Criteria Levels 0.5 through IV, cont.

CRITERIA DIMENSIONS	Levels of Care							
	LEVEL 0.5 Early Intervention	LEVEL I Outpatient Treatment	LEVEL II.1 Intensive Outpatient Treatment	LEVEL II.5 Partial Hospitalization	LEVEL III.1 Clinically Managed Low-Intensity Residential Treatment	LEVEL III.5 Clinically Managed Medium-Intensity Residential Treatment	LEVEL III.7 Medically Monitored High-Intensity Residential Inpatient Treatment	LEVEL IV Medically Managed Intensive Inpatient Treatment
(b) *Interference with Addiction Recovery Efforts*		(b) There is minimal interference.	(b) Mild interference requires the intensity of this level of care to support treatment engagement.	(b) Moderate interference requires the intensity of this level of care to support treatment engagement.	(b) Moderate interference requires limited 24-hour supervision to support treatment engagement.	(b) Moderate to severe interference requires medium-intensity residential treatment to support engagement.	(b) Severe interference requires high-intensity residential treatment to support engagement.	(b) Very severe, almost overwhelming interference renders the adolescent incapable of participating in treatment at a less intensive level of care.
(c) *Social Functioning*		(c) The adolescent evidences minimal to mild impairment.	(c) The adolescent evidences mild to moderate impairment, but can sustain responsibilities.	(c) The adolescent evidences moderate impairment, but can sustain responsibilities.	(c) The adolescent evidences moderate impairment and needs limited 24-hour supervision to sustain responsibilities.	(c) The adolescent evidences moderate to severe impairment and cannot be managed at a less intensive level of care.	(c) The adolescent evidences severe impairment and cannot be managed at a less intensive level of care.	(c) The adolescent evidences very severe, dangerous impairment and requires frequent medical and nursing interventions.

table 5.4 Crosswalk of the Adolescent Placement Criteria Levels 0.5 through IV, cont.

Levels of Care

CRITERIA DIMENSIONS	LEVEL 0.5 Early Intervention	LEVEL I Outpatient Treatment	LEVEL II.1 Intensive Outpatient Treatment	LEVEL II.5 Partial Hospitalization	LEVEL III.1 Clinically Managed Low-Intensity Residential Treatment	LEVEL III.5 Clinically Managed Medium-Intensity Residential Treatment	LEVEL III.7 Medically Monitored High-Intensity Residential Inpatient Treatment	LEVEL IV Medically Managed Intensive Inpatient Treatment
(d) *Ability for Self-Care*		(d) The adolescent is experiencing minimal current difficulties with activities of daily living, but there is significant risk of deterioration.	(d) The adolescent is experiencing mild to moderate difficulties with activities of daily living and requires frequent monitoring or interventions.	(d) The adolescent is experiencing moderate difficulties with activities of daily living and requires near-daily monitoring or interventions.	(d) The adolescent evidences moderate difficulties with activities of daily living and requires limited 24-hour supervision and frequent prompting.	(d) The adolescent evidences moderate to severe difficulties with activities of daily living and requires 24-hour supervision and medium-intensity staff assistance.	(d) The adolescent evidences severe difficulties with activities of daily living and requires 24-hour supervision and high-intensity staff assistance.	(d) The adolescent evidences very severe difficulties with activities of daily living and requires frequent medical and nursing interventions.
(e) *Course of Illness*		(e) The adolescent is at minimal imminent risk, which predicts a need for some monitoring or interventions.	(e) The adolescent's history (combined with the present situation) predicts the need for frequent monitoring or interventions.	(e) The adolescent's history (combined with the present situation) predicts the need for near-daily monitoring or interventions.	(e) The adolescent's history (combined with the present situation) predicts instability without limited 24-hour supervision.	(e) The adolescent's history (combined with the present situation) predicts destabilization without medium-intensity residential treatment.	(e) The adolescent's history (combined with the present situation) predicts destabilization without high-intensity residential treatment.	(e) The adolescent's history (combined with the present situation) predicts destabilization without inpatient medical management.

table 5.4 Crosswalk of the Adolescent Placement Criteria Levels 0.5 through IV, cont.

Levels of Care

CRITERIA DIMENSIONS	LEVEL 0.5 Early Intervention	LEVEL I Outpatient Treatment	LEVEL II.1 Intensive Outpatient Treatment	LEVEL II.5 Partial Hospitalization	LEVEL III.1 Clinically Managed Low-Intensity Residential Treatment	LEVEL III.5 Clinically Managed Medium-Intensity Residential Treatment	LEVEL III.7 Medically Monitored High-Intensity Residential Inpatient Treatment	LEVEL IV Medically Managed Intensive Inpatient Treatment
DIMENSION 4: Readiness to Change	The adolescent is willing to explore how current alcohol or drug use may affect achievement of personal goals.	The adolescent is willing to engage in treatment, and is at least contemplating change, but needs motivating and monitoring strategies.	The adolescent requires close monitoring and support several times a week to promote progress through the stages of change because of variable treatment engagement or a lack of recognition of the need for assistance.	The adolescent requires a near-daily structured program to promote progress through the stages of change because of poor treatment engagement, or escalating use and impairment, or lack of recognition of the role of alcohol or drugs in his or her present problems.	The adolescent is open to recovery, but needs 24-hour supervision to promote or sustain progress.	The adolescent needs intensive motivating strategies in a 24-hour structured program to address minimal treatment engagement or opposition to treatment, or his or her lack of recognition of current severe impairment.	The adolescent needs high-intensity motivating strategies in a 24-hour medically monitored program to address his or her lack of treatment engagement associated with a biomedical, emotional or behavioral condition; or because he or she is actively opposed to treatment, requiring confinement; or because he or she needs high-intensity case management to create linkages that would support outpatient treatment.	The adolescent's problems in Dimension 4 do not qualify him or her for Level IV services.

table 5.4 Crosswalk of the Adolescent Placement Criteria Levels 0.5 through IV, cont.

Levels of Care

CRITERIA DIMENSIONS	LEVEL 0.5 Early Intervention	LEVEL I Outpatient Treatment	LEVEL II.1 Intensive Outpatient Treatment	LEVEL II.5 Partial Hospitalization	LEVEL III.1 Clinically Managed Low-Intensity Residential Treatment	LEVEL III.5 Clinically Managed Medium-Intensity Residential Treatment	LEVEL III.7 Medically Monitored High-Intensity Residential Inpatient Treatment	LEVEL IV Medically Managed Intensive Inpatient Treatment
DIMENSION 5: Relapse, Continued Use or Continued Problem Potential	The adolescent needs to gain an understanding of, or skills to change, current use patterns.	The adolescent needs limited support to maintain abstinence or control use and to pursue recovery goals.	The adolescent needs close monitoring and support because of a significant risk of relapse or continued use and deterioration in his or her level of functioning. He or she has poor relapse prevention skills.	The adolescent needs near-daily monitoring and support because of a high risk of relapse or continued use and deterioration in his or her level of functioning. He or she has minimal relapse prevention skills.	The adolescent understands the potential for continued use and/or has emerging recovery skills, but needs supervision to reinforce recovery and relapse prevention skills, or to limit exposure to substances and/ or environmental triggers, or to maintain therapeutic gains.	The adolescent is unable to control use and avoid serious impairment without a 24-hour structured program because he or she is unable to overcome environmental triggers or cravings; or has insufficient supervision between encounters at a less intensive level of care; or has high chronicity and/or poor response to treatment.	The adolescent is unable to interrupt a high severity or high frequency pattern of use and avoid dangerous consequences without high-intensity 24-hour interventions (because of an emotional, behavioral or cognitive condition, severe impulse control problems, withdrawal symptoms, and the like).	The adolescent's problems in Dimension 5 do not qualify him or her for Level IV services.

table 5.4 **Crosswalk of the Adolescent Placement Criteria Levels 0.5 through IV, cont.**

Levels of Care

CRITERIA DIMENSIONS	LEVEL 0.5 Early Intervention	LEVEL I Outpatient Treatment	LEVEL II.1 Intensive Outpatient Treatment	LEVEL II.5 Partial Hospitalization	LEVEL III.1 Clinically Managed Low-Intensity Residential Treatment	LEVEL III.5 Clinically Managed Medium-Intensity Residential Treatment	LEVEL III.7 Medically Monitored High-Intensity Residential Inpatient Treatment	LEVEL IV Medically Managed Intensive Inpatient Treatment
DIMENSION 6: Recovery Environment	The adolescent's risk of initiation of or progression in substance use is increased by alcohol or drug use (or values relating to such use) by his or her family, peers or members of his or her social support system.	The adolescent's family and environment can support recovery with limited assistance.	The adolescent's environment is impeding his or her recovery, and the adolescent requires close monitoring and support to overcome that barrier.	The adolescent's environment renders recovery unlikely without near-daily monitoring and support or frequent relief from his or her home environment.	The adolescent's environment poses a risk to his or her recovery, so that he or she requires alternative residential containment or support.	The adolescent's environment is dangerous to his or her recovery, so that he or she requires residential treatment to promote recovery goals or for protection.	The adolescent's environment is dangerous to his or her recovery, and he or she requires residential treatment to promote recovery goals or for protection, and to help him or her establish a successful transition to a less intensive level of care.	The adolescent's problems in this Dimension 6 do not qualify him or her for Level IV services.

Note: This overview of the Adolescent Criteria is an approximate summary to illustrate the principal concepts and structure of the criteria.

Reprinted with permission from Mee-Lee D, Shulman G, Fishman M, Gastfriend D, Griffith JH, eds. *ASAM Patient Placement Criteria for the Treatment of Substance-Related Disorders, Second Edition-Revised (ASAM PPC-2R)*. Arlington, VA: American Society of Addiction Medicine; 2001:199-205.

assessment and addiction treatment is recommended. A more practical approach for the busy primary care physician is to establish a working relationship with a trusted and competent counselor or specialist working in the adolescent addiction treatment community. This team approach can be the basis for a strong alliance that connects the adolescent, the family, and the school with treatment professionals in the community. The primary care physician will have the opportunity to continue collaborative observation of the adolescent through the recovery process. (Consents for exchange of assessment and treatment information are rigorously adhered to in the substance abuse field and are enforced by a federal statute[7] prohibiting redisclosure, as for the patient with human immunodeficiency virus [HIV] infection.)

Successful addiction treatment usually involves more than one level of care during a long recovery process. The levels may involve outpatient or inpatient care at the outset with continued care at a level of intensity along the recovery continuum, depending on progress. Most chemically dependent patients in treatment, adult or adolescent, consider themselves "recovering" rather than "recovered" and are involved in sequential treatment levels that usually include a formal structured program, attendance at 12-step self-help groups (eg, Alcoholics Anonymous, Narcotics Anonymous, Al-Anon), and continued self-recovery work that has become part of a "clean" and sober lifestyle. Relapse is neither uncommon nor necessarily permanent but is rather an expected part of the recovery process and can be viewed as a learning opportunity important to the process rather than a failure. Primary care physicians can have an important supportive role during this time or a more active role in a secondary referral process if further formal treatment is required.

Some adolescents and adults are able to terminate a lifestyle of substance abuse or dependence by making a decision to stop drinking or using drugs on the basis of sheer personal commitment and the desire to stop use, with little formal treatment and only the aid of self-help groups or family support. Developmentally, many young people will stop abusing alcohol or drugs by late adolescence. The goals should not be to dictate specific treatment, level of care, or degree of participation but rather to identify the consequences of a drug- and alcohol-based lifestyle and motivate the patient to seek the help needed to initiate and sustain recovery. Motivation is most difficult for the adolescent patient, and there is emerging literature on the role of motivational interviewing to encourage change among nicotine-dependent and other chemically dependent patients.[8,9] Primary care physicians can have an important role in and enhance the motivation of their patients by taking the time to express their concerns and encourage treatment or at least a referral for evaluation. Successful recovery is impossible until the patient overcomes the denial that substance abuse is a primary cause of experienced negative life consequences and not caused by them. Active participation by various health care professionals can assist to break down denial and facilitate entry into the recovery process.

Criteria for the Selection of a Substance Abuse Treatment Program

Not all substance abuse treatment facilities are suitable for adolescent patients. Many facilities have inadequate experience treating adolescents and try to fit them into adult-centered or adult-modeled programs. The following are generic criteria that are included in guidelines recommended by the AAP for evaluating an inpatient or outpatient adolescent substance abuse treatment program[10]:

1. The program views drug and alcohol abuse as a primary disease rather than a symptom of an emotional problem.
2. The program includes a comprehensive evaluation of the patient and is able to manage appropriately any associated medical, emotional, or behavioral problems.
3. The program adheres to an abstinence philosophy. Any use is abuse. Drug use is a chronic disease, and a drug-free environment is essential.

4. There is a low patient-to-staff ratio. Psychiatrists, clinical psychologists, and counselors on staff are knowledgeable about the treatment of chemical dependency and adolescent behavior and development.

5. Professionally led support groups and self-help groups are integral parts of the program.

6. Adolescent groups are separate from adult groups if both are treated at the same facility.

7. The entire family is involved in treatment. The program relates to parents and patients with compassion and concern. The goal is reunification of the family whenever possible.

8. Follow-up and continuing care are an integral part of the program.

9. Patients have an opportunity to continue academic and vocational education and to be assisted in restructuring family, school, and social life.

10. The program administration discusses costs and financial arrangements for inpatient and outpatient care.

11. The program is as close to home as possible to facilitate family involvement even though separation of the adolescent from the family may be indicated initially.

Conclusion

This chapter defines the stages of substance abuse in adolescents and outlines referral guidelines based on the experience of the referring primary care physician and existing diagnostic and treatment criteria. The primary care physician can have an important role in addressing the effects of substance abuse on children and adults in the substance abusing family. Knowledge of the roles, locations, and meeting times of self-help groups, such as Alcoholics Anonymous, Al-Anon, and Alateen groups and Adult Children of Alcoholics groups, as appropriate sources of help is another way the primary care physician can be an important resource for children and families.

As in other complex chronic diseases, the primary care physician can have a role in primary and secondary prevention, screening, assessment, referrals, coordination of care, and long-term follow-up. More active involvement by health care professionals working together with parents, schools, and communities has the potential to make a significant impact on the effects of nicotine, drugs, and alcohol on children and adolescents.

References

1. Comerci GD. Recognizing the five stages of substance abuse. *Contemp Pediatr.* 1985;2:57-68
2. American Academy of Pediatrics, Committee on Substance Abuse. Tobacco, alcohol, and other drugs: role of the pediatrician in prevention and management of substance abuse. *Pediatrics.* 1998;101:125-128
3. American Psychiatric Association. *Diagnostic and Statistical Manual of Mental Disorders, Fourth Edition (DSM-IV).* Washington, DC: American Psychiatric Association; 1994
4. Mee-Lee D. Matching in addictions treatment: how do we get there from here? In: Miller NS, ed. *Treatment of the Addictions: Applications of Outcome Research for Clinical Management.* Binghamton, NY: Harrington Park Press; 1995:113-127
5. American Society of Addiction, Medicine Working Group on Patient Placement Criteria. *ASAM Patient Placement Criteria for the Treatment of Substance-Related Disorders.* 2nd ed. Chevy Chase, MD: The American Society of Addiction Medicine; 1996
6. Center for Substance Abuse Treatment. *Screening and Assessment of Alcohol- and Other Drug-Abusing Adolescents.* Rockville, MD: Substance Abuse and Mental Health Services Administration, US Department of Health and Human Services; 1993. DHHS Publication No. SMA 93-2009
7. Confidentiality of alcohol and drug abuse patient records, 42 CFR §2.1 (1997)
8. Miller WR, Rollnick S. *Motivational Interviewing: Preparing People to Change Addictive Behavior.* New York, NY: Guilford Press; 1991
9. Werner MJ, Adger H Jr. Early identification, screening, and brief intervention for adolescent alcohol use. *Arch Pediatr Adolesc Med.* 1995;149:1241-1248
10. American Academy of Pediatrics, Committee on Substance Abuse. Indications for management and referral of patients involved in substance abuse. *Pediatrics.* 2000;106:143-148

Suggested Readings

Rogers PD, Werner MJ. Substance Abuse. *Pediatr Clin North Am.* 1995;42(theme issue):241-490

Schydlower M, Rogers PD. Adolescent substance abuse and addictions. *Adolesc Med.* 1993;4(theme issue):227-468

Chapter 6

Preventing the Use of Alcohol, Tobacco, and Illicit Drugs

Gilbert J. Botvin, PhD

During the past 3 decades, many local, state, and national programs have been developed and implemented to prevent the use of tobacco, alcohol, and illicit drugs among our nation's youth. The scope of these programs ranges from national media campaigns to school curricula to pamphlets distributed in a physician's waiting room. The effectiveness of these approaches varies considerably.

Substantial time, energy, and resources have been expended to better understand the causes of drug use and abuse and to identify potentially effective intervention strategies. Although significant advances have been made during the past 20 years, dissemination of the results of research to the providers of prevention programs has been slow. As a consequence, the challenge confronting health care professionals has changed recently from identifying and testing potentially effective prevention approaches to bridging the gap between research and practice to increase the use of prevention approaches based on sound science.

For many reasons, health care professionals should be aware of the diverse efforts to prevent drug use as well as the rationale, objectives, and activities of these approaches. First, the familiarity with the problem of drug use and existing efforts to prevent it can provide a health care professional with additional insight into the knowledge, attitudes, and beliefs about drug use of the patient, parents, or both. Second, knowledge of program content enables the health care professional to reinforce the positive messages, attitudes, and skills taught in prevention programs or to balance the effects of programs that provide erroneous or counterproductive information.

Finally, the health care professional is typically viewed as a community expert on health issues. As such, the health care professional should be conversant with the state-of-the-art in drug abuse prevention to provide advice to parents, educators, and government officials. Perhaps even more important, the health care professional should actively advocate for using proven, research-based prevention approaches to upgrade the quality and effectiveness of existing prevention programs.

Overview

This chapter provides a brief review of the current state-of-the-art in drug abuse prevention. First, the nature and importance of prevention are discussed. Next, the hierarchy or levels of prevention approaches are described, along with the terminology used by prevention theorists. Third, a historical overview of the past 3 decades of prevention activities is presented. Fourth, the main types of prevention approaches are briefly described with an emphasis on research-based prevention approaches targeting known causative factors. The chapter concludes with a set of prevention principles derived from prevention research and a summary of the best prevention programs available as determined by the findings of rigorous empirical research.

The modern history of prevention programs begins with initial responses to the "drug epidemic" of the late 1960s. The spread of psychedelic drug use and, to a lesser degree, amphetamine and barbiturate use first on college campuses and later in the youth culture more generally led to often hastily conceived attempts to decrease the number of youths who were "turning on, tuning in, and dropping out."

Nature and Importance of Prevention

The Increasing Prominence of Prevention

Drug use continues to be a major problem in the United States. The most recent data from the *Monitoring the Future Study*[1,2] conducted annually by the University of Michigan indicates small decreases in adolescents' use of alcohol, tobacco, and some illegal drugs, but steady use for many other drugs and sharp increases in use for others, such as 3,4-methylenedioxymethamphetamine (MDMA) or "ecstasy" (see Table 0.1, p ix). The number of young people who are experimenting with or using these substances remains unacceptably high. Consequently, the need to identify and implement the most effective drug use prevention programs remains a national priority, one which health care professionals can help achieve.

The treatment of drug abuse can be difficult and expensive.[3] However, drug treatment has been shown to be cost-effective. It seems preferable to prevent drug use in the first place rather than have to deal with the consequences for an adolescent who becomes harmfully involved. High-quality drug treatment is not only expensive, but it is becoming hard to find and often requires multiple attempts before the adolescent is able to remain abstinent. Prevention offers considerable promise as a natural complement to treatment approaches to drug abuse. An underlying assumption of prevention is that it is likely to be easier to deter the early stages of drug use than to treat such an insidious disorder once it has developed fully. Unfortunately, the conceptual simplicity of prevention belies its complexity. The development of effective prevention approaches has turned out to be far more difficult than was initially imagined by most theorists and prevention advocates. In truth, most efforts to develop effective drug abuse prevention approaches have achieved only limited success—that is, until recently.

Types of Prevention

Prevention approaches are defined in terms of the populations targeted and are referred to as "universal," "selective," or "indicated."[4] Each of these approaches falls along a continuum of prevention activities targeting persons at various points around the beginning of the developmental progression leading to a particular disease, condition, or disorder.

Universal prevention approaches
Universal approaches are designed to target an entire population and are similar to what was previously referred to as "primary" prevention. These approaches are intended to reach potential users before they have developed a particular problem or condition or, in some cases, even before the risk factors associated with the problem or condition have manifested. In fact, by the very nature of universal prevention approaches, risk status is ignored at this stage.

Selective prevention approaches
At the selective prevention level, persons deemed to be at high risk on the basis of a set of screening criteria or risk factors are selected to participate in the prevention program. The approaches are similar to what was previously referred to as "secondary" prevention.

Indicated prevention approaches
The final level in the prevention hierarchy consists of "indicated" prevention approaches. These approaches are designed to be more intensive and include only the persons for whom the intervention is indicated by virtue of some degree of involvement in the early stages of a particular disorder or condition. These approaches are similar to what was previously referred to as "tertiary" prevention. Although all 3 types of prevention are discussed in this chapter, the main emphasis is universal prevention approaches because of their importance and because there is a more extensive scientific literature testing the effectiveness of the universal approaches to substance abuse prevention.

Teaching Drug Information
The earliest prevention programs of the 1960s relied on moralizing or the presentation of overblown and often inaccurate information about the risks of drug use to scare children and adolescents into not using drugs. This approach seemed to do little except impair credibility in the eyes of youth who often knew (or thought they knew) more about drugs and their effects than the adult presenters. However, even presenting drug information about pharmacologic,

physical, psychologic, social, and legal issues in a more objective and less exaggerated way has not been effective.[5,6] Although such programs may have been more credible to youth than programs based on scare tactics, subsequent research has provided convincing evidence that drug information alone does little to discourage use and, in some cases, may be counterproductive. In particular, some data suggested that the programs aroused curiosity or instructed youth in the finer points of drug use, thus encouraging rather than discouraging drug experimentation.[7]

Promoting Personal Growth Through Affective Education

As data on the correlates of drug use became available in the early 1970s, programs began to focus on the psychologic characteristics that seemed to distinguish users from nonusers. The data suggested a relationship between drug use and variables such as low self-esteem, inadequate decision-making skills, and ineffective communication skills, although the direction of causality was unclear. The results of the studies, together with the then pervasive influence of the human potential movement in psychology, sparked the development of prevention programs that focused on "affective education." These programs sought to improve self-esteem, decision-making abilities, and communication and, somewhat later, to help youth clarify values about drug and alcohol use. Although some aspects of the early approaches are included in contemporary prevention programs, neither the methods used to teach affective education approaches nor the programs have been proven effective.[5,6,8]

Providing Alternatives

More or less coincident with the emergence of affective education programs, some drug abuse theorists began to argue that the most effective way of preventing drug use was to provide access to "alternative highs" that would meet the same needs users claimed drugs met (mind expansion, personal growth, excitement, challenge, relief from boredom) in nonpharmacologic ways.

Accordingly, programs were developed that provided youth with a variety of alternatives to drug use, ranging from wilderness challenges to community service to drug-free rock concerts. Although a number of alternative approaches have been tried, only a few have been evaluated carefully. Unfortunately, there is no available evidence that the alternatives approach to substance abuse prevention is effective.[8]

One of the early models for the alternatives approach to substance abuse prevention involved the establishment of youth centers providing a particular activity or set of activities in the community (eg, community service, academic tutoring, sports, hobbies). An underlying assumption of the alternatives approach is that if adolescents were provided with real-life experiences that were as appealing as substance use, their involvement in these activities would replace potential involvement with substance abuse.

Outward Bound programs, an example of an alternatives approach to substance abuse prevention, were organized in the hope that they would alter the affective and cognitive state of a person—in other words, that they would change the way the persons felt about themselves and others and how they saw the world. The programs included a variety of activities generally designed to promote teamwork, confidence, and self-esteem.

Another type of alternatives approach was designed to target more specific individual needs. For persons seeking relaxation or increased energy, these needs might be satisfied through exercise, participation in sports, or hiking. Similarly, the desire for sensory stimulation might be satisfied through activities designed to enhance sensory awareness, such as learning to appreciate the sensory aspects of music, art, and nature. Finally, the need for peer acceptance might be satisfied through participation in sensitivity training or encounter groups.

When considering the alternatives approach, it is important to recognize that although some activities typically included in the programs have been associated with avoidance of substance use, others consistently have been associated with substance use.

Therefore, it is important to select activities carefully. For example, entertainment activities, participation in vocational activities, and certain social activities have been associated with more substance use. Activities associated with avoidance of substance use include academic activities, involvement in religious activities, and participation in sports. Clearly, a difficulty of designing an alternatives program is that the activities most likely to decrease risk of substance use typically are the least interesting to youth at high risk of using drugs.

Although study of the effectiveness of alternatives programs used in isolation has not shown them to be effective, some of the approaches may be effective, particularly when used in combination with other effective prevention strategies. The alternatives concept is still used in many contemporary prevention programs to provide youth with engaging and safe recreation that is drug and alcohol free.

Contemporary Approaches

School-Based Approaches Targeting Social Influences

A major change in the direction of prevention research was triggered toward the end of the 1970s when researchers began testing a prevention approach that focused on the social influences believed to promote cigarette smoking. This approach was developed by Evans et al at the University of Houston and was designed to make students aware of the social pressures to smoke (referred to as psychologic inoculation) that they likely would encounter as they progressed through junior high school.[9] The content of this prevention approach was designed to correct the misperception that everybody was smoking cigarettes and to provide skills for resisting the various social pressures to smoke and information about the immediate physiologic effects of smoking. This prevention approach was tested in a well-designed study that showed smoking rates of the students receiving the prevention program were 50% lower than the rates observed in the control group.[10]

This approach was a dramatic departure from the failures of previous studies testing more traditional information dissemination and affective education approaches to drug abuse prevention. Not surprisingly, it sparked considerable attention and generated a flurry of research to test variations of the approach. A distinctive feature of the variations on the social influence prevention approach was an increasing emphasis on teaching students specific skills for effectively resisting peer and media pressures. Moreover, researchers began testing the extent to which this smoking prevention approach also was effective with other forms of substance use.

As a group, these approaches are referred to as "drug resistance skills training" or "resistance skills training" and have been based on a conceptual model stressing the fundamental importance of social factors in promoting the initiation and early stages of substance use among adolescents.[11] There are 3 major sources of social influence to use drugs: the family (parents and older siblings), peers, and the mass media. Children and adolescents may be inclined toward substance use at least in part because such behavior is modeled by parents or older siblings or because of the transmission of prodrug attitudes within the family. Similarly, persons whose friends use 1 or more substances are more likely to use drugs, alcohol, or tobacco because substance use is modeled by their friends. Finally, media personalities or other persons with high visibility may promote drug use by serving as negative role models using drugs in movies, television shows, rock videos, or in real life. According to social psychologic theory, all social influences are the result of the interaction between individual learning histories and forces in the community and larger society.

Prevention components

Approaches based on the social influence model usually have included several components. The first 3 of these components are referred to as "psychologic inoculation," "normative education," and "refusal skills training," and they have become the central ingredients of many contemporary drug abuse prevention

programs.[12] Many smoking prevention researchers also have
included a fourth component that provides information about the
immediate physiologic effects of cigarette smoking. However,
because this component is specific to cigarette smoking, it usually
has not been included in contemporary drug abuse prevention
programs.

Resistance skills training approaches usually teach students
how to handle situations in which they might experience peer
pressure to smoke, drink, or use illicit drugs.[11,12] The training
involves not only what to say (the specific content of a refusal
message), but also how to refuse an offer to use drugs in the most
effective way possible. Most prevention programs teach specific
techniques to resisting peer pressure or use variations on more
general assertiveness techniques. It is hoped that students will
learn a new repertoire of responses to peer pressure. To facilitate
the learning process, not only are the skills demonstrated to participants, but also an opportunity usually is provided to practice the
skills. Some prevention approaches also include behavioral homework assignments for participants to practice the skills outside the
context of the prevention program to encourage use of the skills
in their everyday lives. The approaches also teach adolescents how
to identify, recognize, and avoid high-risk situations in which they
may likely face peer pressure to use 1 or more psychoactive
substances.

Use of peer leaders
Peer leaders have had a prominent role in many contemporary prevention programs. Indeed, same-age or older peer leaders have
been used in almost all studies testing approaches based on the
social influence model.[11] The rationale underlying the use of peer
leaders is the observation that peers tend to have higher credibility
with adolescents than do many adults, particularly with respect
to lifestyle issues. Furthermore, the use of peer leaders provides
adolescents with opportunities to observe other adolescents demon-
strating the skills in a believable way, thereby increasing the confidence of participants that they can use the skills effectively in
real-life situations involving peer pressure.

However, despite the fact that many prevention studies have used peer leaders, a more careful examination of the studies indicates that peer leaders are rarely the sole program providers. Rather, they typically assist adult providers and usually have specific and well-defined roles. In most of these studies, the primary program provider has been a member of the research project staff, a teacher, or another adult.

Target population and program length

Although most research studies to test approaches based on the social influence model have targeted junior high school students (typically beginning with seventh graders), some studies have involved fourth, fifth, and sixth graders. The prevention programs tested have ranged from as few as 3 sessions to as many as 11 or 12 sessions. Most studies testing prevention approaches based on the social influence model have been conducted in school settings.[11,12] However, several studies also have tested this approach in combination with media and parent components. When considered together, research studies indicate that the inclusion of additional prevention components can produce stronger prevention effects than school-based approaches alone.[13]

Effectiveness

The effectiveness of prevention approaches based on the social influence model has been demonstrated in a number of studies.[14-23] Collectively, study results indicate that this type of prevention approach usually decreases smoking rates by between 35% and 50% after the initial preventive intervention. Some studies have focused on incidence (ie, the transition from nonsmoking to smoking), while others have focused on prevalence (ie, the total number of cases). However, the effects of the best smoking prevention approaches are approximately the same whether results are reported by incidence or prevalence measures. Similar decreases have been reported for alcohol and marijuana use.

To refine and improve current prevention approaches, it is important to identify the relative effectiveness of various program components and the most effective program providers. Some studies have included a public commitment component through which participants publicly state that they will remain drug free. However, evidence from 1 study indicates that a public commitment component may contribute little to the effectiveness of social influence programs.[16] Moreover, a number of programs have used films or videotapes, yet it is unclear what type of media material is most effective or the extent to which media material is necessary as a program component. Finally, more research is needed to determine the optimal age for implementing the prevention programs, the most appropriate program length and structure, and the characteristics of the persons who are the most influenced by these programs.

Studies of the long-term effectiveness of the prevention approaches have produced variable results. In some cases, prevention effects have been maintained for up to 3 years after conclusion of the prevention program.[17,21,22] However, the results of most studies involving long-term follow-up have indicated that the prevention effects usually are not maintained,[24-26] which has led some to conclude that school-based prevention approaches may not be powerful enough to produce lasting prevention effects,[27] whereas others have argued that the prevention approaches tested may have had deficiencies that undermined their long-term effectiveness.[28] For example, it has been argued that the failure of some studies to produce long-term prevention effects may be related to the type of the prevention approach tested or the way in which the programs were implemented.

Accordingly, the absence of long-term prevention effects should not necessarily be taken as an indictment of school-based prevention approaches. There are several possible explanations for the gradual decay of prevention effects: (1) the program may have been too short; (2) "booster" sessions were not included or were inadequate; and (3) the prevention program may not have been implemented with sufficient fidelity or completeness.[28] More recent research suggests that all of these factors may have had a role in the negative findings of many long-term follow-up studies with prevention approaches based on the social influence model.

It is also clear from research with more comprehensive prevention approaches that school-based prevention approaches are powerful enough to produce a meaningful and durable effect on adolescent substance use. Moreover, it has become increasingly clear that to be effective, school-based prevention approaches need to be more comprehensive, have a stronger initial dosage (ie, number of program sessions), must include at least 2 additional years of booster sessions, and must be implemented in a manner consistent with the underlying prevention model.[29]

Adolescent Alcohol Prevention Trial

The Adolescent Alcohol Prevention Trial is an example of a universal school-based prevention program based on the social influence approach. The Adolescent Alcohol Prevention Trial was developed by Donaldson et al for fifth graders, with booster sessions conducted during seventh grade.[30] It includes 2 primary strategies: resistance skills training and normative education. The resistance skills training component is designed to give children the social and behavioral skills they need to refuse explicit drug offers. The normative education component is designed specifically to combat the influences of passive social pressures and social modeling effects. It focuses on correcting erroneous perceptions about the prevalence and acceptability of substance use and on establishing conservative group norms.

In the research testing of the Adolescent Alcohol Prevention Trial, students received information about consequences of drug use only, resistance skills only, normative education only, or resistance skills training in combination with normative education. Results showed that while the combination of resistance skills training and normative education prevented drug use, resistance skills training alone was not sufficient.

Targeting Social Influences and General Personal Competence

Considerable prevention research also has been conducted with a comprehensive school-based prevention model designed to target a broad array of risk and protective factors. Approaches based on this model are more comprehensive than conventional informational approaches, affective approaches, or social influence approaches. This approach emphasizes personal self-management skills and general social skills in combination with elements of the social influence model. Because of its emphasis on personal competence, it is referred to as a "competence enhancement approach."

This prevention approach is based on sound theories of human behavior, such as social learning theory[31] and problem behavior theory.[32] Within the context of this theoretical framework, substance abuse is viewed as a socially learned and functional behavior, resulting from the interplay of social and personal factors. Substance use behavior is learned through a process of modeling and reinforcement and is influenced by a set of cognitions, attitudes, and beliefs.

Program components

Competence enhancement approaches typically teach some combination of the following skills: (1) general problem-solving and decision-making skills; (2) general cognitive skills for resisting social or media influences; (3) skills for increasing personal control and self-esteem; (4) adaptive coping strategies for relieving stress and anxiety through use of cognitive coping skills or behavioral relaxation techniques; (5) general social skills; and (6) general assertiveness skills.

Competence enhancement approaches clearly have a much broader focus than those designed to teach resistance skills or combat social influences to use drugs. These programs are designed to teach general skills for coping with life that have a relatively broad application. Moreover, competence enhancement programs emphasize use of a general set of skills to situations directly related to substance use (eg, the application of general assertiveness skills to situations involving peer pressure to use drugs). However, the same skills can be used for dealing with many of the challenges confronting adolescents in their everyday lives, including the use of tobacco, alcohol, or other drugs.

In contrast with affective education approaches that also embrace personal development, competence enhancement approaches rely on the use of skills training methods rather than experiential classroom activities. Skills are taught using a combination of methods, including demonstration, practice, feedback, praise, and extended practice outside of the classroom through behavioral homework assignments.

Target population and program length

Despite the use of a common prevention strategy, some degree of variation exists for several key program variables, such as the age of a target population, the length of the prevention program, the frequency of program sessions, and the type of program provider. For example, the target population for these prevention approaches has ranged from seventh to tenth graders, although most research studies have focused on seventh graders. The length of the prevention programs also has varied; some programs include as few as 7 sessions, and others include as many as 20 sessions. Variation also has existed in the frequency of prevention sessions. Some sessions were conducted once per week, while others were conducted twice per week or more often. Finally, most studies testing this prevention approach have used adult program providers, including outside health care professionals and regular classroom teachers. Some studies have used peer leaders alone or in combination with adult providers.

Effectiveness

Studies testing competence enhancement approaches have produced impressive results. In general, these studies have shown that competence enhancement approaches to substance abuse prevention decrease new substance use by 40% to 75%.[33-41] Ongoing intervention in the form of booster sessions has shown not only that the preventive gains can be sustained but also that additional booster sessions may increase the magnitude of the initial prevention effects.[34,40] Considered together, the evaluation literature shows that prevention approaches using this model can produce substantial decreases in the onset of tobacco, alcohol, and marijuana use. Long-term follow-up has shown that the prevention effects can be maintained throughout junior high and high school.[40] The main caveat is that, to be effective, prevention programs need to be implemented in a way consistent with the underlying prevention model.[28]

A major weakness in the existing prevention literature is that until recently, research to test the effectiveness of contemporary substance abuse prevention approaches has been limited to predominantly white, middle-class, suburban populations. However, more recent research has shown that prevention approaches that teach drug resistance skills, promote antidrug norms, and foster the development of personal and social skills also effectively decrease substance use among minority youth. Furthermore, although tailoring the prevention approach to the specific culture of the target population can improve effectiveness, the important lesson from a number of prevention studies is that the same prevention approach can be effective with a broad range of adolescents. This finding challenges the widely held view that the causes of substance use are fundamentally different for each different racial and ethnic group and that, as a consequence, prevention approaches must be population-specific.

Life Skills Training Program

The most extensively evaluated and best known example of the competence enhancement approach is a program developed and tested by Botvin et al at Cornell University Medical College called Life Skills Training (LST).[42] This is a universal classroom program designed to address a wide range of risk and protective factors by teaching self-management and social skills in combination with drug resistance skills and normative education. The program consists of a 3-year prevention curriculum intended for middle or junior high school students. It includes 15 classes during the first year, 10 booster classes during the second year, and 5 classes during the third year.

The "drug resistance skills" and "normative education" components provide material that deals directly with social factors promoting drug use. Included is material designed to increase awareness of social influences toward drug use, correct the misperception that everyone is using drugs, promote antidrug norms, teach prevention-related information about drug abuse, and teach drug resistance skills.

The "self-management skills" component provides students with skills for increasing independence, personal control, and a sense of mastery. This includes teaching general problem-solving and decision-making skills, critical thinking skills for resisting peer and media influences, skills for increasing self-control and self-esteem (eg, self-appraisal, goal setting, self-monitoring, self-reinforcement), and adaptive coping strategies for relieving stress and anxiety.

The "social skills" component is designed to enhance students' social competence with a variety of general social skills, including skills for communicating effectively, overcoming shyness, learning to meet new people, and developing healthy friendships. The skills emphasized in the LST program are taught through a combination of instruction, demonstration, feedback, reinforcement, behavioral rehearsal, and extended practice through homework assignments.

The LST program has been extensively tested and refined over the years. Results indicate that this prevention approach decreases the prevalence of tobacco, alcohol, and marijuana use (compared with controls) by 50% to 75%.[33-41] Booster sessions can help maintain program effects.[34] Long-term follow-up data from a randomized field trial involving almost 6000 students from 56 schools found significantly lower smoking, alcohol, and marijuana use 6 years after the initial baseline assessment.[40] The prevalence of cigarette smoking, alcohol use, and marijuana use for students who received the LST program was 44% lower than that for control students, and the regular (weekly) use of multiple drugs was 66% lower.[43]

Although early research with the LST program was conducted with white populations, several recent studies show that it also is effective with inner-city minority youth.[38,41,44-46] It also has been effective when implemented under different scheduling formats and with different levels of project staff involvement. Finally, evaluation studies indicate that this prevention program works whether the program providers are adults or peers.

Programs Focused on the Family

Prevention programs focused on the family view drug and alcohol use and abuse in terms of 1 or more of the following classes of risk factors: (1) family dynamics; (2) socialization or habilitation deficits; (3) negative parental modeling; and (4) lack of social control. These programs can be subdivided into programs concerned largely with parent education and programs concerned with the family unit as a whole, although in practice, this distinction is often blurred, as when members of a parent education group sponsor drug- or alcohol-free parties for youth.

Programs based on "family dynamics theories" appeal to a large body of research that associates increased risk of alcohol and drug abuse with such factors as parental permissiveness or inconsistency, loose family structure, use of harsh physical punishment, and inadequate family communication patterns. Accordingly, these programs seek to improve parenting skills and, thus, indirectly to decrease substance abuse risk among children. Unfortunately, many parent education programs have had difficulty recruiting participants, and it has been suggested that the parents who volunteer for such programs may not be those who most need the program.

Related to programs based on family dynamics are those based on preventing or remediating "socialization or habilitation deficits." These programs are based on the notion that the family is the major socialization agent, especially for young children, and that many modern families fail to effectively inculcate such basic values as self-control, self-motivation, and self-discipline. Accordingly, curricula for parents have been developed under the general rubric "strengthening the family" to teach parents ways of structuring the home environment to increase the likelihood that children will develop these qualities.[47]

A third category of parent education programs includes those that attempt to remedy "negative parental modeling." These programs appeal to concepts from social learning theory that suggest that children's early notions about drugs and alcohol are learned by observing parents' behavior toward alcohol, tobacco, over-the-counter and prescription drugs, and increasingly, marijuana and cocaine. Thus, the goals of these programs are to make parents aware of the effect of their substance-related behavior on their children and, thus, to change "parental behavior" to decrease the drug and alcohol risk for youth. Programmatic interventions based on modeling usually are a part of a larger parent education program and rarely are seen alone, except as public service announcements.

Programs based on social control emerged as 1 component of the activities of concerned parents described in the historical overview. These programs proceed from the assumption that many parents have abdicated their responsibilities for their children's drug and alcohol behavior; thus, the programs seek to empower parents to reinstate social controls to prevent or forestall experimentation with drugs and alcohol. The original core concept of such programs was the parent-peer support group in which parents of children who associated with one another met regularly to institute and enforce a consistent set of rules (eg, for curfews and parties). Although some programs experienced difficulties maintaining parental interest in the parent-peer support group, the groups often have grown into broad-based, community prevention programs (see Chapter 2).[43]

Strengthening Families Program

An excellent example of a successful family-focused program is the Strengthening Families program developed by Kumpfer at the University of Utah. This selective multicomponent program provides prevention programming for 6- to 10-year-old children of substance abusers.[48]

The program includes 3 components: a "parent training program," a "children's skills training program," and a "family skills training program." In each of the 14 weekly sessions, parents and children are trained separately during the first hour. During the second hour, parents and children participate together in the family skills training portion. Afterward, the families share dinner and a film or other entertainment.

Parent training improves parenting skills and decreases substance abuse by parents. Children's skills training decreases children's negative behaviors and increases socially acceptable behaviors through work with a program therapist. Family skills training improves the family environment by involving both generations in learning and practicing their new behaviors.

This approach has been evaluated in a variety of settings and with several racial and ethnic groups. The primary outcomes of the program include decreases in family conflict, improvement in family communication and organization, and decreases in youth conduct disorders, aggressiveness, and substance abuse.

Programs Focused on the Community

Unlike the programs discussed thus far, which tend to rely on psychologic theory, programs focused on community risk factors tend to appeal to sociologic or ecologic models of substance use and abuse; that is, they tend to locate the causes of substance abuse within the organizational characteristics of large social institutions* (eg, the schools, the law enforcement system, and the alcoholic beverage control system).[49,50] These programs usually address 1 or more of the following risk factors: (1) inadequate deterrence; (2) availability; (3) negative social climate; and (4) inadequate social bonding.

"Deterrence-based" programs are probably among society's most ancient preventative responses to substance use problems; severe penalties for the use of certain substances (eg, tobacco) were recorded as early as the 17th century. During the 1970s, deterrence as a method to prevent substance use and abuse fell into disrepute, as many states liberalized drug laws and many

---

*Distinction should be made between programs that address risk factors in the school and community (ie, that focus on risk factors found within the social institution) and school- and community-based programs, which may address risk factors at any level (eg, when a school-based program provides drug information on an individual level or peer pressure resistance skills on a peer level.

localities deemphasized drug enforcement. Recently, however, there has been a resurgence of interest in deterrence-based programs. Of particular interest in the current context is an emphasis on the importance of consistently enforced school drug and alcohol policies that stipulate a no-drug or alcohol campus policy, that articulate penalties for infractions, and that provide for equitable treatment of substance-involved youth. In general, research on deterrence-based programs suggests that such programs can have a dramatic but short-lived effect on use rates. Anecdotal evidence of the effects of school policies abounds, but such effects have not been studied systematically, and long-term effects of such policies are unknown.

Many community-based programs have attempted to decrease the availability of substances to youth. These programs proceed from the assumption that decreased availability will lead to decreased consumption. National enactment of legislation for the 21-year minimum age for purchase of alcohol represents one application of an availability model; local ordinances banning "head shops" (ie, stores that sell drug paraphernalia) represent another. Many communities are attempting to decrease alcohol availability to youth through control of the numbers and types of retail outlets where alcohol can be purchased, through education and monitoring of retail clerks and retail outlet owners, through training of servers in bars and restaurants, and most recently through crackdowns on the availability of fake identification cards. Although the effects of such broad programs are difficult to evaluate, existing data suggest that decreased availability decreases consumption and related problems.

Programs based on "social climate" are perhaps the broadest and most diffuse of prevention efforts. Indeed, rather than being classified as "programs," social climate manipulations are probably best conceptualized as the result of a number of programs acting in aggregate to promote a community-wide message. For example, increased enforcement by police, a strong school policy, the existence of a concerned parent group and "Just Say No" clubs, antidrug editorials in local newspapers, and the institution

of drug education in a community's schools might together con-
stitute a manipulation of the community's social climate related
to drug and alcohol use and abuse. Community organization programs that attempt to involve as many community members as
possible in prevention (eg, parents, youth, health care professionals, schools, police, local government, local media) are the most
common example of programs based on a social climate model.
Like availability programs, social climate programs are extremely
difficult to evaluate, and hence, there is little research evidence
to support or refute the efficacy of such efforts. However, many
theorists have cited social climate models to explain the downturn
in adult smoking, an effect that cannot be attributed to any single
programmatic intervention.

Originally developed by juvenile delinquency theorists, "social
bonding" models stipulate that antisocial behavior (including substance abuse) derives from a failure of some youths to "bond" to
social institutions and their norms, largely because they have not
found (or been provided with) valued roles within those institutions. Thus, the youth have nothing to lose and, hence, no reason to conform to normative proscriptions of antisocial acts.†
Accordingly, substance abuse prevention programs based on social
bonding theories attempt to provide youth with opportunities to
contribute positively to the community and develop positive
social bonds as a result. The earliest of such programs was
"Channel One," jointly sponsored by the National Institute on
Drug Abuse and the Prudential Life Insurance Company, which
provided youth with an opportunity to become involved in community service projects, such as historical restorations, food coop-
eratives for the elderly, and youth job services. More recently, a
variety of alternative activity programs have been developed that
are outgrowths of the social bonding model, and as suggested

---

†Social bonding theorists have criticized the adoption of "no-pass–no-play"
rules in school athletics on the grounds that youth who cannot achieve success
in 1 arena (academics) are then prevented from achieving success in another
arena (athletics), thus further decreasing the probability that positive social
bonding will occur.

earlier, such programs have largely eclipsed alternatives programs. Research on such programs in the substance area is sparse, but evidence from the juvenile delinquency prevention literature suggests that social bonding is a potentially powerful prevention strategy.

Project STAR

Although it departs from the type of community-based interventions described in the preceding paragraphs, Project STAR is important, because it is the most effective community-level prevention approach available. It was developed by researchers at the University of Southern California and has been subjected to rigorous testing by Pentz et al.[13] Project STAR is a universal drug abuse prevention program that reaches the entire community population with a comprehensive school program, mass media efforts, a parent program, community organization, and health policy change. The middle school-based component is a social influence curriculum that is incorporated into classroom instruction by trained teachers during a 2-year period. The mass media component is used to promote and support the overall prevention effort.

The parent program component involves parents in working with their children on Project STAR homework. They also learn family communication skills and become involved in community action. Through the community organization component, the community is mobilized to action, and a general organizational structure is provided for all project-related activities.

The health policy change component is implemented as a task of the community organization to develop and implement policies that affect alcohol, tobacco, and other drug laws as well as other local policies, such as establishing and monitoring drug-free sites in the community.

Research evaluating the effectiveness of Project STAR has shown positive long-term prevention effects.[13] Students who began the program during junior high school and whose results were measured during their last year of high school showed significantly less use of marijuana (approximately 30% less), cigarettes (about 25% less), and alcohol (about 20% less) than children in schools that did not offer the program. The most important factor that affected drug use among students was increased perceptions of their friends' intolerance of drug use.

Programs Focused on the Larger Social Environment

Like programs based on school and community risk factors, programs that address drug and alcohol risk factors in the larger social environment usually cite sociologic or ecologic explanations of substance-related behavior. Indeed, many of the program models described for the school and community programs (eg, deterrence, availability, social climate) have been applied to the larger social environment; the major difference is institutional focus (eg, federal laws as opposed to local ordinances). One area of risk factors, however, clearly belongs to the larger social environment—those associated with mass media.[‡] These risk factors are associated with advertising of psychoactive substances and portrayal of substance use.

Several programs have been developed to counteract the potential negative effects of advertisements to promote the use of tobacco, alcohol, and illicit drugs. First, attempts have been made to limit, decrease, or eliminate cigarette and alcohol advertising.[§] Second, attempts have been made to develop counteradvertising. Counteradvertisements, such as those developed by Doctors Ought to Care, lampoon the format and content of popular advertisements (eg, an attractive model with a cigarette in his nose who claims, "I smoke for smell") or other promotional activities (eg, an "Emphysema Slims Tennis Tournament"). Third, the Partnership for a Drug-Free America has launched a substantial antidrug advertising effort. It has worked successfully with advertising agencies to create interesting and memorable ads designed

---

[‡]Distinction must be made between programs that use mass media as programmatic tools and programs that address risk factors found in the media. As is the case for school and community programs, mass media may be vehicles for prevention programming aimed at any level of risk factor. Indeed, most mass media campaigns are designed to affect the individual, the family, or the peer group.

[§]This strategy is an excellent example of a program that does not fit with traditional definitions of "program."

to counter the pressure to use drugs. The partnership is perhaps best known for the ad that showed an egg in a frying pan with the voice-over, "this is your brain on drugs." More recent ads have focused less on antidrug information and scare tactics and more on the social influence to use drugs. Fourth, the White House Office on National Drug Control Policy launched a 5-year, $1 billion antidrug mass media campaign. Among other things, the campaign involves buying prime-time spots for antidrug ads. Finally, some programs have attempted to educate youth about advertising techniques or aid youth to dissect and critique the persuasive messages in advertisements. For example, the LST program devotes 2 sessions to media influences and advertising techniques. To date, there has been too little research on counter-advertising or advertising education to permit an assessment of their potential as prevention strategies, although the pervasiveness of advertising in our society suggests that further exploration is justified.

Recently, there has been scientific and popular concern about the portrayal of substance use in mass media. These concerns derive in part from the sheer numbers of hours youth devote to watching and listening to mass media (particularly television) and in part from the same social modeling concerns discussed earlier for family and peers (ie, that children learn substance use behaviors by watching and imitating others). For example, content analyses of prime-time television have suggested that the portrayal of alcohol use usually does not provide a balanced view of the positive and negative aspects of drinking. This observation has led some researchers to attempt to educate television writers, producers, and directors about the alcohol messages their products convey and to attempt to aid these media professionals in presenting a more realistic picture of drinking. This approach is exemplified by the "cooperative consultation" process pioneered by Warren Breed and James DeFoe. Similarly, some persons have become concerned about possible prodrug messages in popular music, although the scientific basis for such concerns is murky at best. These persons have supported legislation that would require labeling of records to allow parents some control over the messages to which their children are allegedly exposed.

Drinking and Driving Prevention Program

Programs that seek to prevent drinking and driving and related problems among adolescents fall into 2 broad categories, and significant controversy has arisen among the advocates of each program type.‖ This section describes each program category and discusses the controversy that surrounds them.

The first category views drinking and driving as 1 of a constellation of alcohol-related problems experienced by youth and, thus, may be termed "alcohol-related problem strategies." These programs attempt to decrease drinking and driving by decreasing the amount of adolescent drinking using any of the previously described prevention strategies. An example is Project Graduation, which provides alcohol-free alternative parties during times such as graduation week and the holiday season.

The second category views drinking and driving as 1 of a constellation of traffic safety problems experienced by youth and, thus, may be termed "traffic safety strategies." These programs attempt to decrease drinking and driving by disassociating drinking from driving. Examples of this category of program are Safe Rides, a program which provides free safe transportation for adolescents who have been drinking or who are with a driver who has been drinking, and the Contract for Life, a program in which parents and adolescents agree to provide a ride home or cab fare if the parent or adolescent has been drinking or is with a driver who has been drinking.

As suggested, significant controversy has arisen about these categories of programs. Advocates of the alcohol-related problems

---

‖A third category of program includes those that attempt to decrease the consequences of drinking and driving by making the environment safer, for example, by advocating the use of seat belts, installation of air bags, and the use of breakaway road sign posts. Such programs usually are not defined as prevention programs, although the similarity of their objectives to those of many other drinking and driving prevention programs (eg, the decrease in mortality and morbidity) suggests that they probably should be.

strategies criticize traffic safety strategies on the grounds that they may be misconstrued by youth as sanctioning drinking and also may encourage youth to drink by making drinking safer. Thus, it is argued that although these programs may decrease 1 alcohol-related problem (eg, drinking and driving), they may increase the incidence of others (eg, other accidental trauma, addiction).

Advocates of traffic safety strategies argue that, despite the best efforts to prevent drinking by adolescents, the incidence of such behavior is still significant. Thus, until (or if ever) drinking by adolescents is eliminated, programs that dissociate drinking and driving are needed to decrease mortality and morbidity among adolescents.

Interestingly, the controversy between these positions related to drinking and driving can be resolved empirically, although the data are not available to do so. Specifically, research is needed to determine whether the traffic safety strategies increase drinking by adolescents and, if so, by how much. Such data would allow communities to make an informed comparison between the risks (if any) of increased incidence of other alcohol-related problems and the benefits associated with a decreased incidence of drinking and driving by adolescents. Until these data are available, communities will have to choose between program alternatives (or choose both alternatives) on the basis of programmatic criteria, such as acceptability to community members, acceptability to youth, availability of resources, and program costs.

Summary

The problem of substance abuse has persisted for many years. Efforts to deal with this problem have included a variety of approaches. The most common approaches to substance abuse prevention are those that provide factual information about the adverse consequences of smoking, drinking alcohol, or using illicit drugs with or without the inclusion of scare tactics and moral messages. Other commonly used approaches have relied on affective education and providing adolescents with alternatives to using drugs. However, when carefully evaluated, none of these approaches has effectively prevented substance abuse.

The most effective substance abuse prevention approaches focus on the social and psychologic factors promoting the initiation and early stages of substance use among adolescents. These approaches target the social influences to use drugs alone or in combination with approaches designed to enhance general personal competence by teaching an array of self-management skills and general social skills. Both approaches emphasize skills training methods and deemphasize factual information about drug pharmacology and the adverse consequences of substance abuse. Moreover, these approaches use well-tested behavioral prevention methods to facilitate the acquisition of refusal skills and general life skills. Although prevention efforts with younger populations may be worthwhile, because of the increased risk and vulnerability of the early adolescent period most of the existing research supporting the effectiveness of substance abuse prevention has been conducted with adolescent populations.

Success also has been achieved in decreasing risk factors associated with substance abuse and, in some instances, substance use itself, through family-focused prevention efforts. The most effective approaches provide parent training, teach family management skills, and help parents communicate a clear antidrug message to their children.

Community-based prevention approaches that include elements of the most effective school-based prevention programs along with those of successful community-based prevention initiatives seem to offer considerable promise. Notwithstanding the progress made in prevention research during recent years, future research is needed to further refine the most effective contemporary prevention approaches and to develop new approaches. At the same time, it is vitally important that persons charged with the responsibility of preventing adolescent substance abuse be made aware of what works.

Health care professionals can do several things to help decrease the prevalence of drug abuse. First, they can support and reinforce the no-drug message that underlies almost all current prevention programs and can reinforce the efforts of youth to find activities and cultivate friends that support a drug-free lifestyle. Moreover, health care professionals can validate factual information about the risks of drug and alcohol use when questions are raised by patients and parents.

Second, health care professionals can support community efforts to launch multicomponent prevention programs by promoting the need for a broad-based approach that addresses multiple risk factors. They can be particularly powerful spokespersons for the need for programmatic initiatives that involve community change (eg, restricted availability, increased enforcement) because of their natural roles as community leaders in the area of health.

Finally, health care professionals can help communities and community agencies wade through the often confusing popular and scientific prevention literature and can help communities avoid making a large commitment of money or time to a prevention strategy that, although popular, may have been proved ineffective. By becoming conversant with the growing body of empirical evidence supporting the effectiveness of specific school, family, and community prevention approaches, health care professionals are in an excellent position to help move the field of drug abuse prevention from approaches based on intuition or ideology to approaches based on sound science.

Conclusion

During the past 2 decades, considerable progress has been made in understanding the causes of substance abuse and how best to prevent it. These advances have occurred to a large extent because of an increased emphasis on quality empirical research. The current challenge to the field of substance abuse prevention is to disseminate information about the most effective prevention approaches to health care professionals, educators, prevention specialists, parents, community leaders, and policy makers. For the first time in 2 decades, research-based prevention approaches are available for combating the problem of substance abuse. It is only through the use of these approaches that significant progress can be made toward decreasing the prevalence of substance use among youth.

References

1. Johnston LD, O'Malley PM, Bachman JG. *The Monitoring the Future National Survey Results on Adolescent Drug Use: Overview of Key Findings, 1999.* Rockville, MD: National Institute on Drug Abuse; 2000. NIH Publication No. 00-4690

2. Johnston LD, O'Malley PM, Bachman JG. "Ecstasy" use rises sharply among teens in 2000; use of many other drugs stays steady but significant declines are reported for some [press release]. Ann Arbor, MI: University of Michigan, News and Information Services; December 14, 2000

3. Knight JR. Substance use, abuse, and dependence. In: Levine MD, Carey WB, Crocker AC, eds. *Developmental-Behavioral Pediatrics.* 3rd ed. Philadelphia, PA: WB Saunders Co; 1999:477-492

4. Institute of Medicine, Committee on Prevention of Mental Disorders. *Reducing Risks for Mental Disorders: Frontiers for Preventive Intervention Research.* Mrazek PJ, Haggerty RJ, eds. Washington, DC: National Academy Press; 1994

5. Bangert-Drowns RL. The effects of school-based substance abuse education: a meta-analysis. *J Drug Educ.* 1988;18:243-264

6. Tobler NS. Meta-analysis of 143 adolescent drug prevention programs: quantitative outcome results of program participants compared to a control or comparison group. *J Drug Issues.* 1986;16:537-567

7. Stuart RB. Teaching facts about drugs: pushing or preventing? *J Educ Psychol.* 1974;66:189-201

8. Schaps E, DiBartolo R, Moskowitz J, Palley CS, Churgin S. A review of 127 drug abuse prevention program evaluations. *J Drug Issues.* 1981;11:17-43

9. Evans RI. Smoking in children: developing a social psychological strategy of deterrence. *Prev Med.* 1976;5:122-127

10. Evans RI, Rozelle RM, Mittlemark MB, Hansen WB, Bane AL, Havis J. Deterring the onset of smoking in children: knowledge of immediate physiological effects and coping with peer pressure, media pressure, and parent modeling. *J Appl Soc Psychol.* 1978;8:126-135

11. Botvin GJ, Botvin EM. Adolescent tobacco, alcohol, and drug abuse: prevention strategies, empirical findings, and assessment issues. *J Dev Behav Pediatr.* 1992;13:290-301

12. Hansen WB. School-based substance abuse prevention: a review of the state of the art in curriculum, 1980-1990. *Health Educ Res.* 1992;7:403-430

13. Pentz MA, Dwyer JH, MacKinnon D, et al. A multicommunity trial for primary prevention of adolescent drug abuse. Effects on drug use prevalence. *JAMA.* 1989;261:3259-3266

14. Arkin RM, Roemhild HJ, Johnson CA, Luepker RV, Murray DM. The Minnesota smoking prevention program: a seventh grade health curriculum supplement. *J Sch Health.* 1981;51:611-616

15. Donaldson SI, Graham JW, Hansen WB. Testing the generalizability of intervening mechanism theories: understanding the effects of adolescent drug use prevention interventions. *J Behav Med.* 1994;17:195-216

16. Hurd PD, Johnson CA, Pechacek T, Bast LP, Jacobs DR, Luepker RV. Prevention of cigarette smoking in seventh grade students. *J Behav Med.* 1980;3:15-28

17. Luepker RV, Johnson CA, Murray DM, Pechacek TF. Prevention of cigarette smoking: three-year follow-up of an education program for youth. *J Behav Med.* 1983;6:53-62

18. Perry CL, Killen J, Slinkard LA, McAlister AL. Peer teaching and smoking prevention among junior high students. *Adolescence.* 1980;15:277-281

19. Snow DL, Tebes JK, Arthur MW, Tapasak RC. Two-year follow-up of a social-cognitive intervention to prevent substance use. *J Drug Educ.* 1992;22:101-114

20. Sussman S, Dent CW, Stacy AW, et al. Project towards no tobacco use: 1-year behavior outcomes. *Am J Public Health.* 1993;83:1245-1250

21. Telch MJ, Killen JD, McAlister AL, Perry CL, Maccoby N. Long-term follow-up of a pilot project on smoking prevention with adolescents. *J Behav Med.* 1982;5:1-8

22. McAlister A, Perry C, Killen J, Slinkard LA, Maccoby N. Pilot study of smoking, alcohol and drug abuse prevention. *Am J Public Health.* 1980;70:719-721

23. Shope JT, Dielman TE, Butchart AT, Campanelli PC, Kloska DD. An elementary school-based alcohol misuse prevention program: a follow-up evaluation. *J Stud Alcohol.* 1992;53:106-121

24. Murray DM, Pirie P, Luepker RV, Pallonen U. Five- and six-year follow-up results from four seventh-grade smoking prevention strategies. *J Behav Med.* 1989;12:207-218

25. Flay BR, Keopke D, Thomson SJ, Santi S, Best JA, Brown KS. Six-year follow-up of the first Waterloo school smoking prevention trial. *Am J Public Health.* 1989;79:1371-1376

26. Ellickson PL, Bell RM. Drug prevention in junior high: a multi-site longitudinal test. *Science.* 1990;247:1299-1305

27. Dryfoos JG. Common components of successful interventions with high-risk youth. In: Bell NJ, Bell RW, eds. *Adolescent Risk Taking.* Newbury Park, CA: Sage Publications; 1993:131-147

28. Resnicow K, Botvin G. School-based substance use prevention programs: why do effects decay? *Prev Med.* 1993;22:484-490

29. Botvin GJ. Prevention in schools. In: Ammerman RT, Tarter RE, Ott PJ, eds. *Prevention and Societal Impact of Drug and Alcohol Abuse.* Needham Heights, MA: Lawrence Erlbaum Associates Inc; 1999:281-305

30. Donaldson SI, Sussman S, MacKinnon DP, et al. Drug abuse prevention programming: do we know what content works? *Am Behav Sci.* 1996;39:868-883

31. Bandura A. Social Learning Theory. Englewood Cliffs, NJ: Prentice Hall; 1977

32. Jessor R, Jessor SL. *Problem Behavior and Psychosocial Development: A Longitudinal Study of Youth.* New York, NY: Academic Press Inc; 1977

33. Botvin GJ, Eng A. The efficacy of a multicomponent approach to the prevention of cigarette smoking. *Prev Med.* 1982;11:199-211

34. Botvin GJ, Renick NL, Baker E. The effects of scheduling format and booster sessions on a broad-spectrum psychosocial approach to smoking prevention. *J Behav Med.* 1983;6:359-379

35. Botvin GJ, Baker E, Dusenbury L, Tortu S, Botvin EM. Preventing adolescent drug abuse through a multimodal cognitive-behavioral approach: results of a 3-year study. *J Consult Clin Psychol.* 1990;58:437-446

36. Botvin GJ, Baker E, Filazzola AD, Botvin EM. A cognitive-behavioral approach to substance abuse prevention: a one-year follow-up. *Addict Behav.* 1990;15:47-63

37. Botvin GJ, Eng A, Williams CL. Preventing the onset of cigarette smoking through life skills training. *Prev Med.* 1980;9:135-143

38. Botvin GJ, Schinke SP, Epstein JA, Diaz T, Botvin EM. Effectiveness of culturally focused and generic skills training approaches to alcohol and drug abuse prevention among minority adolescents: two-year follow-up results. *Psychol Addict Behav.* 1995;9:183-194

39. Botvin GJ, Baker E, Botvin EM, Filazzola AD, Millman RB. Prevention of alcohol misuse through the development of personal and social competence: a pilot study. *J Stud Alcohol.* 1984;45:550-552

40. Botvin GJ, Baker E, Dusenbury L, Botvin EM, Diaz T. Long-term follow-up results of a randomized drug abuse prevention trial in a white middle-class population. *JAMA.* 1995;273:1106-1112

41. Botvin GJ, Epstein JA, Baker E, Diaz T, Williams MI. School-based drug abuse prevention with inner-city minority youth. *J Child Adolesc Substance Abuse.* 1997;6:5-19

42. Botvin GJ. Preventing adolescent drug abuse through life skills training: theory, methods and effectiveness. In: Crane J, ed. *Social Programs that Work.* New York, NY: Russell Sage Foundation; 1998:225-257

43. Botvin GJ, Griffin KW, Diaz T, Scheier LM, Williams C, Epstein JA. Preventing illicit drug use in adolescents: long-term follow-up data from a randomized control trial of a school population. *Addict Behav.* 2000;25:769-774

44. Botvin GJ, Dusenbury L, Baker E, James-Ortiz S, Botvin EM, Kerner J. Smoking prevention among urban minority youth: assessing effects on outcome and mediating variables. *Health Psychol.* 1992;11:290-299

45. Botvin GJ, Batson HW, Witts-Vitale S, Bess V, Baker E, Dusenbury L. A psychosocial approach to smoking prevention for urban black youth. *Public Health Rep.* 1989;104:573-582

46. Botvin GJ, Griffin KW, Diaz T, Miller N, Ifill-Williams M. Smoking initiation and escalation in early adolescent girls: one-year follow-up of a school-based prevention intervention for minority youth. *J Am Med Womens Assoc.* 1999;54:139-143, 152

47. Ashery RS, Robertson EB, Kumpfer KL, eds. *Drug Abuse Prevention through Family Interventions.* Rockville, MD: National Institute on Drug Abuse; 1998

48. Kumpfer KL, Alvarado R. Strengthening families to prevent drug use in multi-ethnic youth. In: Botvin GJ, Schinke S, Orlandi MA, eds. *Drug Abuse Prevention with Multiethnic Youth.* Thousand Oaks, CA: Sage Publications; 1995:255-294

49. Pentz MA. Prevention research in multiethnic communities: developing community support and collaboration, and adapting research methods. In: Botvin GJ, Shinke S, Orlandi MA, eds. *Drug Abuse Prevention with Multiethnic Youth.* Thousand Oaks, CA: Sage Publications; 1995:193-214

50. Schinke S, Cole K. Prevention in community settings. In: Botvin GJ, Shinke S, Orlandi MA, eds. *Drug Abuse Prevention with Multiethnic Youth.* Thousand Oaks, CA: Sage Publications; 1995:215-232

Chapter 7

Legal and Ethical Considerations

Nancy Neveloff Dubler, LLB, and M. Max Quinn, JD

In the legally complex world of drug and alcohol use, adolescents exist in a mixed kingdom afforded some of the protections society offers to children and possessed of some of the rights of adults. The resulting uncertainty creates problems for all social and health service professionals and in particular for primary care physicians, who have a special confidential and private relationship with their patients while having certain unspecified obligations to parents.

Two questions are paramount in the minds of many health care professionals. First, what can a primary care physician do to and for a child without parental consent, given the constraints of law, ethics, and practice? Second, under what circumstances could a primary care physician act against the wishes of an adolescent (ie, when is an adolescent out of control or in danger to a degree that trumps the special confidential and private relationship and mandates involving the parent)? This chapter addresses these and other related issues.

Children have been recognized as a separate population and afforded special protections and rights only since the end of the 19th century. Before then, children generally were considered the property of their parents, more correctly of their fathers, to be worked, schooled, apprenticed, or disciplined (even unto death) as the family authority saw fit or deemed necessary. Children were hanged as pickpockets and punished as adults for the crimes they committed.[1]

This singular lack of official sympathy for the plight, special needs, and undeveloped conscience of young people began to change during the late 1800s with the founding of settlement houses and with the passage in Illinois of the first Family Court Act in 1899.[2] The scheme of the first Family Court Act, which was followed in every other state during the next 3 decades, established that children had special rights and protections under the law. It presented the then somewhat bizarre notion that children should be held to different moral and legal standards of conduct, tried in private and closed hearings, and punished separately from adults if found guilty of a crime. It reflected the more sympathetic and enlightened modern notion that moral responsibility evolves with developmental sophistication.

The first Family Court Act established 3 categories of children, which it brought under its jurisdiction. A child could be charged and found to be a juvenile delinquent, a neglected child, or an unruly child (read also ungovernable, incorrigible, or otherwise unmanageable in the varying language of state statutes). A "juvenile delinquent" was a child who committed an act that, if committed by an adult, would be a crime, but because it was done by a juvenile, it was merely juvenile delinquency. A "neglected child" was one not properly provided with food, clothing, education, or medical care by the parents despite their financial ability to do so. An "unruly child" was one opposed to the dictates and behavioral expectations of parents or society, although no crime was committed (staying out past a parentally imposed curfew or not attending school in violation of compulsory attendance laws are examples; neither is a crime if done by an adult). This category of infraction, often called "offenses," has come into disfavor and has been eliminated in some states and is rarely used in others.

Children who use alcohol before the minimum legal drinking age (now 21 years in all states) or who use drugs can be brought to the attention of the family court under any of the 3 jurisdictions. They may be charged with delinquent behavior, may be considered neglected, or may be adjudicated unruly. Despite its sympathetic origins and its understanding of the needs of children, involving the family court in these matters can be problematic. For many families, court is the last resort after informal networks and heartfelt appeals have failed. Some families hope that a judicial reprimand will provide the force for change; sometimes it does—especially when the judge and caregivers can fashion creative supportive and supervisory plans that guide and constrain behavior.

Referral to family court also can be frustrating. Especially in major cities, family courts often are underfunded, understaffed, and overwhelmed by the numbers and complexities of the multi-problem families with which they deal in the context of inadequate social service supports. Referral to the family court under these circumstances may help the child but also may be fruitless. Sometimes the hopes of families for support result only in another demonstration of society's callousness toward or inability to deal with the real needs of poor children and families.

The family court was established at the turn of the 19th century as a reflection of society's judgment that children are different and should not be held to the same standard of behavior as adults when they have neither the moral maturity nor the wisdom to guide independent action. This characterization and the consequent need for different treatment clearly apply to very young children but become less compelling as the child reaches adolescence and approaches maturity. This judgment has resulted during recent decades in the reentry of adolescents into the adult criminal system for certain kinds of crimes. Adolescents are at present granted protections and limited in their rights by statute, common law, and decisions of the Supreme Court. It can be argued that the real start of the reexamination of children's rights began in 1954 with *Brown v The Board of Education,*[3] which decreed that black children were protected by the equal protection clause in the Fourteenth Amendment and were entitled to equality in education. The next landmark case was *In re Gault,*[4] which held that the "protections" of the juvenile justice system justify treating a child differently from an adult only if the different treatment truly benefits the child. Thus, a conviction in a juvenile court based on inadequate protections would not stand. In 1969, the Supreme Court held that the right to free speech applied to children and, hence, protected their right to engage in peaceful political activity and symbolic free speech within the public schools.[5]

Adolescent women also clearly have been brought under the umbrella of constitutional protections as evidenced by their right to an abortion. In a series of cases, the Supreme Court held that parents did not have veto power over a minor's choice to abort.[6,7] Nevertheless, it found constitutional a state requirement that the parents of a minor planning to have an abortion should be notified by the physician if possible and if the adolescent does not offer evidence that she is a mature minor.[8] In addition, the Supreme Court has held that minors have a right to contraceptive privacy and cannot be barred from buying nonprescription contraceptives.[9] The Supreme Court stated in *Carey v Population Services International* that "minors, as well as adults, are protected by the Constitution and possess constitutional right"[9(p692)] and that "State restrictions inhibiting privacy rights of minors are valid only if they serve a significant state interest that is not present in the case of an adult."[9(p693)] Thus, special status for children sometimes is justified, and independent constitutional rights for children often are protected.

In contrast, however, several cases failed to grant constitutional protection to minors in certain circumstances. In *Parham v JR,*[10] the Supreme Court held that if there were an appropriate state statute, it was not a violation of a minor's constitutional rights for the minor to be admitted "voluntarily" to a mental institution by parents even if the minor was not free to leave the institution thereafter. In *Wisconsin v Yoder,*[11] the Supreme Court held that it was constitutionally permissible for Amish parents to exclude their children from secular schooling even if the exclusion would seriously hamper later efforts at independent existence. In the most recent case, *Veronia School District 473 v Wayne Acton,*[12] the Supreme Court held that requiring students who wanted to participate in school athletic activities to be tested for drug use did not violate the students' Fourth Amendment right to protection against unreasonable searches.

These cases are a fair sample of the Supreme Court cases that have ruled on the independent constitutional rights of minors. No clearly unambiguous message emerges.

The Adolescent and Medical Care

Physicians, other health care providers, and health care institutions face ethically thorny and legally complex questions when providing health care to adolescents. On the one hand, the adolescent is still a child for many or most purposes. On the other hand, adolescents possess independent rights in many areas, especially in matters relating to control of their own bodies.

The general rule for children and medical care is that parents have the right to consent to care on behalf of their children but do not have the coequal right to refuse care. The attempt by a parent to refuse care that is deemed by physicians to be necessary for the health and well-being of a child may and should be referred to the family court as a possible instance of medical neglect. If the family court finds medical neglect, it will order treatment despite the opposition of the parents. Under these rules and despite parental objection, children of Jehovah's Witnesses, for example, are regularly provided blood transfusions, and children of self-healing sects are given chemotherapy for cancer.

Parents have the right to consent to care and to refuse care when physician and parent agree. In theory, the parent does not refuse but rather the physician does not propose a treatment that is unlikely to benefit the child and is, therefore, not in the best interest of the child. In an emergency, care should be provided even without parental approval if the child is in pain or if a delay in securing approval might compromise the present or future health or well-being of the child.

Parents have the right and responsibility to supervise their children's care because society assumes that the parents' decision will most naturally reflect the best interest of the child. The law reflects the well-organized perception that parents are the best advocates for and protectors of their child's well-being.

Children, at least very young children, do not have the maturity, skill, education, or wisdom to balance present pain for future benefit. For example, they do not have the benefit of understanding the mechanism of an immunization; they do not have the ability to appreciate that the present momentary pain is outweighed by the decreased risk of acquiring a future illness that is likely to be much more painful and perhaps permanently disabling. Almost every very young child will be deterred merely by the presence of the needle. Young children cannot puzzle out complex personal cost-benefit analyses and weigh the sorts of risks and benefits that informed consent requires.

Many of the assumptions about children and parents, however, are far from self-evident when the child enters adolescence. By common law tradition and in some states by statute, 2 categories of adolescents can provide consent to care—the mature minor and the emancipated minor. Symmetry would seem to demand that they therefore be accorded a similar right to refuse care, although that right is somewhat in doubt, especially if the refusal would have serious long lasting health consequences or might lead to death. The "mature minor" is one who, subjectively in the judgment of another, possesses the adult cognition and judgment for making health care decisions. The "emancipated minor" is one who has joined the armed services, is married, is living separate from and financially independent of parents, or has otherwise demonstrated clear patterns of singular existence. Mature minors and emancipated minors can consent to their own medical care.

Another way to think about the mature minor is suggested by an analysis of cases specific to medical care. In this context, the cases demonstrate that a physician has never been found liable for providing health care to a minor without parental consent and solely on the consent of the minor under the following circumstances[13]:

1. The treatment was undertaken for the benefit of the minor rather than a third party.
2. The minor was near majority (or at least 15 years of age) and was considered to have sufficient mental capacity to fully understand the nature and importance of the medical steps proposed.
3. The medical procedures could be characterized by the court as less than "major," or "serious."[13(p134)]

The doctrine of the mature minor exists in the intersection of a child's cognitive and judgmental ability and the nature and quality of the medical intervention.

By law, therefore, adolescents are similar to but not entirely like younger children, even if both share a condition of minority. Needless to say, there is nothing magical about the age of majority. It is largely a societal convenience. It was formerly 21 years, but when the constitution was amended to lower the voting rights age from 21 to 18 years, most markers of majority followed suit. In addition, many states have enacted "minor treatment statutes" that stipulate ages younger than 18 years (now the age of majority in all states) at which a child can consent to care.[13(p129)]

Emergency treatment of a child of any age without parental consent is legally permissible, and in many cases is also an ethical imperative. A broken bone or other painful condition requires immediate attention to alleviate current pain and avoid complications (including death) that could ensue from delay brought about by taking time to locate a parent for consent to the child's treatment.

The last 2 decades have thrown into disarray some assumptions about the relationships of parents and children. Adolescents have become progressively more visible as an independent group within American society, for example, as a sizable consumer market or as a growing segment of the criminal population. Adolescents' independence and singular lifestyles reveal at the least a potential for conflict of interests between the parent and the adolescent. For many of the adolescents who are estranged and alone, it may no longer make sense to require parental involvement in medical care. Yet, it could be argued that it is precisely these children who may need a more wise and mature review of complex decisions.

In recognition of these differences in lifestyle and of changing sexual mores and, in the light of the epidemiology of sexually transmitted diseases (STDs) and the public health interest in providing care, all states now permit minors to secure medical care and treatment for STDs without parental consent.[13(p130)]

Legislators reasoned that the sensitive nature of the disease and the fear of parental disapproval would discourage children from seeking care, thus endangering themselves and others. Even if treatment of STDs were not singled out, providers likely would be protected for providing care without parental consent by the emergency doctrine, given that the dangers of not treating are substantial.

In this context, drug and alcohol abuse presents a problem. More than half of the states now have specific statutes permitting treatment for substance abuse without parental consent.[14] In jurisdictions without specific legislative empowerment, the emergency doctrine or the emancipated minor category may apply. One authority states[13(p131)]:

> *Even in the absence of statute, however, a child with a drug problem who flatly refuses to tell his parents that he needs treatment or to permit the physician to do so, undoubtedly would be held competent by a court to give consent to such treatment, since the social and personal consequences to the child of the addiction are so profound and since continuing to make illegal purchases of drugs will subject the child to serious risks of arrest and punishment.*

To summarize, physicians are not liable for the nonnegligent provision of care to a minor without parental consent under the following 3 circumstances: (1) an emergency; (2) the child is a mature minor or an emancipated minor; or (3) the care is for an STD or substance abuse. Whether the parents could be held financially liable without their previous consent is questionable, and the physician must be ready to absorb the cost of care provided without parental consent. Moreover, the attempt to collect payment from the parent could present a breach of the confidential physician-patient relationship.

Confidentiality

Confidentiality and protection for the fact of treatment and the conditions of treatment is considered a basic element of health care provision and a linchpin of the physician-patient relationship. All professional oaths for physicians state that it is the ethical obligation of the physician to guard the communications of a patient as private and to protect secrets shared between physician and patient.[15] These oaths are incorporated by most state licensing statutes. In addition, all states have codified the preexisting common law by enacting privilege statutes that protect communications between physician and patient, husband and wife, priest (clergy) and penitent, and lawyer and client. These statutes permit the patient to raise the "privilege" of confidentiality in court to exclude otherwise relevant and permissible testimony, especially testimony that may describe the content of the physician-patient interaction. Needless to say, judges do not favor these statutes as they impede the free flow of otherwise relevant testimony. They therefore tend to construe such statutes narrowly.

A substantial number of affronts are arrayed against these fragile supports for confidentiality, including (1) third-party payer contracts, which require reports on conditions and treatment; (2) narrow constructions of the legal protections; (3) the computerization of medical information and record keeping; (4) gossip; (5) mandatory reporting laws for specific circumstances; and (6) presentation of a danger to the public or the imminent risk of harm to the patient. Mandatory reporting regulations now require notification of the local health department for a range of illnesses, including in all states STDs and in some states AIDS. Certain nonreportable behaviors also may require breaching confidentiality and warning a specifically endangered third party. This last exception, called the Tarasoff rule (after the California case[16] that established it), requires psychotherapists, and perhaps by extension all physicians, to warn possibly endangered strangers that they may be harmed by a patient. Such warnings are required if the patient has specifically identified a potential victim, has a feasible plan to cause harm, and in the judgment of the therapist, possesses the clear intent to act according to the plan. The case caused much consternation when decided but has not, in fact, been followed by many other states. Accordingly, health professionals should review their own state statutes regarding their obligation to report under applicable state law. The local or state medical society should know whether the jurisdiction has a so-called Tarasoff rule. Even when warning an endangered third party may not be required legally, a physician may feel morally bound to act.

For adolescents who are substance abusers, issues of confidentiality are even more complex. The basic contract between or among the adolescent, parent (if involved), and physician must acknowledge the possibility of breach from outset. The physician should make clear to the child or to the parent and child (in the case in which they meet together with the physician) that the statements given and history told by the adolescent and the treatment plan agreed to are confidential and will not be shared with the parent or with any other except under certain circumstances. Exceptions are as follows: (1) the patient requires parental involvement; (2) the patient consents specifically to a parent's request for information; or (3) the physician concludes that the adolescent's behavior may harm the adolescent or someone else. This contract shared openly with parent and child makes all parties knowing participants in the same game played by the same rules.

If an adolescent comes alone to the physician, requests care, and refuses to tell the parent, the physician must decide whether to accept the adolescent's consent as a sufficient basis for treatment, considering the factors to which the adolescent, parents, and physician agreed. Even if the physician is so willing, he or she might stipulate to the minor some limit to confidentiality under an exception relating to direct and immediate harm. A contract about confidentiality at the outset has the usefulness and the virtue of providing not only a clear basis for present medical practice but also a guideline for future behavior, which should resolve many of the moral uncertainties inherent in the relationship between health care professionals and their adolescent patients.

In general, confidentiality is owed to the adolescent patient, because it is the adolescent who stands as the patient in the physician-patient dyad. However, even the most sophisticated and mature adolescent is likely to have areas of less adult behavior, especially if the adolescent is engaged in self-abusive or self-destructive behavior involving drugs and alcohol.

The Model Act of the American Academy of Pediatrics provides that[13(p143)]:

> *Any minor who has physical or emotional problems and is capable of making rational decisions and whose relationship with his parents or legal guardian is in such a state that by informing them the minor will fail to seek initial or future help may consent to the health professionals for health services...After the professional establishes his rapport with the minor, then he may inform the patient's parents or legal guardian unless such action will jeopardize the life of the patient or the favorable result of the treatment.*

There are no well-known cases in which a child has sued a physician for breach of confidentiality because the physician revealed information to a parent or guardian without the child's permission or despite the child's objection. To our knowledge, there are also no cases discussed in the literature in which a physician was held liable for nondisclosure to a parent when a parent requested information. In contrast with education records, which are specifically available for parent review (Family and Educational Rights Privacy Act of 1974[17]), medical records remain private and subject to the specific contract and practice exceptions noted. It would be bad practice for a physician to shield a suicidal patient behind a wall of confidentiality or to report an alcohol experimenter or an inquisitive but responsible sexual beginner. If either of these hypothetical patients developed into an adolescent with a regular pattern of drunk driving or one who was promiscuous and committed to unsafe sex in a locality heavily involved in the AIDS epidemic, however, it would no longer be acceptable to guard confidentiality and exclude from notice of the potentially destructive or lethal behavior of the patient. Even in these cases, the physician should attempt to involve the patient and secure permission for the parental contact. Should all attempts at provider-patient agreement fail, the parent or guardian should be informed.

The physician is never forbidden by law or by the application of ethical principles from sharing information with the parent under circumstances in which the patient is a danger to his or her self or others. In general, confidentiality is a positive good to be encouraged and supported, although it is never an absolute barrier to communication.

If confidentiality were not strongly supported, it is feared that adolescents would be less likely to seek continuous care from one health care professional. If confidentiality were not assured, some adolescents would not seek care at all; those who sought care might do so in distant localities and provide false histories and incorrect family information, thus making adequate care difficult or impossible.

Some confidential treatment for drug and alcohol abuse is protected specifically by state and federal statutes. Thus, more than 35 states and the District of Columbia specifically give juveniles the right to obtain alcohol or other drug treatment without requiring parental consent.[17,18] In addition, there are federal alcohol and drug confidentiality regulations[19] that apply to any program or individual providing diagnosis, treatment, or referral for alcohol or drug problems and receiving federal funds or any program with a tax-exempt status. These regulations specify that information about a minor patient in such a program can be released only with the patient's written and informed release.

However, even when the ethical and legal protections for the patient are strong, they are not absolute. The health care professional always should be aware that specific planned destructive behavior or self-destructive behavior (suicide) should be evaluated as a potential basis for parental notification.

Physicians should be quite comfortable about the improbability of liability and about the propriety of protecting the secrets of the patient when doctrines of confidentiality seem to require exclusion of the parent from the treatment. The guidelines and specific protections are quite clear. But what of the converse? What of a physician asked to screen for substance abuse or requested to treat despite objections of the patient? Decisions about screening or treatment despite objections by the patient are appropriately made by the state governments; they are not appropriate decisions for physicians (see Chapters 2 and 4).[20]

Two of the powers of government in the Anglo-American tradition are the *parens patriae,* in which the state intervenes to protect persons incapable of protecting themselves, and the police power under which the state intervenes to protect others. Both require some formal determination that the person is incapable of recognizing, defining, and acting responsibly in the pursuit of self-interest and, as a result, is a possible danger to self or others. Thus, involuntary commitment and involuntary treatment for psychiatric illness require a petition, argument, and court review. Before an adolescent can be compelled to submit to treatment for drug and alcohol abuse, some comparable formal process should be required if argument, persuasion, and cajoling fail.

It would be practically impossible and generally a bad idea for physicians to attempt diagnosis or treatment despite the adolescent's objection. The adolescent is the patient and, although denial of their condition may exist, diagnosis and treatment cannot and should not proceed without the patient's consent. However, a physician might push heavily for the adolescent to seek care but not surreptitiously take blood or urine for one purpose and use it for another. This would, of course, be a substantial breach of the trust underlying the physician-patient relationship (see Chapter 2).

The parents may seek a court order or the intervention of police to impose medical care. Even in these circumstances, however, the physician would be under no obligation to comply unless specifically ordered by a judge.

Parents may seek to have their children found delinquent or unruly so that they may be segregated from society. Once so confined, the medical providers in a juvenile detention setting are obligated to provide constitutionally adequate care and the right to test within very expanded guidelines. It is unclear, however, whether they may impose care without specific court authorization.

Physicians dealing with younger children regularly impose care. Even the most reasonable 2-year-old will resist the pain of immunization; many must be held for the treatment, which is clearly in their best interest. Older children may have irrational fears of necessary surgery. Some adolescents refuse care because of the oppositional stage of development, not on preference or considered judgment. Thus, there may be limited circumstances in which it is necessary and appropriate to treat despite the objections of a child and rarely despite the objections of the adolescent.

It is difficult to imagine this analysis applying to treatment of substance abuse. Because all use of alcohol by a minor is illegal and all illicit drug use is illegal, any child engaged in these behaviors is exhibiting delinquent behavior.[14(p21)] If a court so finds, the child may be segregated and ordered to participate in treatment. Without this intervening judicial finding, however, coerced treatment is inappropriate.

Conclusion

Diagnosis and treatment of substance abuse is a real and growing problem for society (see Table 0.1, p ix). Consumption of alcohol by adolescents remains problematic. Although the overall use of illicit drugs is on a slight decline, there is presently an increased use of some drugs, such as "Ecstasy," and greater availability of purer forms of heroin. The number of young people experimenting with or using these substances remains unacceptably high. Physicians need to recognize that substance abuse is no different than other chronic diseases similar to asthma or diabetes. Determinants of substance abuse may have much more to do with socioeconomic status and community characteristics. Physicians can be catalysts for treatment if they are accepted and trusted by the patient. Physicians thus are likely to be more useful as allies of and advocates for rather than opponents of the patient's position and wishes.

References

1. Aries P. *Centuries of Childhood: A Social History of Family Life.* New York, NY: Vintage Books; 1965
2. Platt AM. *The Child Savers: The Invention of Delinquency.* Chicago, IL: The University of Chicago Press; 1969
3. *Brown v The Board of Education of Topeka,* 347 US 483 (1954)
4. In re *Gault,* 387 US 1 (1967)
5. *Tinker v Des Moines Independent Community School District,* 393 US 503 (1969)
6. *Bellotti v Baird,* 443 US 662 (1979)
7. *Planned Parenthood of Central Missouri v Danforth,* 428 US 52 (1976)
8. *H. L. v Matheson,* 450 US 398 (1981)
9. *Carey v Population Services International,* 431 US 678 (1977)
10. *Parham v JR,* 442 US 584 (1979)
11. *Wisconsin v Yoder,* 406 US 205 (1972)
12. *Vernonia School District 47J v Acton,* 115 S Ct 2386 (1995)
13. Holder AR. *Legal Issues in Pediatrics and Adolescent Medicine.* 2nd ed. New Haven, CT: Yale University Press; 1985
14. Evans DG. *Kids, Drugs and the Law.* Center City, MN: Hazelden Foundation; 1985
15. Seigler M. Confidentiality and medicine: a decrepit concept. *N Engl J Med.* 1982;307:1518-1521
16. *Tarasoff v The Regents of the University of California,* 551 P 2d 334 (Cal 1976)
17. Family and Educational Rights Privacy Act, 20 USC §1221 (1974)
18. Rosoff AJ. *Informed Consent: A Guide for Health Care Providers.* Rockville, MD: Aspen Systems Corporation; 1981:211-231. Cited by: Evans DG. *Kids, Drugs and the Law.* Center City, MN: Hazelden Foundation; 1985:37
19. 52 *Federal Register* 21809 (1987) (codified at 42 CFR §2)
20. American Academy of Pediatrics, Committee on Substance Abuse. Testing for drugs of abuse in children and adolescents. *Pediatrics.* 1996;98:305-307

Chapter 8

Specific Drugs

Susan M. Coupey, MD, FAAP

This chapter is designed as a reference to assist the health care professional in understanding the pharmacologic, behavioral, and somatic consequences of particular drugs of abuse. Literally hundreds of psychoactive drugs may be abused. The slight decrease in use of any illicit drug during the past 30 days by twelfth graders in 2000 from a peak in 1999 still reflects an unacceptably high number of young people who have recently used drugs (see Table 0.1, p ix).[1-3] This chapter includes only the drugs (or classes of drugs) that are abused by significant numbers of children and adolescents. Presented are the following: tobacco (cigarettes and smokeless); marijuana; alcohol; cocaine, amphetamine, and other stimulants; hallucinogens (lysergic acid diethylamide [LSD], phencyclidine [PCP], and designer hallucinogens); anabolic-androgenic steroids; opiates, including heroin, and designer opiates; sedative-hypnotics; tranquilizers; and inhalants. The National Institute on Drug Abuse has recently included several of these drugs among those categorized as "club drugs," as noted on p 263.[4]

Tobacco

Epidemiology

Tobacco was smoked or taken as snuff by the natives in North and South America for centuries and was introduced in Europe as a medicinal herb during the 16th century.[5(p183-205)] Soon, however, the use of tobacco became a widespread social practice, and it remains so today. A significant part of American history revolves around the lucrative tobacco trade from the colonies in Virginia to England. During the 19th century, most of the tobacco used by Americans was chewing tobacco; few people smoked. However, by the "roaring 20s," smoking had overtaken chewing, and by the

1950s, fueled by the returned veterans of World War II, cigarette smoking became a national habit. As the health dangers of smoking began to be documented and publicized during the 1960s and 1970s, a return to the use of chewing or smokeless tobacco was noted.

The smoking behavior of adolescents tends to be similar to that of adults, although nicotine addiction is identified as a pediatric disease.[6] Children and adolescents are the primary source of new smokers; more than 1 million youth each year become regular smokers. Few persons initiate smoking after reaching adulthood.

The prevalence of smoking within the past 30 days by twelfth graders, as measured in the annual *Monitoring the Future* studies, decreased from 1975 through 1992, when it reached its lowest level, 27.8%.[7] However, the prevalence began to increase again in 1993, a trend that continued until 1999. In 2000, there was an encouraging decrease to 31.4%.[1-3] A similar percentage of twelfth graders were current smokers (within the past 30 days) in 1997 (36.5%) as in 1975 (36.7%). However, the data indicate that after 6 years of steady increases in prevalence of current smoking, there was a leveling off in 1997, with 19.4% of eighth graders and 29.8% of tenth graders indicating that they had smoked within the past 30 days. Adolescent girls in grades 8 and 10 are more likely than boys in those grades to be current smokers, but by grade 12, more boys than girls are smokers.

The Centers for Disease Control and Prevention's 1997 *Youth Risk Behavior Survey* found that 48.2% of US high school boys and 36% of girls reported any current (within the past 30 days) use of tobacco (cigarettes, smokeless tobacco, or cigars).[8,9] Findings from the survey indicated that among US high school students in 1997, 70% had tried cigarette smoking, and of those, just over one third became daily smokers. Smokeless tobacco use was quite prevalent, particularly among US high school boys, with 15.8% reporting current use in 1997, compared with only 1.5% of girls. Similarly, 31.2% of boys reported current cigar use, whereas only 10.8% of girls indicated cigar use. The prevalence of daily cigarette smoking was higher among white students

(19.9%) than among Hispanic (10.9%) and black (7.2%) students. White male (19.8%) and female (20.1%) students were more likely to be daily smokers than black male (10.1%) and female (4.3%) students. The 1997 *Youth Risk Behavior Survey* found little difference in the prevalence of ever having smoked among ninth graders (67.7%), tenth graders (70.0%), eleventh graders (68.8%), and twelfth graders (73.7%), but the prevalence of daily smoking increased from 13.1% among ninth graders to 19.4% among eleventh graders.

A study of almost 1000 third through sixth graders in a semi-rural community in the southern United States found that 15% of the children had tried cigarettes and 7.4% currently used a tobacco product (cigarettes, 1.2%; chewing tobacco, 4.3%; snuff, 2.2%; cigars, 1.3%; pipes, 0.3%). Of the children, 40% first tried cigarettes with a family member, and 46% obtained their first cigarette from a family member or at home.[10]

The *Childhood Antecedents of Smoking Study,* a prospective longitudinal study conducted in a suburban school district in the Minneapolis-St Paul area documented predictors of smoking behavior among seventh and eighth graders who had not yet become regular smokers.[11] The predictors included peer influence (having friends who smoke), having siblings who smoke, having less educated parents (especially for girls), being more independent and rebellious, and being less concerned about the health consequences of smoking. The latter finding was considered encouraging by the authors, because it suggests that for younger adolescents, "there may yet be value in communicating messages about the health consequences of smoking." A retrospective study of the cognitive and school performance characteristics preceding the onset of smoking found that cigarette smoking in high school was associated with significantly more school absence in elementary school and high school, lower grade-point averages in grades 4 and 6 and in high school, lower IQ in grade 6, and lower scores on Stanford achievement tests in grades 3 and 5.[12] The associations suggest that smoking behavior may be part of lifestyle differences among children and adolescents and that smoking prevention efforts must begin early and "address general values and lifestyles rather than only the practice of smoking."[12]

Clinical Pharmacology

The active ingredient of cigarette smoke and chewed or snorted tobacco is nicotine,[13] which is a naturally occurring alkaloid that is well absorbed in the lungs by inhalation or through the mucous membranes of the mouth and nose. Nicotine is deactivated in the liver and excreted by the kidneys. Tolerance develops with continued use, at least partially because of increased activity of the liver microsomal enzyme systems responsible for deactivation of the drug, and an abstinence syndrome ensues when the drug is discontinued. Nicotine has a central role in the dependence-producing process of cigarette smoking and smokeless tobacco use. Tobacco use fits all the criteria of drug dependence or addiction and differs from other compulsive behaviors, because the addiction is determined primarily by the effect of nicotine on the brain.[13] Thus, treatment strategies should address pharmacologic and behavioral factors.

In the peripheral nervous system, nicotine blocks cholinergic synapses and also has a sympathomimetic effect via stimulation of the release of epinephrine. Nicotine is highly toxic. Symptoms of low-level poisoning—dizziness, nausea, and generalized weakness—commonly are noticed by beginning smokers. A toxic overdose can lead to tremors, seizures, paralysis of the respiratory muscles, and death. In the central nervous system (CNS), nicotine shifts the electroencephalogram into an arousal pattern. However, most smokers claim that the net effect is relaxation and relief of tension.

Other components of cigarette smoke have a key role in the toxic effects of smoking. Carbon monoxide is one such component. Regular smokers have a higher than normal amount of carboxyhemoglobin, which impairs the oxygen-carrying capacity of the blood and often contributes to dyspnea on exertion in smokers and impairs oxygen transfer to the fetus via the placenta in pregnant women who smoke. Tars and other carcinogens in smokeless tobacco and cigarette smoke are responsible for the association between tobacco use and malignant neoplasms.

Health Consequences

The contribution of cigarette smoking to excess morbidity and mortality attributable to heart disease, emphysema, and lung cancer in older adults is well known and will not be restated.[14] Instead, the focus is the health consequences of smoking and tobacco use for pediatric patients, including the fetus, neonate, infant, child, and adolescent.

The fetus of the pregnant woman who smokes will have chronic hypoxia; the result is generalized growth retardation marked by decreased birth weight, length, and circumference of the head, chest, and shoulders.[14] A longitudinal study of the effects of tobacco use during pregnancy on the offspring of adolescent mothers (mean age, 16 years) found that adverse growth effects on the infants of adolescent mothers were prominent despite lower levels of tobacco exposure than for infants of adult mothers in the same clinic, suggesting that young maternal age may increase vulnerability of the fetus to the toxic effects of tobacco.[15] Because of the varied effects, the neonate of a pregnant woman who smokes is at increased risk of death.[14]

Infants and young children of parents who smoke are at increased risk of serious respiratory illnesses, such as bronchitis and pneumonia. One study found that children whose mothers smoked had a hospital admission rate for respiratory illness 28% higher than that of children of mothers who did not smoke.[14] Other studies have documented that asthma, persistent middle-ear effusions, and sudden infant death syndrome are more common in children of smokers than of nonsmokers.[14] Although the statistical associations do not prove cause and effect, the evidence that passive inhalation of smoke (exposure to second-hand smoke) impairs the health of children is compelling. Significantly increased amounts of nicotine and its metabolite, cotinine, have been measured in the urine and saliva of infants who were exposed to parental tobacco smoke,[16] providing definite evidence that infants passively absorb the constituents of smoke from their environment.

A number of studies have found measurable impairment of small airways in adolescent smokers. One longitudinal study in Boston documented a significant decrease in forced expiratory volume in 1 second and in the middle half of forced vital capacity in adolescents who became smokers compared with their nonsmoking peers.[17] The pulmonary function test results of these children were not different from those of their peers before the onset of smoking. The Berlin-Breman study of seventh and eighth graders documented a linear decrease in the ratio of forced expiratory volume in 1 second to forced vital capacity as carbon monoxide levels in expired air (a measure of recent smoking) increased.[18] The study also showed an inverse relationship between smoking by adolescents and high-density lipoprotein cholesterol that was evident within 2 years of beginning to smoke. A meta-analysis comparing serum lipids in 8- to 19-year-old smokers and nonsmokers found significant changes in the direction of increased risk of coronary artery disease in children and adolescents who smoked.[19]

Smoking has long been identified as a risk factor for cancer of the cervix in women, and nicotine and its metabolite, cotinine, are found in increased concentrations in the cervical mucus of women who smoke. A study of a group of young women who did not smoke documented a significant association between passive exposure to environmental tobacco smoke and nicotine levels in cervical lavage specimens.[20] Exposure in the home resulted in the highest nicotine levels, suggesting that parents who smoke may put their adolescent daughters at higher risk of cancer of the cervix. Thus, accumulating data suggest that abnormalities known to be precursors of smoking-related disease are measurable in young people within a few years of initiation of the behavior.

Laboratory Evaluation

Methods commonly used to verify smoking behavior include measuring saliva or urinary cotinine and nicotine concentrations, the carboxyhemoglobin or thiocyanate concentration in the blood, and the concentration of carbon monoxide in expired air. These measures are used primarily in research studies.

Treatment

The most effective treatment for cigarette smoking is prevention of the onset of the behavior. Prevention is particularly important for the child and young adolescent. The most successful smoking prevention programs are school based, target the sixth or seventh grader, use peer counselors, emphasize positive health behaviors rather than dwelling on risks, discuss risks that are immediate and applicable to the age group, and teach skills for resisting the social pressures to smoke.[21-23] However, clinical practice guidelines issued in 1977 by the US Department of Health and Human Services state, among other recommendations: "Efforts to prevent tobacco use should be conducted by many types of individuals and groups and in diverse venues."[24]

Discussions of tobacco use should begin before adolescence when the child is in the elementary grades and continue through high school. Health care professionals have a significant role; they should seize every opportunity to discourage smoking among the parents of infant and child patients, among school-aged patients, and especially among adolescent patients.[25,26] A study of a stratified random sample of California physicians inquired how often the physicians asked adolescents about smoking.[27] Overall, physicians screened younger adolescents (11-14 years of age) during 71% of routine visits and older adolescents (15-18 years of age) during 85% of visits. Pediatricians had the lowest rates of screening, compared with internists, adolescent medicine specialists, and family physicians. Physician counseling about the health hazards of tobacco use can be effective, even if it occurs at only 1 visit.

For adolescents who are already smokers and want to quit, there are myriad smoking cessation programs of variable effectiveness. The 1997 *Youth Risk Behavior Survey* found that of US high school students who had ever been daily smokers, 73% had tried to quit, but only 13.5% were former smokers.[9] Sargent et al[28] studied factors associated with smoking cessation in a cohort of more than one thousand 12- to 18-year-olds surveyed annually for 3 years.[28] Of the study participants, 27% reported failed attempts to quit smoking, and 26% wanted to quit at the time of the survey. The smoking cessation rate was 46% among occasional smokers, 12% among daily smokers of 1 to 9 cigarettes, and 7% among daily smokers of 10 or more cigarettes. These data indicate that adolescents who are less addicted are more likely to quit than daily smokers whose quit rates are comparable to those of adult smokers. Unlike adults, for adolescents in the study, experience with quitting was not associated with a higher likelihood of cessation. These data emphasize the prominent role of nicotine addiction in the maintenance of smoking behavior. Health care professionals should focus on preventing occasional smokers from progressing to daily smokers, thus preventing addiction.[29] Nicotine patch therapy as an adjunct to smoking cessation treatment has been studied in adolescents and seems to be safe and well tolerated.[30] Nicotine patches (nicotine transdermal systems) are easier to use than nicotine gum. There are 4 patches on the market; 2 are sold over the counter, NicoDerm CQ (SmithKline Beecham Consumer Healthcare, Pittsburgh, PA) and Nicotrol (McNeil Consumer Products, Fort Washington, PA), and 2 require a prescription, Habitrol (Novartis Consumer Health, Summit, NJ) and Prostep (Lederle Laboratories, Pearl River, NY). The patch should be used for 8 weeks, and there seems to be little difference among the brands. A nicotine nasal spray and a nicotine inhaler also are available. The use of sustained-release bupropion hydrochloride (Zyban [Glaxo Wellcome, Research Triangle Park, NC]) may be helpful, although no studies have been done in adolescents.

The Food and Drug Administration (FDA) issued regulations restricting the sale, distribution, promotion, and advertising of nicotine-containing cigarettes and smokeless tobacco to minors.[31] The regulations are based on the emerging evidence of the addictive quality of nicotine, the vulnerability and exploitation of youth, and growing knowledge about the tobacco industry's intent to promote tobacco to children and adolescents and their awareness of the addictive properties of nicotine. It will be several years before the full effect of the regulations on the initiation of smoking by children and adolescents will be evident.

See Chapter 9 for an expanded discussion of tobacco use and abuse.

MARIJUANA

Epidemiology

More than 50 million Americans have tried marijuana. Among twelfth graders in the United States, half reported using marijuana at least once in their lifetime, and 38.5% reported use within the last year, making marijuana the most common illicit drug chosen by adolescents.[7] With the exception of cigarettes, marijuana is the substance chosen most often by adolescents for regular use; 6.0% of twelfth graders and 3.8% of tenth graders use it daily.[1] Use of marijuana by adolescents increased steadily during the 1990s; the prevalence of use within the past 30 days for eighth, tenth, and twelfth graders was 3.2%, 8.7%, and 13.8%, respectively in 1991 and 10.2%, 20.5%, and 23.7%, respectively in 1997.[1,7] The almost tripled use during the decade by eighth graders who are approximately 14 years old is most disturbing, although 1997 data indicated a leveling off of the increase. Recent use (within the past 30 days) by twelfth graders decreased to 21.6% in 2000 from a high of 23.7% in 1997 (see Table 0.1, p ix).[1-3]

Pharmacology

Marijuana is obtained from the hemp plant. During the 1970s, the marijuana smoked in the United States was made from leaves and flowering shoots of *Cannabis sativa,* but during the 1980s, growers began cultivating the more potent *Cannabis indica.* During the 1990s, the 2 varieties were crossed, resulting in the modern hybrid American marijuana plant—*Cannabis sativa,* x *indica*—combining the most desirable traits of both varieties.[32] Although during the 1970s both leaves and buds were smoked, currently only the seedless buds of female plants, sinsemilla, are considered worth smoking. The pharmacologic effects are related to the content of Δ^9-tetrahydrocannabinol (THC) and other cannabinoids. THC is the constituent primarily responsible for the neurophysiologic, biochemical, and behavioral manifestations of marijuana. During the 1970s, the THC content of marijuana was between 0.5% and 2%. The average THC content for indoor-grown sinsemilla during the 1990s was between 8% and 10%.[32]

Thus, there have been exponential increases in the potency of marijuana during the past 2 decades. The concentration of THC and, accordingly, the dose delivered from any individual marijuana supply may vary enormously. Awareness of this variation in potency is essential for comparing the results of studies of the effects of marijuana and for managing the intoxicated patient.

Effects begin within seconds to minutes after inhalation of the smoke or within 30 to 60 minutes after oral ingestion. Smoking routes the cannabinoids directly from the lungs to the brain and other organs, with minimal opportunity for dilution or metabolism. Thus, higher concentrations are delivered to the brain more rapidly when marijuana is inhaled than when it is ingested orally or injected intravenously. The drug is a euphoriant and is used to produce feelings of relaxation and well-being, although in high doses, it is a hallucinogen. Although the smoker experiences the effects almost immediately and can stop further inhalation at any time, the oral user experiences effects that begin more slowly, last longer, and are more variable, making unpleasant reactions more likely.

Although the initially high blood levels of THC decrease rapidly during the first 30 minutes, the drug and its metabolites are highly lipid soluble and are stored in fatty tissue and released slowly. The serum half-life is approximately 19 hours.[33] Although repeated use results in an accumulation of cannabinoids, blood levels do not accurately reflect concentrations present in the brain or other organs, because cannabinoids are distributed readily into tissues throughout the body, a situation that is quite different from that for alcohol, in which blood levels accurately represent concurrent levels in the brain. THC also differs from other psychoactive drugs, such as caffeine and nicotine, which are metabolized rapidly and eliminated completely, thereby making detection impossible only a few hours after intake. Elimination of THC and its metabolites occurs primarily in feces but also in urine, and complete elimination may require up to 1 month.

A cannabinoid receptor has been found in the brain, and the gene for the receptor has been cloned.[34] Isolation of the receptor led to the discovery of an endogenous ligand, anandamine, a fatty acid compound possessing pharmacologic properties similar to THC.[35,36] The behavioral effects of marijuana probably are mediated by specific cannabinoid receptors and interaction with other neurochemical systems. Like other drugs with addictive potential, such as heroin and nicotine, in rat experiments, THC resulted in the release of dopamine in the brain's "reward" pathway in the nucleus accumbens.[37] An antagonist of central cannabinoid receptors in addition to the opiate antagonist, naloxone hydrochloride, each will prevent the THC-stimulated increase in dopamine levels, indicating that marijuana and opiates separately and individually elevate dopamine levels by activating opiate receptors, but marijuana presumably elevates dopamine levels indirectly by stimulation of an endogenous opioid compound. Recent animal experiments also have shown that long-term cannabinoid administration alters the limbic system in the brain in a manner similar to other drugs of abuse.[38,39] Administration of a cannabinoid antagonist precipitates a profound withdrawal syndrome in THC-tolerant mice and rats and activates corticotropin-releasing factor in the rat amygdala.[39,40] Activation of corticotropin-releasing factor mediates the stress-like and negative-affective components of withdrawal from other abused drugs, such as heroin and cocaine. These findings indicate that marijuana behaves in the brain like other addictive drugs of abuse.

Health Consequences

Although the major effects of marijuana are on behavior, the use of marijuana is not without physiologic consequences.[41] Acute cardiovascular effects of marijuana include transient increases in heart rate and blood pressure and peripheral vasodilation and, in large doses, orthostatic hypotension. These effects, most likely attributable to THC-induced changes of autonomic function, are temporary and usually have no deleterious effects on the healthy person. In healthy or asthmatic persons, the immediate pulmonary effect of the inhalation of marijuana smoke is bronchodilation. For some smokers, however, the particles in the inhalant act as an irritant, causing bronchoconstriction. Furthermore, in long-term users, significant functional airway impairment can occur.[42] Pharyngitis, sinusitis, bronchitis, and asthma have been reported in heavy smokers.[43] Some evidence indicates that smoking marijuana results in much higher carbon monoxide levels in the blood and tar deposition in the lungs than use of a similar quantity of tobacco.[43] Unfortunately, most studies that have attempted to determine the long-term effects of marijuana use in humans have been confounded by the use of tobacco cigarettes by most subjects. However, some recent studies have attempted to address this issue,[44,45] and precancerous bronchial epithelial abnormalities have been found in marijuana smokers who do not use tobacco.[44,45] The adverse effects of marijuana and tobacco on bronchial epithelium seem to be additive, however, making smokers of both substances at especially high risk of neoplastic transformation. One study demonstrated that smoking more potent marijuana to the desired level of intoxication resulted in exposure to a decreased amount of tar than smoking less potent preparations, presumably because of decreased intake of smoke.[46]

Concern about the effect of marijuana on fertility arises from studies of men who are heavy users; the studies demonstrated diminished sperm motility and sperm counts, both of which are reversible effects.[47] In addition, marijuana decreases serum testosterone levels in males. A study of pubertal development and hormones in adolescent boys enrolled in a drug rehabilitation program compared with controls who did not use drugs found no differences in heights, weights, or sexual maturity ratings, but the boys who abused drugs had mean testosterone levels of less than half those of the control subjects as well as significantly lower gonadotropin levels.[48] Serum testosterone levels increased 7 to 12 months after drug withdrawal. The boys who abused drugs frequently were exposed to marijuana and alcohol, and none used opiates; thus, much of the sex steroid decrease was likely attributable to marijuana use. Animal data show that marijuana interferes with ovulation in females and causes a decrease in circulating pituitary gonadotropins.[49]

In a multicenter study of a cohort of more than 7000 pregnant women, 11% reported using marijuana during pregnancy; use of the drug was not associated with preterm delivery, low birth weight, or abruptio placentae.[50] A study of Jamaican neonates exposed to marijuana prenatally, compared with nonexposed neonates, found no differences on the Brazelton Neonatal Assessment Scale at 3 days of age.[51] Thus, marijuana apparently has few if any adverse effects during pregnancy.

The major deleterious health effects of marijuana are behavioral. The extent of behavioral effects usually is related directly to the concentration of marijuana used, although the personality of the user, the user's expectation of the effect, and the milieu in which the drug is used also have a contributing role. The popularity of marijuana arises from the euphoria, sense of relaxation, and increased visual, auditory, and taste perceptions produced at low or moderate doses in most young people. Unpleasant effects may occur with larger doses. The dysphoric reactions tend to occur more often in adults, especially the elderly, but they can occur at any age, particularly in novice users and when intoxication occurs unexpectedly. Dysphoric reactions range from mild fear to distortions in body image, depersonalization, disorientation, paranoia, and acute panic reactions. Although delirium and hallucinations also have been reported, these extreme reactions should raise suspicion that PCP has been mixed with the marijuana, often without the user's knowledge.[52]

Marijuana has a major effect on the performance of tasks related to coordination. Lack of hand steadiness, decreased postural stability manifested by increased body sway, and inaccurate execution of various movements are observed with doses commonly used in social settings. Time perception is altered so that subjects under the influence of moderate doses of marijuana consistently overestimate the amount of time that has elapsed. The capacity to follow a moving object (tracking) is affected adversely by even low doses and may persist after the sensation of intoxication has passed.[53] One study demonstrated an increased reaction time and diminished ability to detect a brief flash of light, effects that may be attributable in part to a lack of sustained attention.[54] A study using neuropsychologic tests of attention performed on college students who were heavy marijuana smokers (smoked a median of 29 of the last 30 days) or light marijuana smokers (smoked a median of 1 of the last 30 days) after a supervised period of abstinence of at least 19 hours found no significant residual differences overall in the 4 subtests of attention.[55] However, when results for women were analyzed separately from those for men, investigators found marked and significant differences on the subtest measuring visual-spatial memory between women who were heavy and light smokers; the heavy smokers showed worse performance. The results of the study emphasize that residual effects of marijuana may be different for men and women, and earlier studies that were performed almost exclusively on men should be interpreted with caution. Even minor impairment in tracking ability, reaction time, sense of time, and visual-perceptual functioning have obvious and important implications for everyday tasks, such as driving an automobile or operating complicated machinery.

Marijuana also seems to exert a major effect on learning and memory. Short-term memory, especially when it is heavily dependent on attention, such as during information acquisition and storage, is significantly affected by even a single moderate dose. A double-blind, placebo-controlled study of the acute effects of marijuana smoking on cognition that measured learning, associative processes, abstraction, and psychomotor performance found that marijuana impaired all capabilities except abstraction and vocabulary.[56] Problem-solving skills that are acquired while using the drug are decreased, learning occurs more slowly, and "state-dependent" learning occurs. The latter phenomenon is an interesting situation in which material that is learned while under the influence of the drug is best remembered in the state of drug intoxication in which it was originally learned. Although information acquisition occurs, the quality of the learning experience is diminished because the data or skills learned in the drug-intoxicated state are decreased or impaired.

Data support the existence of residual effects on attention, psychomotor tasks, and short-term memory in the 12- to 24-hour period after marijuana use, but evidence is insufficient for long-term effects.[57] A study comparing performance of adult marijuana users (n = 144) and nonusers (n = 72) matched on intellectual functioning before the onset of drug use (on the basis of standardized tests given in grade 4) found that heavy marijuana use (7 or more times per week) was associated with deficits in mathematical skills, verbal expression, and selective impairments in memory retrieval.[58] Light (1-4 times per week) and intermediate (5-6 times per week) marijuana use was not associated with cognitive deficits. Pope and Yurgelun-Todd[59] studied 2 groups of college students, heavy marijuana users (smoked a median of 29 of the last 30 days) and light users (smoked a median of 1 of the last 30 days), in their laboratory after 19 hours of supervised abstinence and found significant residual neuropsychologic deficits in heavy users compared with light users, but they caution that whether the impairment is attributable to a drug withdrawal effect, a residue of drug in the brain, or a neurotoxic effect of marijuana is unclear. A study of marijuana-dependent adolescents that evaluated auditory-verbal and visual-spatial memory and compared test scores with those of IQ- and age-matched controls found significant short-term memory deficits in the marijuana abusers that persisted for 6 weeks after the last dose.[60] The finding of persistent memory deficits in adolescents who had been drug-free for several weeks has serious implications for the school performance of regular marijuana smokers.

An "amotivational syndrome" consisting of loss of energy, apathy, absence of ambition, loss of effectiveness, inability to carry out long-term plans, problems with concentrating, impaired memory, and a marked decrease in school or work performance has been described.[61] The evidence for a causative relationship between marijuana and the amotivational syndrome remains equivocal, as evidence is available only from case reports, and similar symptoms also are seen in persons who have not used marijuana. Furthermore, many troubled adolescents use drugs to escape from their problems; thus, marijuana use may be a result of preexisting behavioral problems rather than the cause. A study of 133 cannabis users selected through random urine testing of Army draftees identified comorbid psychiatric disorders by using the Structured Clinical Interview from the *Diagnostic and Statistical Manual of Mental Disorders, Third Edition, Revised (DSM-III-R)*[62] after 2 to 5 days of abstinence.[63] The prevalence of comorbid psychiatric disorders varied with the pattern of marijuana use as defined by *DSM-III-R;* 83% of young men with cannabis-dependence disorder, 46% of those with marijuana abuse, and 29% of occasional users received at least 1 *DSM-III-R* comorbid psychiatric diagnosis. Thus, long-term marijuana use in this sample of young men was associated with a high prevalence of comorbid psychiatric disorders.

As mentioned, marijuana produces pharmacologic tolerance after several days of regular use, and a clinical withdrawal syndrome characterized by a flulike illness and drug craving occurs within 24 to 48 hours of discontinuing the drug.[64] Adolescents who are heavy marijuana users report withdrawal symptoms, including malaise, irritability, agitation, insomnia, drug craving, shakiness, diaphoresis, night sweats, and gastrointestinal disturbance.[65] The intensity of the symptoms peaks by the fourth day, and symptoms gradually resolve in 10 to 14 days. The most persistent symptoms seem to be insomnia and irritable mood and, to a lesser extent, drug cravings. The insomnia is treated effectively with trazodone hydrochloride.[65] One study of more than 200 adolescents with substance use disorders, 79% with cannabis dependence, found that two thirds of the cannabis-dependent adolescents reported withdrawal symptoms.[66] It is important to appreciate the magnitude of the cannabis withdrawal syndrome described by today's adolescents who are smoking much more potent marijuana than the adults who described mild withdrawal symptoms 20 years ago. Given the new understanding of the neurochemistry of cannabis addiction, it is not surprising that the withdrawal syndrome is similar to that seen with opiate dependence.

Laboratory Evaluation

Marijuana and its metabolites may be detected in the urine by the enzyme-multiplied immunoassay technique (EMIT [Behring, San Jose, CA]) within 1 hour after marijuana has been smoked; however, results from urine testing are variable and subject to misinterpretation. For an infrequent user, the urine assay usually remains positive for up to 10 days and for heavy users, up to 1 month after cessation of use (see Chapter 4). Some urine tests for cannabinoid metabolites are so sensitive that they will detect exposure by passive inhalation of secondhand smoke. The standard cutoff level for detection of cannabinoids is 20 ng/mL of urine, but using a cutoff level of 50 to 100 ng/mL of urine eliminates most false-positive results.[41] Urine testing is not reliable for determining the quantity of marijuana used or the time interval since use.

Treatment Considerations

Prevention of marijuana use is a desirable goal for health care professionals caring for adolescents, but failing that, prevention of escalation from occasional use to abuse and cannabis dependence should be pursued vigorously. Educating parents and adolescents about the addictive potential of the drug and the role of the drug in exposing the adolescent to injuries while intoxicated can be helpful. In addition, pointing out that regular marijuana smoking impairs learning, socialization, and sexual function may impress young people. Regular screening for a history of marijuana use and withdrawal symptoms helps identify the adolescents who need further evaluation and treatment for chemical dependency. There is no specific treatment recommended for acute reactions to marijuana other than reassurance for adolescents who become anxious or undergo a panic reaction. Talking to the adolescents in a calm, nonthreatening manner in a tranquil milieu often can be helpful.

Alcohol

Epidemiology

Aside from caffeine, alcohol is used by more people and in larger quantities than any other psychoactive substance. Alcoholic beverages have been consumed by humans since the dawn of time (Neolithic man drank berry wine in 6400 BC), and efforts to regulate consumption have gone on for centuries.[5(p145-182)] In 1839, England imposed penalties for selling spirits to persons younger than 16 years, and currently in the United States, the national minimum legal drinking age is 21 years. Despite efforts at regulation, a large number of adolescents consume alcohol. The prevalence of drinking among adolescents has not changed much during the 1990s. In 1997, 82% of American twelfth graders had tried alcohol, 53% had consumed it within the past 30 days, and 34% reported being drunk within the past 30 days. Comparable percentages for eighth graders are 54%, 25%, and 8%, respectively. Among twelfth graders in 1997, 3.9% drank alcohol daily, 2% got drunk daily, and 31% had consumed 5 or more drinks in a row during the last 2 weeks (binge drinking).[7] Recent use of alcohol (within the past 30 days) by twelfth graders decreased to 50% in 2000, compared with 52% in 1998; however, one third continued to report having been drunk at least once within the past 30 days over the same period (see Table 0.1, p ix).[1-3] In the past, men were much more likely to be heavy drinkers than were women, but at least in the adolescent and young adult populations, these differences seem to be lessening.[67] Among college freshmen, approximately 30% of men and 14% of women are binge drinkers, and almost half reported being drunk twice or more during the past 30 days, in contrast with 5% or fewer of the nonbinge drinkers.[67] Increased levels of drinking on college campuses are associated with higher levels of campus vandalism, assault, and rape.[68] Violent behavior has been linked with the use of alcohol as well as binge drinking and drinking while driving. Male and female high school students report the influence of alcohol and drugs commonly in their unwanted sexual experiences.[69]

Children of alcoholic parents are more likely to become alcoholics themselves. It is widely acknowledged that there is some genetic component to alcoholism, especially for men (see Chapter 1). In addition, family life with an alcoholic parent often is disruptive and sometimes abusive and can lead to a wide variety of problem behaviors in adolescent children, including alcohol and drug abuse.

Pharmacology

Ethanol (C_2H_5OH) is produced by fermentation of the starch or sugar in various fruits and grains by the action of yeast. Fermentation alone will not produce a beverage with greater than 15% alcohol, because the yeast dies at higher concentrations. More potent alcoholic products must be produced by distillation from the fermented mash. Alcohol is consumed in the form of beer, made from barley and hops and containing approximately 5% alcohol; wine, made from grapes and containing approximately 15% alcohol; and spirits or "hard liquor" (eg, scotch, rum, vodka, gin) distilled from barley, corn, or sugar cane and containing approximately 45% alcohol.

Alcohol is absorbed quickly and efficiently from the gastrointestinal tract and requires no digestion. The rate of absorption depends on the concentration of alcohol, the amount and type of food in the stomach, and whether the liquid is carbonated. Diluted alcohol is absorbed more slowly than a highly concentrated "shot" of liquor. However, if the diluent is carbonated or the alcoholic product is effervescent (eg, champagne), the alcohol will pass more rapidly into the small bowel and be absorbed even faster than from the stomach. Eating foods containing fat or protein before or while drinking alcohol delays absorption.

Drug effects are noticed approximately 10 minutes after consumption and peak at approximately 40 to 60 minutes after ingestion. To be excreted, alcohol must be oxidized by the enzyme alcohol dehydrogenase. The metabolism occurs primarily in the liver but also in the gastric mucosa, the so-called "first-pass" metabolism.[70] The activity of the enzyme, not the concentration of alcohol in the blood, is the rate-limiting step in alcohol excretion. Because alcohol cannot be stored in the body and very little can be excreted by lungs or kidneys, it remains in the bloodstream unchanged until metabolized. If a person consumes alcohol at a faster rate than it can be metabolized, the blood alcohol concentration will increase. The initial metabolic product is acetaldehyde, a compound that may have a central role in the toxic effects of alcohol. Women have higher blood alcohol concentrations than do men after consuming comparable amounts of alcohol; evidence suggests that the higher concentration results in part from decreased first-pass metabolism related to decreased activity of gastric alcohol dehydrogenase in women.[71] Thus, girls and women are more vulnerable than boys and men to acute complications of drinking and may have greater deterioration in their ability to drive and perform other psychomotor tasks.

The precise mechanism responsible for alcohol intoxication is unknown, but it is unlikely that it reacts with specific receptors in the brain like marijuana or opiates. Most likely, ethanol acts at the site of the membrane proteins containing a receptor for the inhibitory neurotransmitter γ-aminobutyric acid (GABA) and modifies GABA-activated neurotransmission.[72] Tolerance to alcohol develops with frequent moderate to heavy consumption. Some of this tolerance can be explained by the induction of enzymes in the liver, which permits faster metabolism of the drug, and some by brain tolerance, an adaptation to the neuropsychologic effects of alcohol. Barbiturates and benzodiazepines also interact with receptor sites linked to the GABA receptor, and cross-tolerance among these 3 drugs occurs whenever any one of them is administered for a long period.[72] Physical dependence develops after frequent consumption of alcohol for prolonged periods, resulting in withdrawal syndromes of varying severity. The most common withdrawal symptoms include nausea, vomiting, insomnia, autonomic hyperactivity, and a mild confusional state.[72] Symptoms begin within hours of stopping the drug and peak at 24 to 36 hours. Administration of benzodiazepines or resumption of drinking suppresses the symptoms. Delirium tremens, the most serious alcohol withdrawal syndrome, can lead to seizures and death. This serious withdrawal syndrome has not been described in an adolescent.

Health Consequences

Alcohol is a CNS depressant. At high blood levels, it leads to respiratory depression, arrest, and death. At low blood levels, alcohol impairs regulatory and inhibitory control mechanisms in the brain. Complex and poorly learned behaviors, such as driving in young people, are impaired. Individuals often become generally disinhibited and engage in behaviors that ordinarily would embarrass them. Anxiety is decreased, judgment is poor, and attention, short-term memory, and thought processing are impaired. As blood alcohol levels increase, motor coordination becomes impaired and reaction time becomes quite prolonged. If drinking continues, stupor, coma, and death can ensue.

For most adolescents, the adverse physical health consequences of alcohol consumption result primarily from injuries incurred while intoxicated. Of patients 13 to 19 years of age (mean, 14.8 years) admitted to the trauma service in a pediatric emergency department, 34% had a toxicology screen positive for alcohol (12%) or other drugs of abuse, and this positive rate was significantly higher than the percentage of positive screens in the control group of asthmatic patients (2%).[73]

Alcohol-related motor vehicle crashes are the leading cause of death for 15- to 24-year-old American drivers and passengers. A study of the effect of the legal drinking age on fatal injuries in 15- to 24-year-olds in the United States found that a higher legal drinking age was associated with fewer deaths of motor vehicle drivers and pedestrians, unintentional injuries, and suicides.[74] A decrease in the number of deaths of 0.7% was observed for each year that the legal drinking age was increased.[74] The results indicate that the net benefit of a higher legal drinking age is found for other categories of violent death for adolescents as well as for motor vehicle drivers. For adolescents, other types of mishaps, such as drownings, falls, or fire-related deaths, also have been associated commonly with alcohol intoxication.[75] In addition, elevated blood alcohol levels are found in a substantial percentage of adolescent suicide and homicide victims. Physical complications of acute intoxication, such as coma, gastrointestinal bleeding, aspiration pneumonia, and acute pancreatitis, are relatively rare in adolescents and usually result from the ingestion of a large quantity of alcohol during a short period. Complications of chronic alcoholism, such as cirrhosis of the liver or Wernicke encephalopathy, are virtually unknown in adolescents.

Psychosocial and emotional problems commonly are associated with alcohol use by adolescents. It is often difficult to differentiate whether this emotional ill health is a cause or an effect of the alcohol use. One study of 171 acutely intoxicated 12- to 18-year-olds brought to the emergency department of a large hospital found that alcohol intoxication was the predominant initial problem for 88%.[76] Extensive psychosocial examination of the patients and their families led to the conclusion that alcohol or another drug was the primary problem for 41% of the adolescents. Of the adolescents studied, 19% had a primary emotional or psychologic problem, 17% had a family problem, 3% had peer relation problems, and 20% had no serious psychosocial problems. Of the 171 intoxicated adolescents, 28% had alcohol-dependent fathers.

A study of 103 adolescents with depression found 30 with comorbid alcohol and substance abuse disorders; 23 (77%) of those with substance abuse disorders had alcohol dependence or abused alcohol, and 15 (50%) had a diagnosis of cannabis abuse or dependence.[77] Half of the adolescents who abused marijuana also abused alcohol. Factors that discriminated depressed adolescents with substance abuse disorders from depressed adolescents without substance abuse disorders included the presence of conduct disorder and schoolwork impairment for girls and boys and longer depressive episodes for girls. The study could not determine causality but highlighted the high prevalence of comorbid alcohol and depressive disorders and suggested a clinical profile of the adolescents.

Because alcohol use by adolescents is so prevalent, it is important to define alcohol abuse in this age group. Relatively few adolescents—less than 5%—could be considered alcoholics, that is, addicted to alcohol. Adolescents who drink daily, have a family history of alcoholism, have blackouts or withdrawal symptoms, and continue drinking despite many negative family, school, and social consequences should be considered alcoholics. A much larger group of adolescents, however, should be considered problem drinkers.[78] Most of the 31% of twelfth graders who reported binge drinking would be in this category.[7] Problem drinkers have been drunk 6 or more times per year and experience negative consequences from alcohol use 2 or more times per year. The negative consequences include driving after drinking and troubles with family, friends, teachers, police, or dates because of drinking. Adolescent problem drinkers are at especially high risk of motor vehicle crashes or unintentional injuries and for significant developmental, educational, and emotional difficulties. Finally, adolescents who are neither alcoholics nor problem drinkers but who, nevertheless, drink occasionally and become intoxicated are still at some risk of motor vehicle crashes, injuries, and acute overdose.

Alcohol is a known teratogen and seems to have its greatest effect on the developing fetus if consumed in large doses early in pregnancy. During the early 1970s, fetal alcohol syndrome was identified and recognized as a leading cause of mental retardation.[79] Many sexually active adolescent girls fail to use adequate contraception, and unintended undiagnosed pregnancy is endemic in this age group. Thus, many fetuses of adolescent girls are exposed to the harmful effects of alcohol and to the secondary additive effects of inadequate nutrition and multiple drug abuse. In addition, fetal alcohol syndrome should be considered as a diagnosis for adolescents with low intellectual functioning who have short stature.[80] The characteristic facial features seen in infants and young children are less prominent in adolescents and adults with the syndrome.

Laboratory Evaluation

Behavioral effects and the toxic effects of alcohol correlate well with blood alcohol levels, which are expressed as g of alcohol per 100 mL of blood. A blood alcohol level of 0.05% usually is associated with a "high" feeling; a level of 0.20% is associated with marked intoxication; at 0.30%, the person is usually stuporous; and death can occur at blood alcohol levels beginning at 0.35%. The concentration of alcohol in the breath is directly related to blood alcohol levels, a fact used by law enforcement agencies as the basis for a noninvasive method for determining blood alcohol levels. Most agencies define alcohol intoxication as a blood alcohol level of 0.10% or higher. Among 16- to 19-year-olds who had been drinking and were involved in fatal motor vehicle crashes, blood alcohol levels of 0.10% to 0.14% occurred most often.[81] Only 16% of the adolescents had levels less than 0.10%, and 28% had levels more than 0.14%.

Treatment Considerations

Acute ethanol intoxication should be treated with protective and supportive therapy, including maintenance of the airway and respiratory support with a ventilator, if necessary, until the alcohol is metabolized and the patient recovers. Large overdoses may cause hypoglycemia, particularly in children, and blood glucose levels should be monitored. When present, hypoglycemia should be corrected rapidly by administering an intravenous glucose solution.

All adolescent patients should be screened for alcohol abuse by history, and anticipatory guidance about injuries and other risk behavior related to intoxication should be provided by the health care professional.[82] Adolescents who might be considered alcoholics by psychosocial criteria or, in rare instances, by physiologic addiction, may require treatment in a residential treatment facility staffed by persons with experience and training in the management of adolescent drug abuse. Disulfiram (Antabuse [Wyeth-Ayerst Laboratories, Philadelphia, PA]), a drug that causes headache, nausea, vomiting, and vertigo when alcohol is consumed, may be a useful adjunct to the treatment of the adolescent alcoholic.

For the large number of adolescents who are problem drinkers, community programs, peer support groups, and individual and family counseling by mental health professionals can be helpful. Community-based programs, such as Alcoholics Anonymous, that have a history of success treating adults are used less commonly by adolescents, who may find little in common with older group members. Programs specific to adolescents (eg, Alateen) are available in some communities.

Cocaine

Epidemiology

Cocaine is a stimulant drug derived from the leaves of the coca plant, *Erythroxylon coca,* and has been used by humans in various forms for thousands of years.[83] The tropane alkaloid cocaine was first extracted and purified during the latter half of the 19th century by German chemists and initially was perceived to be harmless. The first epidemic of cocaine abuse in the United States occurred during the 1890s, shortly after the isolation of the drug, and the next was during the 1920s. The 1950s and 1960s also had a resurgence of stimulant abuse, but this time, the abused drugs were amphetamine and methamphetamine. The most recent epidemic of cocaine abuse peaked during the mid to late 1980s, fueled by the development and marketing of a smokable form of the drug called "crack."

Prevalence of ever having used cocaine among twelfth graders increased dramatically from 9% in the class of 1975 to a peak of 17.3% in the class of 1985, decreased through the late 1980s, and leveled off during the early 1990s to approximately 6%.[7] In 1996, cocaine use increased to 7.1%, and in 1997, 8.7% of twelfth graders reported using cocaine at least once. The prevalence of cocaine use within the past 30 days by eighth, tenth, and twelfth graders in 1997 was 1.1%, 2.0%, and 2.3%, respectively. Fewer than 1% of students reported using crack within the past 30 days, and only 0.2% of twelfth graders reported daily cocaine use. Recent use of cocaine (within the past 30 days) by twelfth graders decreased to 2.1% in 2000, compared with 3.4% in 1988 (see Table 0.1, p ix).[1-3] Among a largely white, middle class group of almost 500 adolescent drug abusers from 8 US cities surveyed in 1990, 28% had smoked crack. The adolescents reported rapid loss of their ability to modulate use of the drug, preoccupation with thoughts of crack, and rapid development of tolerance.[84] Increasing knowledge of the rapid addiction potential of crack is, in part, responsible for the decrease in cocaine use by adolescents during the 1990s.

Pharmacology

Cocaine hydrochloride powder is a white crystalline substance typically sold on the illicit drug market in units of a g. Heavy users may purchase cocaine supplies in larger quantities and at decreased prices by the oz (approx 28 g), "quarter" (approx 7 g), or "eighth" (approx 3.5 g).[85]

Cocaine powder is absorbed readily into the bloodstream via the nasal mucosa. Thus, nasal inhalation or snorting is an effective and popular route of cocaine administration. Because it is soluble in water, cocaine powder can be administered intravenously. When cocaine and heroin are mixed in the same syringe, the drug combination is known as a "speedball."

Cocaine powder is not smokable, because the active drug decomposes at the temperatures achieved by a match or lighter. However, by using a simple chemical procedure, the powder can be transformed readily into a smokable form of the drug known as "freebase" or crack.[86] The procedure can be performed quickly and cheaply by using baking soda, heat, and water. Crack is not a new drug but a new way of packaging and selling freebase cocaine. Before the appearance of crack, anyone who wanted to smoke cocaine freebase had to buy cocaine powder and perform the chemical conversion process. The selling of crack on the illicit drug market made the smokable cocaine freebase directly available to the consumer. Crack (and the way it is packaged) is especially attractive to adolescents for several reasons. Smoking generates an instantaneous and extremely intense euphoria, or "rush," which stems directly from the rapid and efficient absorption of cocaine by the pulmonary route of administration. Crack is sold in very small dose units of ready-to-smoke "rocks," placing the drug within financial reach of almost any adolescent. The rocks are dispensed in tiny plastic vials that are concealed easily and convenient to carry. During the 1980s, smoking cocaine was perceived by potential users as less invasive, "sick," or dangerous than injecting it, although there are few differences in absorption, magnitude of drug effects, and addiction potential of the 2 methods of administration. By the 1990s, however, most adolescents became aware of the highly addictive nature and destructive effects of smoking crack.

Cocaine has 3 principal pharmacologic actions: it is a local anesthetic, a peripheral sympathomimetic, and a potent CNS stimulant.[87,88] The psychoactive use of cocaine by humans stems from the drug's ability to chemically alter brain function and thereby induce feelings of stimulation and euphoria. The effects of cocaine on the CNS are complex, and its mechanism of action is not well understood. When used intermittently, cocaine stimulates the release and inhibits the reuptake of dopamine and norepinephrine in selected areas of the brain. Long-term use leads to depletion of dopamine and other neurotransmitters. The neurochemical changes caused by long-term use may be the physiologic substrate of compulsive cocaine use and addiction.[89]

Health Consequences

The mood-altering effects of cocaine are especially appealing to adolescents. Cocaine produces intense feelings of euphoria, energy, and confidence. In the early stages of cocaine involvement, users often feel more talkative, sociable, adventurous, and sexual. Cocaine can instantly overcome shyness, awkwardness, boredom, stress, sexual inhibitions, and low self-esteem. For many, it is the ultimate escape from negative mood states. Cocaine use often is referred to as "partying" by those who have come to expect good feelings and decreased inhibitions from cocaine. These are highly attractive benefits to many adolescents, particularly those who seek any opportunity to celebrate and "let loose."

A pattern of escalating cocaine use and dependency is promoted to some extent by the unique pharmacologic properties of cocaine. The high is extremely pleasurable but short-lived, leading to a pattern of repeated dosing at short intervals to maintain the desired mood state. As use becomes regular and intensified, the brief euphoria is followed immediately by an unpleasant rebound dysphoria, or "crash," that leaves the user feeling uncomfortable and desiring an immediate return to the euphoric state. The crash from cocaine typically leads to the abuse of alcohol and other sedative-hypnotics as the user attempts to alleviate the unpleasant feelings. As tolerance to cocaine develops, many users find themselves "chasing" the original high, which is vividly remembered.[90]

Tolerance and dependence occur with long-term cocaine use. Decreased intensity or disappearance of the cocaine-induced euphoria usually occurs with repeated doses, particularly when there is a pattern of intensive use. Larger doses may temporarily override an existing tolerance to these effects, but at a certain point, most intensive users become resistant to the cocaine-induced euphoria, irrespective of the amount of drug taken. Dependence on cocaine is evidenced by a loss of control over use, urges and cravings for the drug, and continued use despite adverse medical and psychosocial consequences. There is usually no dramatic physical withdrawal syndrome associated with abrupt cessation of long-term cocaine use. Nevertheless, cocaine is considered physically addictive, because it produces significant biochemical changes in brain activity that seem to cause cravings and urges that propel compulsive drug-taking behavior. The greatest danger of cocaine, by far, is its high addiction potential. Even in reasonably stable, well-functioning adolescents, cocaine may acquire control of the user's behavior.

Serious physiologic consequences tend to be uncommon in cocaine users, even in high-dose, long-term users. Death rates attributable to cocaine use are low, despite publicity suggesting the contrary. However, potentially fatal toxic reactions to cocaine occur, including seizures, stroke, respiratory arrest, cardiac arrhythmias, myocardial infarction, and hypertension.[91] Deaths attributable to cocaine are more likely to occur on days when the temperature exceeds 31.1°C (88°F), reflecting the powerful sympathomimetic and thermogenic properties of the drug.[92] The most common types of medical problems stemming from cocaine use usually are related to the route of drug administration. Intranasal users may experience rhinorrhea, sinus headaches, nasal congestion, nasal sores, and nasal bleeding. Long-term crack smokers may experience chest congestion, wheezing, and sore throat from inhaling the hot cocaine vapors. Adolescent crack smokers report high rates of fatigue, insomnia, anorexia, weight loss, and chronic cough, and 10% of abusers had a seizure due to cocaine.[84] Crack smokers in poor, inner-city neighborhoods, particularly women who exchange sex for drugs, are at high risk of human immunodeficiency virus (HIV) infection; of 1137 young adult crack smokers in 3 different cities, 15.7% had HIV infection, compared with 5.2% of the non-smokers.[93] Intravenous users tend to experience drug-related medical problems resulting from their use of needles. As with other intravenously abused drugs, the problems include abscesses at injection sites, hepatitis, endocarditis, and exposure to HIV.

The most obvious and severe consequences of long-term cocaine use are behavioral, psychologic, and social dysfunction. Unfortunately, cocaine use often is not evident until the problem has progressed to serious abuse and dependency. Early warning signs are rarely present or recognized, except when the adolescent is actually observed using or possessing cocaine. Common symptoms in regular or intensive users include mood swings, irritability, short temper, depression, memory impairment, chronic lassitude, erratic sleep patterns (insomnia, excessive sleeping, or both), social withdrawal, and loss of interest in school, hobbies, sports, and family.[94] More severe symptoms include paranoia, suicidal ideation, and violence. As the user becomes increasingly obsessed with cocaine, all other aspects of functioning tend to deteriorate.

Cocaine abuse during pregnancy has been associated with an increased rate of spontaneous abortions and stillbirths related to abruptio placentae. Although teratogenicity has been demonstrated in mice, the relationship of cocaine to congenital abnormalities in humans remains unclear. Some studies have found that infants born to cocaine-abusing mothers demonstrate depressed interactive behavior, difficulty with arousal, and irritability once aroused, but other studies have not found such differences between exposed and unexposed infants.[95-97] A well-controlled study of cocaine-exposed neonates that quantified exposure on the basis of radioimmunoassay of cocaine in maternal hair found a dose-response effect on head circumference and neurologic abnormalities; newborns with higher levels of prenatal cocaine exposure had smaller heads and higher rates of neurologic impairment.[98] To date, no specific neonatal withdrawal syndrome requiring pharmacologic therapy has been described.

Laboratory Evaluation
Cocaine can be detected in urine and blood. However, because cocaine is metabolized rapidly, reliable detection of the drug requires sophisticated testing methods, such as enzyme immunoassay or radioimmunoassay procedures, that can yield accurate results for up to 48 to 72 hours after cocaine use.

Treatment Considerations
Treatment of severe overdose reactions may require respiratory assistance and a life-support system. Physiologic compromise often is complicated by the presence of other drugs. No specific pharmacologic antagonist to cocaine is available.

Treatment of cocaine addiction is best conducted within the context of a highly structured chemical dependency treatment program.[99] The program should include the following: (1) immediate total abstinence from cocaine and all other mood-altering substances; (2) individual, group, and family counseling; (3) supervised urine testing at least 2 to 3 times per week; and (4) the application of specific relapse-prevention techniques. Most cocaine abusers do not require hospitalization, because there is no withdrawal syndrome that necessitates intensive medical management. However, inpatient treatment may be needed when there is physical dependency on sedative-hypnotics or alcohol; suicidal, violent, or psychotic behavior; or inability to achieve abstinence despite outpatient treatment. There is no known effective pharmacotherapy for cocaine dependence.[100,101] Experimental trials with a variety of agents, including antidepressants, lithium, bromocriptine, and others have yielded inconsistent and unimpressive findings. None of the trials have been conducted in adolescents. The most effective treatment programs combine professional interventions with self-help, focusing on behavioral and attitudinal change, development of a drug-free lifestyle, and maintenance of long-term sobriety.

Amphetamines and Other Stimulants

Epidemiology
Amphetamines first achieved widespread therapeutic use in the United States during the early 1950s, when they were prescribed for common conditions, such as obesity, mild depression, and fatigue. Now, however, their high potential for abuse is recognized, and they have been classified under Schedule II of the Controlled Substances Act. The only uses for which they are considered effective and medically indicated are for treatment of narcolepsy and attention-deficit/hyperactivity disorder. Concurrent with the introduction of amphetamines as therapeutic agents was a surge in their popularity as drugs of abuse. Such abuse has ranged from occasional self-medication for obesity or fatigue to prolonged amphetamine binges. Crystal methamphetamine, also known as "ice," is a smokable form of the drug like crack cocaine. Abuse of ice has been widespread in California and the southwestern states since the early 1990s, and it spread to the Midwest during the latter half of the decade (see **Club Drugs,** p 263). Street names for amphetamines include "speed," "crank," "black beauties," "BAM" (crushed tablets injected intravenously, sometimes with heroin), "mollies," "bennies," "plash," and "uppers."

Among twelfth graders in 1997, 16.5% reported using stimulants (mostly amphetamines) at least once (this percentage includes only use of a drug not prescribed by a physician), and 4.4% reported the use of ice.[7] However, only 0.3% reported using amphetamines and 0.1% reported using crystal methamphetamine daily. The prevalence of stimulant use within the past 30 days for eighth, tenth, and twelfth graders in 1997 was 3.8%, 5.1%, and 4.8%, respectively. The prevalence of ice use within the past 30 days was measured only for twelfth graders and was 0.8% in 1997 and 1.0% in 2000.[1-3] The use of amphetamine stimulants increased gradually among high school students during the early 1990s, began to level off in 1997, and increased again in 2000. Recent use of amphetamines (within the past 30 days) by twelfth graders has increased markedly to 5.0% in 2000, compared with a low of 2.8% in 1992 (see Table 0.1, p ix).[1-3] As the dangers of cocaine and crack use became widely known during the late 1980s, many adolescents switched to amphetamines as their stimulant of choice, because they believed that amphetamines were safer to use. The slogan during the last amphetamine epidemic, "speed kills," has been forgotten.

Another group of drugs, the amphetamine look-alikes, have become problematic in recent years. The drugs, which contain phenylpropanolamine hydrochloride, ephedrine, pseudoephedrine, ma huang (an ephedrine-like herbal drug), and/or caffeine, are sold over the counter or through mail-order houses and, thus, are widely available.[102] They are promoted as treatments for weight loss and are more likely to be abused by adolescent girls than boys. When taken in large enough doses, they are capable of producing the high and the adverse effects associated with amphetamines. In addition, methylphenidate (Ritalin [Novartis Pharmaceuticals, East Hanover, NJ]) is sold on the illegal market and can be abused by adolescents. The FDA has recently issued an advisory to remove phenylpropanolamine from all drug products because of a possible risk of hemorrhagic stroke.[103]

Pharmacology

Amphetamine, the name of a specific chemical [(±)α-methylphenethylamine] is the parent compound for the class of stimulants known as amphetamines, including combinations of neutral salts of dextroamphetamine and amphetamine with isomers (Adderall [Shire Richwood Inc, Florence, KY]), dextroamphetamine sulfate

(Dexedrine [SmithKline Beecham Pharmaceuticals, Philadelphia, PA]), and methamphetamine hydrochloride. Amphetamine has effects similar to cocaine, but the high lasts much longer; the effective half-life of cocaine is 45 minutes, whereas that of amphetamine is 4 to 8 hours.[88] A number of amphetamine analogues also exist, including fenfluramine hydrochloride, phendimetrazine tartrate, and others. All have properties similar to those of the amphetamines, and many are marketed for treatment of obesity. The over-the-counter amphetamine look-alikes are actually sympathomimetic agents with a chemical structure quite different from that of the amphetamine analogues.

Although the mechanism of action of amphetamines is not understood entirely, it is clear that the norepinephrine- and dopamine-mediated systems of the brain are involved. Amphetamines may exert their effects by preventing catecholamine reuptake or by facilitating release of catecholamines from the presynaptic neuron. An alternative explanation is that they directly affect catecholamine receptors by inhibiting monoamine oxidase. In any case, clinical manifestations are produced from a direct effect on adrenergic receptors in muscles and glands and from stimulation of the medullary respiratory center and the cerebrospinal axis.

The amphetamines are well absorbed from the gastrointestinal tract, after which they undergo deamination and hydroxylation in the liver. Accumulated hydroxylated metabolites have been implicated in the development of the psychosis sometimes associated with amphetamine use. Finally, the unchanged amphetamines and the metabolized forms are excreted through the kidneys. They can be detected in the urine between 3 hours and 3 days after ingestion.

Health Consequences

Within approximately 30 minutes of oral ingestion or 5 minutes after subcutaneous injection, amphetamines begin to exert their effects. Effects begin almost instantly after intravenous administration or smoking, and they are intense.

Amphetamine use results in an initial rush or feeling of extreme exhilaration that is followed by a more sustained period of euphoria, greater ability to concentrate, wakefulness, depressed appetite, self-confidence, and excitement.[104] Preexisting fatigue or depression are abolished immediately. Tolerance quickly develops, and in long-term users, confusion, paranoia, headache, and depression develop. Many long-term users have a history of weight loss and may seem to be agitated or paranoid. Dilated pupils, hypertension, and tachycardia are among the more common physical findings.

Manifestations of mild toxic effects of amphetamine include restlessness, irritability, insomnia, tremor, hyperreflexia, diaphoresis, dilated pupils, and flushing. With increasing doses, the adolescent experiences confusion, hypertension, tachypnea, and mild temperature elevation. With more severe toxic effects, delirium, hypertensive crisis, dysrhythmias, seizures, coma, cardiovascular collapse, and death may occur.[104] Among 18 young adults admitted to an emergency department with acute toxic effects of methamphetamine, 5 died and 13 survived.[105] The manifestations in the patients who died were coma, shock, seizures, oliguria, and hyperthermia. The most common complication in the fatality group was rhabdomyolysis with acute renal failure. Intracerebral hemorrhage can occur even with small doses of amphetamines.[106] Phenylpropanolamine has been reported to cause hypertension, seizures, psychosis, and cerebral vasculitis and hemorrhage.[103,107] As with other drugs, intravenous use of amphetamines may be associated with risk of HIV infection and other infectious complications resulting from sharing unsterile needles.

Methamphetamine use impairs driving ability. A study of 28 cases in which drivers who had positive test results for amphetamines were arrested or killed indicated typical driving behaviors of drifting out of the lane of travel, erratic driving, weaving, speeding, drifting off the road, and high-speed collisions.[108] Behaviors in those arrested included rapid or confused speech, rapid pulse, agitation, paranoia, dilated pupils, and violent or aggressive attitude.

Tolerance and physical dependence occur with regular heavy use of amphetamines, and a withdrawal syndrome occurs on cessation of use.[104] Depression is the most prominent manifestation of stimulant drug withdrawal. It reaches its peak 2 to 3 days after the last dose is taken. The mood swing may be so severe that it is accompanied by suicidal or homicidal ideation. Exhaustion, prolonged sleep, and voracious appetite also occur, as does severe drug craving.

Amphetamine psychosis, which usually occurs in long-term users, also has occurred after a single large dose. This drug-induced psychosis may be confused with schizophrenia. The hallucinations that occur with use of amphetamines are most often visual, tactile, or olfactory, compared with the auditory hallucinations associated with paranoid schizophrenia. Repetitive, stereotyped, compulsive behaviors that are probably dopamine-related also are observed in long-term users. Symptoms of psychosis begin to fade within a few days after cessation of drug use. The amphetamine analogues also have been associated with a drug-induced psychosis. Prenatal exposure to amphetamines and methamphetamines increases the risk of cleft lip or palate, cardiac anomalies, fetal growth retardation, and fetal and infant death.[109,110] A long-term follow-up study of children born to mothers who abused amphetamine indicated that growth deficits and school problems continued for the children into adolescence.[111] Furthermore, a neonatal withdrawal syndrome consisting of diaphoresis, irritability, hypoglycemia, tremulousness, and seizures has been reported.

Laboratory Evaluation
Urine and blood assays for amphetamines are widely available and are able to detect the drugs for 2 days after the last dose (see Chapter 4).

Treatment Considerations
Manifestations of amphetamine overdose are often severe and life threatening. If the drug has been taken orally and the patient is awake, ipecac syrup, followed by activated charcoal and a cathartic, such as magnesium citrate, should be administered. A quiet environment with minimal external stimuli should be provided while hyperthermia and hypertension are treated. The CNS stimulant effects may be treated with chlorpromazine hydrochloride or droperidol. Chlorpromazine should be used only when the

diagnosis of toxic effects of amphetamine is certain, because it is contraindicated in the treatment of the psychosis induced by PCP or hallucinogens.

Treatment of amphetamine addiction is similar to that of cocaine addiction and should be conducted in a specialized chemical dependency program. Hospitalization usually is not necessary, as the withdrawal syndrome is not life threatening; however, close monitoring with frequent urine testing as an adjunct to relapse prevention may be necessary.

Hallucinogens: LSD and Naturally Occurring Hallucinogens

Epidemiology

Naturally occurring hallucinogenic substances have been used in certain cultures for thousands of years, mainly in religious ceremonies.[5(p145-182)] Members of the Native American church use peyote, a cactus plant containing mescaline, because they believe it enables them to commune more easily with God. In a similar fashion, native populations of Mexico use mushrooms containing the hallucinogen psilocybin in their religious rites. LSD or "acid," a potent hallucinogenic drug that became popular in the United States during the psychedelic era of the 1960s, has had a resurgence of popularity among adolescents during the 1990s.[112] LSD does not occur naturally and was first synthesized in 1938 at Sandoz Laboratories in Switzerland. PCP or "angel dust" is a more dangerous type of hallucinogen that first came into widespread abuse during the late 1970s (see p 231). The newest hallucinogenic substance to be abused by adolescents is the designer hallucinogen 3,4-methylenedioxymethamphetamine (MDMA) or "ecstasy," a derivative of amphetamine (see page 234). MDMA is also recognized as a stimulant (see **Club Drugs,** p 263).[4]

When widespread use of hallucinogenic substances began during the mid 1960s, a small but significant number of adolescents used them daily or almost daily. Today, however, hallucinogens are used largely on an intermittent basis (see **Club Drugs,** p 263).[4] After several years of steadily increasing use of LSD and other hallucinogens, reported use by US high school students may have leveled off in 1997.[7] From 1985 to 1997, prevalence of ever having used LSD among twelfth graders increased approximately 80%, from 7.5% to 13.6%. During the early 1990s, LSD-related arrests and seizures of large quantities of the drug alsoincreased.[112] Recent use (within the past 30 days) by twelfth graders decreased to 1.6% in 2000 from a high of 4.0% in 1995.[1-3] In 1997, prevalence of ever having used a hallucinogen among eighth, tenth, and twelfth graders, respectively, was 5.4%, 10.5%, and 15.1%, and prevalence of use within the past 30 days was 1.8%, 3.3%, and 3.9%, respectively.[7] Only 0.3% of twelfth graders reported daily hallucinogen use.[7] Recent use (within the past 30 days) of all hallucinogens by twelfth graders decreased to 2.6% in 2000 from a high of 4.4% in 1995 (see Table 0.1, p ix).[1-3] An analysis of the *National Household Survey on Drug Abuse* indicated that use of hallucinogens during the past year was highest at 19 years of age, and onset of use was most likely between 15 and 19 years of age.[113] Prevalence of hallucinogen use was highest among whites and persons with high family income.

Pharmacology

Hallucinogens exert their effects by modifying neurotransmitter pathways in the brain. The chemical structure of the neurotransmitter serotonin is based on the indole nucleus, and LSD and psilocybin contain an indole ring in their chemical structures. LSD and psilocybin increase serotonin levels in the brain by binding with specific serotonin receptors, producing inhibition at presynaptic and postsynaptic sites.[114,115] Mescaline contains a catechol nucleus similar to that found in the catecholamine-type neurotransmitters, such as norepinephrine.[116] MDMA and 2,5-dimethoxy-4-methylamphetamine (also known as DOM and STP) are synthetic catechol-type hallucinogens. Other hallucinogens act on the neurotransmitter acetylcholine. A number of plants, such as the deadly nightshade, contain cholinergic hallucinogens. Jimsonweed ("loco") contains atropine and scopolamine, potent acetylcholine blockers, and is used by some adolescents for its mind-altering properties.[117]

Of the hallucinogens, LSD is the most potent. It is effective orally in minute doses (approximately 20-50 μg per dose) and has a wide therapeutic index in terms of lethality; doses hundreds of times greater are not associated with death.[118] Mescaline is 4000 times less potent, and psilocybin is approximately 100 to 200 times less potent than LSD.[5(p145-182)] Most of the indole- and catechol-type hallucinogens are sold as tablets or powders. However, LSD, which dissolves easily, usually is sold absorbed onto a piece of blotting paper ("blotter acid") and is ingested, paper and all. Psilocybin can be ingested in the form of mushrooms that have been gathered in the wild or cultivated indoors.[119]

The initial effects of LSD, which begin within 10 to 15 minutes of ingestion, are sympathomimetic, including tachycardia and anxiety. Effects on the brain begin 30 to 60 minutes after ingestion and peak in approximately 3 or 4 hours. Effects of the drug may last up to 12 hours. The most striking effect of LSD and similar hallucinogens is a dramatic alteration in visual perception. Colors seem brighter and often are split into the full spectrum so that objects seem to have rainbows around them. The shape and size of objects are distorted, and their boundaries seem to shift and dissolve. Synesthesia, a mixing of senses, may occur (eg, visualizing music as a series of colors and shapes). Most users realize that the perceptual changes are caused by the drug and can remember them when the "trip" is over. Thus, they are not true hallucinations but rather pseudohallucinations or illusions. Very high doses of LSD, however, can produce frank visual hallucinations. Accompanying the visual-perceptual distortions are mood changes, feelings of depersonalization, and some usually minimal somatic symptoms, such as tremors, dizziness, nausea, and tingling. The emotional reactions to the drug experience can vary from panic to a transcendental feeling of union with the universe. Tolerance seems to develop with frequent use of any indole- or catechol-type hallucinogen, but the tolerance is short-lived, disappearing after 1 to 2 weeks of abstinence.

The anticholinergic types of hallucinogens, such as jimsonweed, produce a different syndrome of intoxication, with many more physiologic disturbances attributable to their peripheral and central effects.[117] Users experience true visual hallucinations and have no concurrent awareness that they are drug induced. Therefore, panic, combative behavior, and disorientation are much more common than with LSD. In addition, signs of peripheral anticholinergic effects are prominent, including mydriasis, flushed face, dry mucous membranes, tachycardia, and in some cases fever, hypertension, urinary retention, and seizures.

Health Consequences

The toxic effects of the indole- and catechol-type hallucinogens seem to be mainly psychologic. When used under controlled conditions, such as religious ceremonies or laboratory experiments, the hallucinogens seem to be quite safe from a physiologic standpoint. However, the purity of street drugs is always in question. The naturally occurring hallucinogens, such as mescaline, are expensive, and on the illicit drug market, misrepresenting such substances with the less costly and more potent LSD or PCP is the norm. Mushrooms may be toxic. A case of acute renal failure after ingestion of mushrooms misrepresented as psilocybin-containing mushrooms but probably a *Cortinarius* species has been reported.[120] Several cases of acute renal failure after eating *Cortinarius* species mushrooms have been reported in the literature.[120]

The adverse psychologic effects of the hallucinogens occur in 3 areas. Panic attacks during the height of the drug experience (a "bad trip") are common. Users can become quite distraught and are at risk of injury unless they are supervised and protected by lay or medical caretakers. Psychotic reactions may be precipitated by drug experience, often in persons with clinically significant psychiatric difficulties before drug ingestion.[121] The psychoses often require long-term treatment. Occasional suicides during drug-induced psychosis have been reported. A disturbing effect that has been reported with hallucinogens is the "flashback," an unwanted repetition of the drug experience without the ingestion of drugs. Flashbacks seem to occur during times of psychologic stress, and the frequency and intensity diminish the longer the person refrains from use of hallucinogenic drugs.

LSD has not been shown to be a teratogen in humans despite the "chromosome breakage" publicity of the late 1960s. Nevertheless, it is prudent to recommend abstinence from any "recreational" drug during pregnancy.

The anticholinergic hallucinogens have more potential for physiologic harm for several reasons: 1) effects may last for days rather than hours; 2) the intoxicated person is disoriented, cannot be reasoned with, and usually must be physically restrained; and 3) large overdoses can cause seizures, severe hypertension, or coma with respiratory depression.

Treatment Considerations

Acute intoxication with LSD or other indole- or catechol-type hallucinogens should be treated by removing the person to a quiet, nonthreatening environment and "talking down," that is, repeatedly reassuring the person that the experiences are drug-related and eventually will disappear. Agitation and panic can be treated with a benzodiazepine or haloperidol. Flashbacks often require only reassurance or a mild tranquilizer. The adolescent with flashbacks should be cautioned to avoid not only hallucinogens but also marijuana and antihistamines, which can trigger flashbacks. It has been reported that the LSD flashback syndrome also can be precipitated by antidepressant therapy with selective serotonin reuptake inhibitors, such as sertraline hydrochloride and paroxetine hydrochloride.[122] Prolonged psychotic reactions require psychiatric intervention.

Treatment of anticholinergic-type hallucinogen intoxication requires hospitalization because of the long-lasting mental effects of this type of hallucinogen. Gastric lavage is indicated in all cases, even if the ingestion occurred hours or days before medical treatment, because of the markedly decreased gastric motility associated with atropine poisoning. Intravenous fluids and urinary catheterization may be required. Sedation can be achieved with benzodiazepines or barbiturates. Phenothiazines should be avoided because of their additive anticholinergic effects. Physostigmine should be reserved for life-threatening overdoses.

Hallucinogens: PCP

Epidemiology

It is difficult to quantify the use of this illicit hallucinogenic substance, because many users do not know that they have taken it. On the street, PCP often is sold as mescaline, THC, or psilocybin, and it is commonly used as an adulterant in other illicit products. In 1997, approximately 4% of twelfth graders reported ever using PCP; only 0.7% reported use during the past 30 days.[7] A study of 202 general adolescent clinic patients at an urban children's hospital found 18 patients with a positive urine test for PCP.[52] Recent use (within the past 30 days) by twelfth graders was 0.9% in 2000.[1-3] All of the adolescents also had cannabinoid metabolites in their urine. None of the 128 patients without cannabinoid metabolites in their urine had a positive urine screen for PCP. The concordance between a self-reported history of use and confirmatory urine test was higher for marijuana use than for PCP (91% vs 11%), suggesting the possibility that adolescents were smoking PCP without knowing it.

PCP was first used illicitly in 1967 in the Haight-Ashbury district of San Francisco, where it was sold as the "peace pill." It soon developed a bad reputation because of its propensity to cause bad trips, and use decreased. During the mid 1970s, new marketing strategies, such as dusting PCP onto a leaf mixture for smoking and misrepresenting PCP as other less available substances, led to greatly increased use, especially in large cities. By the early 1980s, PCP was being described as the most commonly used hallucinogen in the United States. PCP is sold on the street as PCP, "angel dust," "elephant (monkey) tranquilizer," "hog," "super grass," "angel mist," "peace weed," and many other names. In addition, users often purchase PCP under the assumption that they are obtaining mescaline or another hallucinogen.

Clinical Pharmacology

Phencyclidine hydrochloride, or 1-(1-phenycyclohexyl)piperidine hydrochloride, was developed during the late 1950s by Parke-Davis, Morris Plains, NJ as an anesthetic agent with the brand name Sernylan. Initially, the drug seemed promising, because it produced analgesia and sleep without causing respiratory or cardiovascular depression. A related drug, ketamine hydrochloride, often is used in pediatric anesthesia and is now identified as a club drug by the National Institute on Drug Abuse (see **Club Drugs,** p 263).[4] The psychotoxic effects of PCP, however, made it unsuitable for use in humans, and for some time it was used legitimately only in veterinary medicine as a primate anesthetic. This drug was taken off the market in the late 1970s, and all PCP now available is illegally manufactured. It is easily and inexpensively made by anyone with a rudimentary knowledge of organic chemistry. Phencyclidine is available as a white crystalline powder that is readily soluble in water or alcohol. It can be dissolved and injected intravenously; snorted intranasally; ingested in food or beverages or as pills; or, most commonly, sprinkled (dusted) in powdered form over dried parsley, oregano, or marijuana leaves and smoked.

The route of administration determines the timing of onset of drug effects. Effects are felt within seconds of an intravenous dose, within 2 to 5 minutes after smoking or snorting the drug, and within 30 minutes of ingesting it. The maximum effect of the drug usually occurs 15 to 30 minutes after smoking or 2 to 5 hours after ingestion. The effects of PCP can last 12 hours or more, and drug-induced psychosis can last up to a month.

PCP is a weak base with a dissociation constant of 8.5, and it is absorbed rapidly in the alkaline environment of the small bowel.[123] Most of the drug is rapidly metabolized to apparently inactive substances and excreted in the urine. More than 50% of an ingested dose is excreted in the urine as hydroxylated and glucuronidylated metabolites within 12 hours. If the urine is acidified from pH 7 to pH 5, the PCP clearance rate increases 100-fold.[123]

Health Consequences

In low doses (1-5 mg), PCP produces euphoria and disinhibition with emotional lability much like drunkenness. Moderate doses (5-10 mg) lead to a bodywide anesthetic effect with supersensitivity to sensations and impaired perceptions often resulting in panic reactions. Large doses (more than 10 mg) can produce a toxic psychosis indistinguishable from schizophrenia, with paranoia, auditory hallucinations, and excitement or stupor.[124] Massive overdoses can result in coma, seizures, rhabdomyolysis, and very rarely, apnea. Smoking or snorting the drug produces rapid effects and allows the user to control the dose better, thus increasing the chance of avoiding toxic complications. Toxic reactions requiring medical attention more commonly follow ingestion rather than inhalation of PCP. However, passive (ie, infants and children of abusers) and active smokers of the drug occasionally require treatment for acute short-term psychosis and also may require medical attention for accidental injuries that occurred during an altered state of consciousness.[125] PCP is a potent analgesic; even if severely wounded, intoxicated persons feel no pain.

The major effects of PCP other than the effects on the mind are sympathomimetic (tachycardia, hypertension, and hyperreflexia), cholinergic (miosis, flushing, and diaphoresis), and cerebellar (vertical and horizontal nystagmus, dysarthria, and ataxia). Mental status can vary widely, from an excited, delirious, violent state; to an unresponsive, calm, blankly staring state; to coma. The intoxicated person experiences altered stereognosis and proprioception, numbness and analgesia, auditory or visual hallucinations, dysphoria, paranoia, and disorientation. Very high doses of PCP have been associated with coma, cardiac arrhythmias, muscle rigidity, decerebrate rigidity or opisthotonic posturing, and rhabdomyolysis, leading to acute renal failure, seizures, and death.

PCP crosses the placenta and has been detected in the urine of newborn infants whose mothers had taken the drug up to 3 weeks before delivery.[126] Neonatal symptoms are similar to those occurring in infants of mothers who have used opiates and include jitteriness, hypertonicity, and vomiting. Teratogenicity of the drug has been suggested but has not been proven. Accidental intoxication in infants and young children has been reported.[127] Hypertension and hyperreflexia are uncommon in children younger than 5 years. The most frequent symptoms of PCP intoxication in young children are lethargy, nystagmus, and opisthotonos.

Laboratory Evaluation

The best method of screening for PCP intoxication is a urine assay. The concentration of PCP in the urine bears little relation to the degree of impairment in the user, however, because the rapidity of excretion of the drug is variable and depends on the pH of the urine. Blood levels of PCP correlate more closely with symptoms and degree of toxic effects, but this test is not as widely available.

Treatment Considerations

Acute transient toxic psychosis caused by smoking or snorting PCP should be treated by protecting the person from harm and minimizing the environmental stimuli. The patient should be placed in a dimly lit, quiet room. Talking down should be avoided. Benzodiazepines, such as diazepam, may be given for agitation; however, antipsychotic drugs should be avoided, because they may add to complications, and their effectiveness has not been proven. If the patient has ingested PCP, induction of emesis or gastric lavage is indicated, because the drug is poorly absorbed from the acidic stomach. Acidification of the urine with ascorbic acid or ammonium chloride promotes more rapid excretion of the drug and may help shorten the duration of symptoms.[128] Acidification of the urine should not be attempted in neonates because of the dangers of inducing metabolic acidosis. Newborns are best treated with phenobarbital and observation.

Hallucinogens: Designer Hallucinogens (MDMA)

Epidemiology

A popular synthetic hallucinogen, MDMA (called "ecstasy") is a modification of the phenethylamine molecule that forms the backbone of the structure of amphetamine and methamphetamine. Legal use by psychiatrists to facilitate psychotherapy began during the 1970s.[129] During the early 1980s, it became a recreational drug popular on college campuses; it was used in small groups to enhance communication. In July 1985, MDMA became a controlled substance and was classified under Schedule I of the

Controlled Substances Act by the US Drug Enforcement Agency because of reports of neurotoxic effects in animals. However, it is readily available on the illicit market, and use increased greatly during the 1990s.[7,130] Surveys at a private southern university documented increased prevalence of the use of MDMA, from 16% of students in 1986 to 24% in 1990.[130] Use of MDMA has been included in the *Monitoring the Future* studies of US high school students since 1996, which was likely too late to document the upsurge in use by this age group.[130] In 1997, 3.2% of eighth graders, 5.7% of tenth graders, and 6.9% of twelfth graders reported they had ever used MDMA.[7] Approximately 4% of tenth and twelfth graders reported using the drug within the past year, and 1.6% reported use within the past 30 days. Recent use (within the past 30 days) by twelfth graders increased sharply to 3.6% in 2000 (see Table 0.1, p ix).[1-3]

Pharmacology

MDMA and its congener 3,4-methylenedioxyethamphetamine (MDEA) or "eve" are ingested in pill form. Doses of 1 to 2 mg/kg of body weight are reportedly safe, but many adolescents take several pills at once or mix it with marijuana, LSD, or "herbal ecstasy" (look-alike ephedrine-containing tablets).[131] Initial effects occur within 30 minutes to 1 hour and peak at about 90 minutes; effects may last up to 8 hours. Tolerance occurs with frequent use. About two thirds of the dose is excreted unchanged in the urine.

In oral doses of 100 mg, MDMA reportedly induces euphoria and enhanced self-awareness. MDEA reportedly has effects similar to but milder than those of MDMA. Intoxicated persons complain of muscle aches, sweating, difficulty concentrating, and sometimes intense dysphoria. They show signs of sympathetic activation, tachycardia, and widely dilated pupils.

Health Consequences

MDMA is a stimulant and a hallucinogen.[4] MDMA is used preferentially at "raves," all night dance parties held at clubs with loud synthesized electronic rock music (see **Club Drugs**, p 263).[83] Raves began in Britain during the late 1980s, and the craze spread to large American cities on the East and West coasts during the early 1990s. This new way of using MDMA as a party drug has been associated with increasing toxic effects. Initially, recreational users and psychotherapists thought MDMA was quite safe, but combining drug use with prolonged vigorous dancing has resulted in severe toxic reactions and death.[132-135] The mechanism for the toxic effects is thought to be hyperthermia. The drug can induce hyperthermia (as shown in rat studies), and in combination with dehydration and increased ambient temperatures in dance halls, lethal reactions can occur even with recreational doses of MDMA.[132-134] A study of 48 consecutive patients treated in a London emergency department who had taken MDMA found that all patients were 15 to 30 years of age, and all incidents occurred during the early morning hours on weekends.[132] Half of the patients also had taken another illicit substance, most commonly stimulants (cocaine, amphetamines, or both). Toxic signs included sympathetic overactivity, disturbed behavior, and increased temperature. Serious complications, including delirium, seizures, and coma, were more common when MDMA was used in combination with other substances. Rhabdomyolysis and acute renal failure have been reported when MDMA was used at raves.[133] A study in Dallas documented 5 deaths in association with MDMA and MDEA.[134] The patients ranged in age from 18 to 32 years and included 4 men and 1 woman.[134] In 3 of the deaths, the drugs may have contributed to the induction of arrhythmias in the presence of underlying cardiac or pulmonary disease. One death apparently was attributable to bizarre and risky behavior that resulted in a fatal injury. For the fifth person, MDMA was thought to be the immediate cause of death. Recently, MDMA has been shown to have hepatotoxic effects.[135] Of 62 patients admitted to an intensive care unit with acute hepatic failure, 5 (8%) had disease related to use of MDMA, and MDMA was the second most common cause of hepatic injury in patients younger than 25 years.[135] Full recovery was observed in all cases. One case of fulminant hepatic failure related to MDMA use by an 18-year-old girl in Germany was treated successfully with liver transplantation.[136]

Study of the long-term effects of regular use of MDMA is just beginning. A study measuring cognitive task performance in 3 groups of adolescents, 10 regular users (had taken MDMA 10 times or more), 10 novice users (had taken MDMA 1-9 times), and 10 control subjects who had never taken MDMA, found that both groups of users showed memory deficits on immediate and delayed word recall, suggesting possible lasting effects.[137] Long-term damage is a concern; studies in animals have shown that MDMA can lead to serotoninergic neurodegeneration.[138]

Laboratory Evaluation
Routine urine toxicology screens do not detect MDMA unless very large quantities were ingested, in which case the test result will be positive for amphetamines.[131] Confirmation by gas chromatography/mass spectrometry is recommended whenever results of a routine urine drug screen are positive for amphetamines.

Treatment Considerations
Education of adolescents about the toxic effects of MDMA use in conjunction with intense physical activity is required to prevent occurrence in the United States of the morbidity documented in Europe. Adolescents should be told that the use of other drugs, in particular stimulants, must be avoided with use of MDMA. Treatment of acute toxic reactions should address the specific physiologic dysfunctions and provide life-support measures as well as emotional support until drug effects wear off.

Anabolic-Androgenic Steroids

Epidemiology
Anabolic-androgenic steroids are synthetic derivatives of testosterone. They are prescription drugs that are used therapeutically for the treatment of certain anemias, gynecologic conditions, male hypogonadism, wasting syndromes, and other conditions and as an adjunct to growth hormone therapy.[139] Nonmedical use of anabolic-androgenic steroids to increase skeletal muscle mass and enhance strength by adults involved in power weight lifting

and bodybuilding was first reported in the United States during the 1960s, and use spread to athletes engaged in other sports during the 1970s and 1980s. Since 1990, anabolic-androgenic steroids have been classified under Schedule III of the Controlled Substances Act, making it illegal under federal law to distribute and possess anabolic-androgenic steroids without a prescription. Many of the drugs used for nonmedical purposes are obtained on the black market.[139] A large proportion are imported from other countries where they are readily available by prescription, and many are specifically manufactured for the black market by clandestine laboratories.

Reporting of steroid use by adolescents began at the end of the 1980s. The *Monitoring the Future* studies first began tracking the use of anabolic-androgenic steroids by high school students in 1989, when 3% of twelfth graders reported using steroids.[7] Although the prevalence of ever having used steroids decreased to 2.1% in 1991 and remained relatively stable during the following 5 years, the prevalence increased in 1997 to 2.4% of twelfth graders. An analysis of trends in the use of anabolic-androgenic steroids among adolescents that combined data from 3 large national surveys found a significant decrease between 1989 and 1996 in the prevalence of male and female adolescents ever having used steroids.[140] For female adolescents, however, the low point was in 1991, and there were significant increases in use in later years. In 1997, the annual prevalence of the use of anabolic-androgenic steroids was 1%, 1.2%, and 1.4% for eighth, tenth, and twelfth graders, respectively.[7] In 2000, there was a rise in the annual prevalence of use by tenth graders to 2.2%. Recent use (within the past 30 days) by twelfth graders has remained relatively constant and was 0.8% in the same year.[1-3]

Boys are more likely than girls to use steroids. A study of more than 3000 Chicago high school students found that overall, 4.4% of students reported using steroids, 6.5% of boys and 2.5% of girls.[141] Analysis of the 1991 *Youth Risk Behavior Survey* of US ninth through twelfth graders found that 4.1% of boys and 1.2% of girls reported using anabolic-androgenic steroids.[142]

This analysis also indicated that students in the South (3.5%) reported significantly higher steroid use than students in the West (2%) and Northeast (1.7%).

Anabolic-androgenic steroid use is most prevalent among male and female adolescents who participate in sports.[141] Sports with the highest incidence of steroid use include football and wrestling, whereas those with the lowest incidence of use include track, swimming, and soccer. A substantial number of nonathletic adolescents also use anabolic-androgenic steroids, presumably to enhance their body image and improve appearance.

Pharmacology

Anabolic-androgenic steroids can be administered orally or by intramuscular injection. Injectable steroids are formulated in water or in oil, and the oil-based steroids have a longer half-life. When used for performance enhancement, steroids are taken in high doses, 10 or more times the recommended therapeutic dose.[143,144] A regimen combining 2 or more oral and parenteral drugs ("stacking") is used most often.[143,144] The steroids commonly are used in cycles of 4 to 18 weeks with drug-free rest periods between cycles.[143,144]

Common injectable steroid drugs used by adolescents are nandrolone decanoate (Deca-Durabolin [Organon Inc, West Orange, NJ]) and testosterone cypionate (Depo-Testosterone [Pharmacia & Upjohn Company, Bridgewater, NJ]) as well as some veterinary steroids, such as boldenone undecylenate and stanozolol.[143] Commonly used oral anabolic steroids include oxandrolone (Oxandrin [BTG Pharmaceuticals, Iselin, NJ]), oxymetholone (Anadrol [Unimed Pharmaceuticals Inc, Buffalo Grove, IL]), methandrostenolone, and methenolone. Anabolic-androgenic steroids effectively increase muscle mass, strength, and training capacity. In addition, when combined with proper training and diet, they enhance performance. Thus, there is a powerful motivation for competitive athletes to use steroids and for trainers and coaches to intentionally or unintentionally encourage such use.

Although there are no immediate euphoric or biobehavioral effects of taking anabolic-androgenic steroids, there is evidence of dependence in long-term users.[144] Adolescents who have used steroids for 5 or more cycles have great difficulty quitting, and in some, withdrawal symptoms of depression and disabling fatigue develop.[145] A study of the abuse liability of testosterone in adult male volunteers measured ratings of subjective mood changes and physiologic responses after daily intramuscular injections of up to 200 mg for 5 consecutive days.[146] The study found none of the usual pharmacologic effects that are associated with abuse. However, anabolic-androgenic steroids have been shown in animal experiments to have direct effects on certain CNS receptor complexes, including benzodiazepine-binding sites, and there is speculation that behavioral effects may be mediated through regulatory systems in the brain.[147] Another study in male rats found that treatment for 15 weeks with a "cocktail" of testosterone cypionate, nandrolone decanoate, and boldenone undecylenate did not seem to alter the rewarding properties of brain stimulation but seemed to increase the sensitivity of the brain's reward system to a known drug of abuse, amphetamine.[148] Thus, the effects of anabolic-androgenic steroid abuse may be more severe in adolescents who also abuse other drugs.

Health Consequences

Long-term use of anabolic-androgenic steroids is associated with potentially serious adverse effects.[139,149] Hepatic function is impaired, and cholestatic jaundice, hepatomas, and hepatic malignant neoplasms may develop. Serum lipid levels are altered to patterns that facilitate atherogenesis, and triglyceride levels also may be elevated, increasing the risk of cardiovascular disease. Sharing needles for parenteral injection puts the user at risk of infectious complications, including hepatitis and HIV infection as well as local skin infections. A national study of more than 16 000 Canadian sixth graders and above found that 2.8% of respondents reported using anabolic-androgenic steroids during the year before the study, and of those who reported using steroids, almost a third reported injecting them.[150] Within the group of students who reported injecting steroids, 29% reported sharing needles.

In men who use anabolic-androgenic steroids, testicular atrophy, prostate changes, decreased sperm counts, accelerated male pattern baldness, and gynecomastia may develop. In women, menstrual irregularities, clitoral hypertrophy, low-pitched voice, hirsutism, and male-pattern baldness may develop. In both sexes, acne, fluid retention, hypertension, and thickened skin may develop.

There are many reports of severe behavioral alterations among steroid users, including mood fluctuations, increased aggression ("roid rage"), increased or decreased libido, and depression or mania. The results of studies on the effects of steroid abuse on personality are conflicting and are confounded by the inability to control for premorbid personality. One well-designed study of 88 steroid-using athletes compared with 68 athletes who did not use steroids using the Structured Clinical Interview from the *DSM-III-R* found that 23% of steroid users reported major mood disorders (mania, hypomania, or depression), and the frequency of mood disorder was significantly higher than in athletes who did not use steroids.[151] A double-blind, placebo-controlled study of supraphysiologic doses of testosterone ethanate on healthy men who were not competitive athletes and did not have psychiatric disorder and whose spouse or significant other also provided data found that angry behavior was not increased.[152]

Adolescents who use anabolic-androgenic steroids engage more often in other risk behaviors. Analysis of data from the 1993 Massachusetts *Youth Risk Behavior Survey* of high school students found that the prevalence of ever having used anabolic-androgenic steroids was significantly associated with all other risk behaviors measured, including driving after drinking alcohol, carrying a gun, having a higher number of sexual partners, not using a condom at last sexual intercourse, engaging in a physical fight that resulted in an injury requiring medical attention, and suicide attempts.[153] The data suggest that anabolic-androgenic steroid use among adolescents is a component of the "problem behavior syndrome." Among college students, when compared with nonusers, steroid users have higher rates of binge drinking and use of tobacco, marijuana, cocaine, amphetamines, sedatives, hallucinogens, opiates, inhalants, and designer drugs.[154]

Laboratory Evaluation

Almost 100 000 samples of athletes' urine are tested annually in laboratories accredited by the International Olympic Committee. The major urinary metabolites of anabolic-androgenic steroids can be detected by gas chromatography/mass spectrometry.[155] High-resolution mass spectrometry improves detection. Use of testoster-one must be determined by calculating the testosterone-epitestosterone ratio.[156] This ratio normally is about 1:1, and a ratio greater than 6:1 indicates probable exogenous testosterone use.

Treatment

Prevention of anabolic-androgenic steroid use by athletes is best addressed by team-based interventions. One such program, the Adolescents Training and Learning to Avoid Steroids (ATLAS) program was conducted and evaluated with high school football teams from 31 schools in the Portland area.[157] The intervention consisted of a 7-week program of weekly 50-minute class sessions led by coaches and peer educators, weight-room sessions led by trainers, and 1 evening session for parents. When intervention participants were compared with controls, decreases in intent to use anabolic-androgenic steroids, greater knowledge, more negative attitudes toward steroid use, and greater perception of personal vulnerability to the harmful effects of steroids were noted. Programs that emphasize only the risks of steroid use (scare tactics) are ineffective; the presentation of balanced information about risks and benefits seems more effective.[158]

Opiates

Epidemiology

Opiates are naturally occurring or synthetic sedative analgesic drugs that have effects similar to opium, a compound derived from the poppy plant *Papaver somniferum*. Morphine is an alkaloid that is isolated from opium, and heroin is produced in clandestine laboratories by acetylation of morphine. Other drugs in this class include codeine, methadone hydrochloride (Dolophine [Roxane Laboratories, Columbus, OH]), fentanyl citrate, meperidine hydrochloride (Demerol [Sanofi Pharmaceuticals Inc, New York, NY]), hydromorphone hydrochloride (Dilaudid [Knoll Laboratories, Mount Olive, NJ]), oxycodone hydrochloride (ingredient in Percodan and Percocet [Endo Pharmaceuticals Inc, Chadds Ford, PA], Tylox [Ortho-McNeil Pharmaceutical, Raritan, NJ], and others), propoxyphene hydrochloride (Darvon [Eli Lilly & Co, Indianapolis, IN]), diphenoxylate hydrochloride (ingredient in Lomotil [GD Searle & Co, Chicago, IL]), and pentazocine (Talwin [Sanofi Pharmaceuticals Inc, New York, NY]).

Opiates, particularly heroin, were major drugs of abuse among adolescents and young adults during the 1960s and early 1970s. Use dramatically decreased during the 1980s, coincident with increasing knowledge of the addictive potential of the drugs and the health risks of injection drug abuse. Throughout the 1980s and early 1990s, prevalence of ever having used heroin among twelfth graders ranged from 0.9% to 1.3%, and prevalence of use within the past year ranged from 0.4% to 0.6%.[7] However, in 1995, heroin use by twelfth graders markedly increased, and this increase continued through 1997. In 1997, prevalence of ever having used heroin among twelfth graders was 2.1%, and the prevalence of use within the past year was 1.2%, an approximately 100% increase since 1993.[7] The prevalence of use within the past year by twelfth graders increased further to 1.5% in 2000. Recent use (within the past 30 days) by twelfth graders has remained relatively constant since 1996 and was 0.7% in 2000 (see Table 0.1, p ix).[1-3] The increased use by adolescents coincides with a heroin epidemic among adults in the United States, as documented by the *National Household Survey on Drug Abuse,*[159] which found that the number of current heroin users more than tripled from 68 000 in 1993 to 216 000 in 1996.

Most adolescents now use heroin by nasal inhalation (snorting, sniffing) rather than by injection. Heroin production worldwide increased during the 1990s, and the purity of the available drug is much higher than in the past, permitting those using by nasal inhalation to achieve the desired rush that formerly was achieved only by intravenous injection. During the 1970s, the heroin sold on the streets was less than 5% pure, but now, drug purity of 80% to 90% is available.[159] Many adolescents mistakenly believe that heroin is less addictive by nasal inhalation, and in addition, barriers to use by intravenous injection, such as fear of AIDS and social stigma, are eliminated by using the nasal inhalation route. The use of other opiates besides heroin also has increased by high school students. In 1997, 9.7% of twelfth graders reported that they had ever used an opiate other than heroin, compared with only 6.6% in 1991.[7] Prevalence of ever having used heroin among twelfth graders increased further to 10.6% in 2000.[1-3]

"Designer drugs" are synthetic chemical modifications of extant drugs of abuse that are designed and manufactured in makeshift laboratories and sold at great profit for recreational use.[160] Modifications of the opiates meperidine and fentanyl came to attention on the West Coast during the late 1970s, when several unexplained deaths were traced to overdose of 2-methylfentanyl,[161] a compound that is a synthetic analogue of fentanyl citrate and an exceedingly powerful opiate. Another derivative found on the illicit market is 3-methylfentanyl ("China white"), a drug that is 2000 times as potent as morphine.[161] It was responsible for at least 12 deaths in San Francisco in 1986 and 16 deaths in Pennsylvania in 1988.[160,162]

Pharmacology

The range and intensity of the pharmacologic effects of each opiate drug depend largely on the relative binding affinity to the major CNS receptors called mu (μ), kappa (κ), delta (δ), sigma (σ), and epsilon (ε).[163] Of these, μ, κ, and δ receptors mediate analgesia. Opiates bind to the μ opioid receptors at several anatomic locations in the brain, including the nucleus accumbens, where they activate the brain's reward pathways and, thus, foster dependence and addiction. Tolerance develops after repeated dosing, necessitating higher doses to achieve the same effects, and dependence develops within approximately 3 to 4 weeks of regular use of heroin or morphine. Dependence can develop very rapidly with frequent use of very short-acting opiates, such as fentanyl.

Opiates can be used orally, intranasally, subcutaneously, intramuscularly, and intravenously. In addition, opium and heroin freebase can be smoked. Taken orally, the opiates are readily absorbed from the gastrointestinal tract; however, first-pass extraction and metabolism by the microsomes in the endoplasmic reticulum of the liver result in less intense effects, compared with administration by the parenteral or intranasal route.[164] Intravenous use ("shooting up" or "mainlining") produces a very intense effect almost immediately. Instillation via the intranasal route, or snorting, also results in intense, rapid effects. "Skin popping," or subcutaneous use, produces less intense effects beginning in about 15 minutes.

Heroin, or diacetylmorphine, is a bitter crystalline powder that is imported from 3 areas of the world: southwest Asia, southeast Asia, and Mexico. Heroin from each of these areas has distinctive additives or contaminants; brown heroin from Mexico usually contains lactose, procaine, quinine, and acetylprocaine, whereas white heroin from the Far East contains quinine, mannitol, starches, and sucrose.[165] An epidemic of acute onset of hallucinations and agitation approximately 1 hour after snorting heroin among users in large East Coast cities was traced to scopolamine adulteration of the heroin, causing anticholinergic toxic effects.[166]

Heroin is metabolized through hydrolyzation to 6-monoacetyl morphine and then to morphine, which is conjugated with glucuronic acid in the liver. It is excreted in the urine as free and conjugated morphine. Detoxification occurs rapidly; 90% of heroin is cleared from the body within 24 hours after administration. The effects of methadone, a long-acting opiate that usually is taken orally, begin within 30 minutes, and peak blood levels are reached in 4 to 6 hours. It is excreted slowly and has a plasma half-life of approximately 22 hours.

Health Consequences

Although the major indication for the therapeutic use of opiates is analgesia, the high potential for abuse of opiates is related to their capacity to produce euphoria. In addition to a direct analgesic effect, the opiates produce an altered psychologic response to pain, suppression of anxiety, and sedation, all of which contribute to their abuse.

Acute effects of opiates include respiratory depression, a result of suppression of the medullary response to carbon dioxide, that causes a decrease in the respiratory rate, minute volume, and tidal exchange. With overdose, there is the potential for respiratory arrest. The cough center, also located within the medulla, is similarly depressed, explaining the therapeutic use of opiates as antitussives but representing an additional danger of aspiration in stuporous or comatose persons. Among the gastrointestinal effects of opiate abuse is delayed gastric emptying time attributable to the increased tone of the antral portion of the stomach and the proximal duodenum. Although the delayed gastric emptying time is accompanied by decreased production of hydrochloric acid and biliary and pancreatic secretions, the net effect facilitates the formation of duodenal ulcers. Constipation is common because of a decrease in the propulsive contractions of the small and large intestine and increased tone of the ileocecal valve and anal sphincter. Tolerance to the gastrointestinal effects does not develop.

The classic triad of acute opiate overdose is CNS depression, respiratory depression, and miosis. Possible cardiopulmonary effects include bradycardia, hypotension, and noncardiogenic pulmonary edema.[163] A rapid response to intravenous naloxone, an opiate antagonist, is diagnostic of acute opioid overdose.

Sloppy and uncontrolled manufacturing processes pose great dangers to consumers of designer opiates. 1-Methyl-4-phenyl-4-propionoxypiperidine is a designer modification of meperidine.

If the chemical synthetic process is not strictly controlled, however, a substantial amount of a contaminant, 1-methyl-4-phenyl-1,2,3,6-tetrahydropyridine (MPTP), is formed. Irreversible Parkinson disease is caused by MPTP, a neurotoxin with a predilection for the substantia nigra of the brain.[167,168] The first designer drug catastrophe was identified in 1982, when severe parkinsonism caused by MPTP suddenly developed in a group of young drug addicts in California.

The consequences of long-term opiate abuse are related not only to the pharmacologic action of the drug but also and even more often to the method of drug administration and the lifestyle of the abuser. Intravenous use is associated with the most serious complications. Lack of aseptic technique, the sharing of needles and syringes, and the presence of adulterants result in a number of common and often quite serious complications. Cellulitis, skin abscesses, thrombophlebitis, endocarditis, intracranial and pulmonary abscesses, pneumonia, and hepatitis are among the infectious complications commonly encountered. During the 1980s, HIV infection became the infectious complication of greatest concern. Intranasal use of heroin may be associated with acute bronchospasm. Peripheral neural complications include transverse myelitis and brachial and lumbosacral plexitis, which have been reported after reexposure to heroin after a period of abstinence.

Although opiates actually decrease libido, increased rates of sexually transmitted diseases are noted in drug-abusing adolescents because of a lifestyle that often includes trading sex for drugs or money to purchase drugs. A positive result of a reactive serologic test for syphilis may be attributable to true infection or may be a biologically false-positive result, which can occur with heroin abuse. The female opiate user may experience amenorrhea and anovulatory cycles, which may account for the low pregnancy rate despite sexual activity.

Abuse of opiates during pregnancy is associated with serious complications, including increased risk of spontaneous abortion and stillbirth, infants who are small for their gestational age, and newborn abstinence syndrome. Maternal drug withdrawal during pregnancy, particularly during the third trimester, may increase the risk of fetal demise. Newborn abstinence syndrome begins from several hours to 6 weeks after delivery. The time of onset and severity of the symptoms depend on the specific drug used (methadone withdrawal occurs later than heroin withdrawal), the total daily dose used, duration of addiction, and the time of the last maternal dose. Symptoms range from mild irritability and feeding difficulty to seizures. A large number of female opiate addicts are HIV infected and, thus, risk passing the infection on to their infants. Those who receive methadone maintenance treatment are more likely to be treated with zidovudine and to obtain prenatal care, resulting in decreased obstetric and fetal complications.[169]

Addiction to opiates is a function of the amount of drug abused and the frequency and duration of the abuse. Although no exact formula can be defined for the development of addiction, an abstinence syndrome may develop even after discontinuation of the daily therapeutic use of opiates for a period of weeks. In the heroin addict, withdrawal symptoms begin to occur approximately 6 hours after the last dose. In contrast with methadone, withdrawal symptoms do not begin until more than 24 hours after the last dose.

The opiate abstinence syndrome begins with yawning, restlessness, increased lacrimation, insomnia, and rhinorrhea and progresses to mydriasis, piloerection, diaphoresis, flushing, tachycardia, hypertension, tremors, and twitching and later muscle cramps, fever, nausea, vomiting, and intestinal hyperactivity with diarrhea. Seizures, one of the most severe manifestations of opiate withdrawal, are rare in adolescents.

Laboratory Evaluation

Urine testing for the presence of opiates is widely available in most medical centers. Thin-layer chromatography and radioimmunoassay techniques detect opiate metabolites for several days after the last use (see Chapter 4).

Treatment Considerations

As noted, acute opiate overdose may result in respiratory depression, pulmonary edema, and cardiopulmonary arrest;

thus, aggressive respiratory and cardiovascular support is necessary. The acute toxic effects of an opiate may be antagonized by the administration of naloxone, beginning with intermittent doses of 0.4 to 2.0 mg intravenously given as often as every 2 to 3 minutes.[170] Bolus doses as high as 8 mg may be required. A continuous infusion may be necessary, especially in cases of methadone intoxication in which the duration of toxic effects may be prolonged. Because the duration of action of naloxone is much shorter than that of methadone, therapy should not be discontinued as soon as the patient regains consciousness. Relapse into coma may occur if naloxone therapy is discontinued prematurely. Radiography of the chest should be performed to determine whether pneumonia or pulmonary edema is present. Antibiotics are given when either of these is present, as secondary infection commonly occurs with the latter.

Many adolescents briefly experiment with heroin without becoming addicted; nevertheless, heroin must be considered highly addictive, and the long-term prognosis of addiction to opiates is poor. Adolescents who become addicted face a prolonged and even lifetime battle to achieve abstinence in which detoxification is but the first step. Treatment of the abstinence syndrome is aimed at maintaining patient comfort and preventing rare but severe effects, such as seizures. Detoxification should be viewed as preparation for entrance into a dependency treatment program. Few patients will continue to abstain from opiate use after detoxification without the benefit of therapeutic support. A variety of detoxification methods have been used, including acupuncture, pharmacologic withdrawal, and abrupt cessation of drug use with behavioral support. The most common method of detoxification involves the administration of methadone in a single daily dose of 30 to 40 mg; the dose is decreased in 5-mg aliquots per day. By this method, abstinence can be attained in 7 to 10 days. An alternative method is the administration of diazepam in a dose of 10 to 15 mg every 4 to 6 hours for 3 or 4 days. Although this method avoids the use of a substitute opiate and provides more rapid detoxification, it is less likely to ablate all symptoms of withdrawal and, hence, is less well tolerated by adolescent addicts. Clonidine hydrochloride, a centrally acting α_2-adrenergic agonist, decreases many of the autonomic signs and symptoms of opiate withdrawal and produces mild sedation and a sense of well-being that facilitates withdrawal.[171] It is a useful drug for opioid detoxification. Naltrexone, a specific μ opioid receptor antagonist, has a long half-life that permits once-a-day dosing and effectively blocks the cognitive and behavioral effects of opioids.[169] It is used in rapid detoxification regimens.

The long-term treatment of opiate addiction primarily has involved 2 modalities: drug-free therapeutic communities and methadone maintenance treatment programs. Drug-free therapeutic communities vary in their approaches but most often share common themes of total drug abstinence, behavior modification, and self-help directed by ex-addicts rather than by behavioral therapy professionals. A typical treatment course would require 12 to 18 months of residence within the therapeutic community, followed by day treatment support after "graduation." Few adolescents are able to tolerate prolonged confinement in a therapeutic community, and even for those who stay, the prognosis after discharge is not good.

An alternative method of treatment for opiate addiction is methadone maintenance. The treatment programs administer a daily dose of a substitute opiate, methadone, in combination with supportive services and behavioral intervention. Methadone can be taken orally once a day and has a more prolonged and a less intense effect than heroin, and clients in the programs can resume normal activities and pursue educational and vocational goals. The original hope that opiate addicts could thereby stabilize their lifestyles and eventually undergo detoxification and remain abstinent has not been realized. Although many adolescents achieve some success in remaining relatively drug-free while receiving methadone maintenance, eventual detoxification and abstinence have been overly optimistic goals. Methadone maintenance must be viewed as a potential lifelong therapy.

Sedative-Hypnotics

Epidemiology

The most common sedative-hypnotic drugs subject to abuse are the barbiturates. The drugs were first used in medical practice at the beginning of the 20th century for their CNS depressant and sleep-inducing effects.[172] Presently, however, they are used legitimately primarily as anesthetic agents and anticonvulsant agents. Treatment of insomnia and anxiety now is accomplished using the much safer benzodiazepine class of drugs. Commonly abused barbiturates include secobarbital (Tubex [Wyeth-Ayerst Laboratories, Philadelphia, PA], "reds," "red devils," "F-40s"), pentobarbital sodium (Nembutal [Abbott Laboratories, North Chicago, IL], "yellow jackets," "Mexican yellows"), and amobarbital sodium ("downers," "blue heavens"). Abuse of barbiturates by adolescents peaked during the 1970s and decreased thereafter as prescription use decreased.[7] Methaqualone ("quaaludes," "ludes," "soapers") is another sedative drug that has potential for toxic effects, addiction, and abuse. Although methaqualone is now a Schedule II drug and most manufacturers have suspended production, bootleg forms may be available.

In 1997, the prevalence of ever having used sedatives (only use that was not ordered by a physician was reported) among twelfth graders was 8.7%.[7] This percentage represents a significant increase from a low of 6.1% in 1992 but is nowhere near the approximately 18% prevalence of use in 1975.[7] Illicit barbiturate use increased gradually among US twelfth graders during the 1990s, from 6.2% in 1991 to 8.1% in 1997. However, the prevalence of use within the past 30 days was only 2.1%, and daily use was 0.1% in 1997. Recent use (within the past 30 days) by twelfth graders has shown an increasing trend, from 2.1% in 1997, to 2.6% in 1998, to 3.0% in 2000 (see Table 0.1, p ix).[1-3] Adolescents who are not in school and those who abuse other drugs are more likely than twelfth graders to have used barbiturates and other sedatives, as this class of drugs is often used to treat unwanted effects of illicit stimulant drugs. Prevalence of ever having used methaqualone was reported by approximately 1% or fewer twelfth graders throughout the 1990s.[7]

Pharmacology

Barbituric acid, a substance with no CNS activity, is the parent compound for all barbiturates. The barbiturates exert their action on the CNS by enhancing the action of GABA, the primary inhibitory neurotransmitter.[172] All barbiturates are absorbed rapidly after oral ingestion. Barbiturates also are effective when administered intramuscularly or intravenously and occasionally are abused by these routes. They are detoxified in the liver or excreted unchanged in the urine. Elimination is delayed in infants, pregnant women, and patients with diminished renal or hepatic function.

Barbiturates are classified as long acting, intermediate acting, short acting, and ultrashort acting. Phenobarbital is a long-acting barbiturate with a duration of action of 24 hours. It has a low potential for abuse, because after absorption into the bloodstream, some hours are required for phenobarbital to enter the CNS and affect the brain. Thus, a person who ingests phenobarbital does not feel intoxicated. Short-acting barbiturates, such as secobarbital and pentobarbital, are more lipid soluble and, thus, cross the blood-brain barrier relatively quickly. They produce sedation and a decrease in anxiety within 15 to 30 minutes of ingestion and have a high potential for abuse. Ultrashort-acting barbiturates, such as thiopental sodium and methohexital sodium, are so highly lipophilic that they are used intravenously for anesthesia. They are quickly taken up by the gray matter of the brain and induce sleep within 30 seconds. Short-acting barbiturates are highly protein bound and rapidly redistributed out of the circulation into body fat; thus, they are not easily dialyzable in cases of overdose.

Regular use of barbiturates causes induction of hepatic microsomal enzymes, and pharmacokinetic tolerance develops because the drug is deactivated more rapidly. In addition, other drugs ingested concomitantly, such as anticoagulants and oral contraceptives, also are metabolized more rapidly, resulting in decreased effectiveness. Tolerance to barbiturates also develops through receptor desensitization (pharmacodynamic tolerance) as the dose increases.

However, no tolerance to the lethal dose develops, so the therapeutic index becomes narrower in barbiturate addicts, and overdose is common.

Methaqualone is absorbed rapidly and completely after oral ingestion, reaching peak levels within 1 to 2 hours. It is metabolized in the liver to inactive forms that are excreted in the urine.

Health Consequences

The sedative-hypnotic drugs produce effects that may be mistaken for alcohol inebriation. Users may have slurred speech, an unsteady gait, impaired judgment, and inadequate impulse control. All sedative-hypnotics produce some drowsiness, although tolerance to drowsiness develops over time. The drug effect depends partially on the setting in which it is taken; when barbiturates are taken at a party to get high, the person often experiences excitement and disinhibition rather than sedation.

Mild toxic effects are manifested by nystagmus, ataxia, emotional lability, and mental confusion. Large overdoses result in coma, which may be followed by respiratory and cardiovascular collapse and death.[173] Pulmonary edema and aspiration pneumonia are encountered occasionally. Miosis, diminished or absent pupillary and corneal reflexes, abnormal temperature regulation (hypothermia occurring early and hyperthermia occurring later), and decreased gastrointestinal motility with delayed gastric emptying time also are seen with barbiturate overdose.

Overdose with methaqualone may cause features quite different from those produced by the other sedative-hypnotics, including increased deep tendon reflexes, muscular hypertonicity, myoclonus, generalized muscle twitching, shivering, and occasionally seizures.[174] Severe toxic effects include coma, respiratory depression, and increased vascular permeability, resulting in effusions and pulmonary edema.

The sedative-hypnotic drugs are highly addictive. The dose and period of use necessary to induce tolerance and addiction vary with each barbiturate. On average, however, addiction develops within 1 to 2 months of regular daily use of 500 mg or more. Addiction to methaqualone has been reported in adults after the use of 2 g daily for as little as 1 month.

The sedative-hypnotic abstinence syndrome produces serious and possibly life-threatening effects. Symptoms are similar to those of delirium tremens, the severe alcohol abstinence syndrome. Anxiety, restlessness, tremors, insomnia, abdominal cramps, nausea, and vomiting are the earliest symptoms. The symptoms usually begin between 12 and 16 hours after the last dose of a short-acting barbiturate. By 24 hours, the patient has hyperactive reflexes and orthostatic hypotension. If untreated, symptoms peak at 48 to 72 hours, with the onset of hallucinations, delirium, hyperthermia, and generalized seizures. The longer-acting barbiturates are associated with the same reaction pattern, but the symptoms are delayed; for example, seizures may not occur until 1 week after the last dose of phenobarbital.

Barbiturates freely cross the placenta, resulting in equal maternal and fetal plasma concentrations. Because elimination is increased during pregnancy, however, lower plasma levels result. Fetal abnormalities have been reported with barbiturate use during pregnancy, but no pattern has emerged. Prenatal exposure to phenobarbital has been associated with lower verbal intelligence in adults.[175] An abstinence syndrome may occur in neonates born to women who use barbiturates during the third trimester of pregnancy. Abstinence symptoms in infants may not begin until 4 to 7 days after birth and include overactivity, restlessness, insomnia, tremors, hyperphagia, hypertonicity, and vasomotor instability.

Laboratory Evaluation

Plasma and urine testing is widely available for the qualitative and quantitative detection of barbiturates. Most medical facilities routinely use such testing to determine therapeutic levels of barbiturates and are able to supply the information needed to diagnose suspected abuse or a drug overdose (see Chapter 4).

Treatment Considerations

Barbiturate overdose is often lethal despite the best treatment; barbiturates often are used for suicide. The objective of the initial management of a patient who has taken a toxic overdose of a sedative-hypnotic drug is to prevent further absorption of the drug.[173] Prevention of further absorption is important, because barbiturates decrease gastrointestinal motility, allowing continued absorption for hours or days. An alert patient who is treated soon after an ingestion may be given ipecac syrup to induce vomiting. This treatment is followed by administration of a slurry of activated charcoal and then a saline cathartic, such as magnesium citrate. The stuporous or comatose patient or a patient with any respiratory embarrassment requires intubation with a cuffed endotracheal tube to prevent aspiration and maintain a patent airway before administration of activated charcoal. Doses of charcoal should be administered every 2 to 4 hours or given continuously via nasogastric tube until substantial improvement of the patient's condition is noted.

Monitoring of serum electrolytes, blood gas, urinary output, and plasma barbiturate levels helps guide fluid replacement and other aspects of supportive therapy. For all barbiturates, increasing urinary output is beneficial; alkalinization of the urine also is helpful for the treatment of overdoses with long-acting barbiturates. Hemodialysis or hemoperfusion may be considered for the treatment of severe toxic effects, but such treatment may not be effective with the short-acting barbiturates because of protein binding.[173] For the treatment of methaqualone intoxication, fluid therapy must be judicious, because pulmonary edema may accompany poisoning. Vasopressors may be needed to treat hypotension.

Anticipation and treatment of the abstinence syndrome are essential. Any person who has used 500 mg or more of barbiturates daily for at least 1 month and all patients with a history of a seizure disorder who use any amount of sedatives regularly should undergo detoxification in an inpatient unit.[176] Phenobarbital is used in gradually tapered doses until the patient is drug free.[177] When seizures occur as a result of barbiturate withdrawal, phenytoin usually is ineffective, and seizures must be treated with barbiturates. Chlorpromazine is contraindicated because of its tendency to lower the seizure threshold. The person addicted to methaqualone also should undergo detoxification with phenobarbital, which can be accomplished over a briefer period, usually within 3 to 5 days.

Tranquilizers

Epidemiology

Tranquilizers, primarily the benzodiazepines, are the most prescribed group of drugs in the United States. Trends in illicit use by US high school students have remained fairly consistent during the 1990s, although there is some evidence of increased use since 1995.[7] Among eighth, tenth, and twelfth graders in 1997, 4.8%, 7.3%, and 7.8%, respectively, reported ever using tranquilizers. Approximately 2% of tenth and twelfth graders reported using tranquilizers within the past 30 days. However, only 0.1% twelfth graders reported using such drugs daily. Recent use (within the past 30 days) by twelfth graders has remained relatively stable at 2.4% in 1998 and 2.6% in 2000 (see Table 0.1, p ix).[1-3] Although diazepam has been one of the most widely abused tranquilizers, flunitrazepam (Rohypnol, manufactured by Roche Pharmaceuticals Inc outside the United States), a drug that is not licensed for sale in the United States but is sold legally in 64 other countries including Mexico, rapidly is becoming the benzodiazepine of choice for abuse by adolescents. A study of almost 1000 young women in Texas found a prevalence of ever having used flunitrazepam of 5.9%.[178] Flunitrazepam, also known as the "date rape drug," "rophies," "R2s," "RIP," "Mexican Valium," "ruffles," "roches," "the forget pill," and "pantydroppers," is 10 times more potent than diazepam and often is used at parties to heighten the effect of alcohol and other drugs (see **Club Drugs**, p 263). The small white pills dissolve easily in liquid and are odorless, colorless, and tasteless; hence, they also are used to spike the drinks of unsuspecting young women for the purpose of rape.

Pharmacology

Although the pharmacokinetics of the benzodiazepines vary considerably, their other pharmacologic and toxic properties are similar.[179] After oral ingestion, benzodiazepines are absorbed readily and rapidly from the stomach. Whether they are used orally, intramuscularly, or intravenously, all benzodiazepines become bound to plasma proteins once they enter the systemic circulation. The extent to which the drugs bind varies somewhat depending on their degree of lipid solubility; however, they tend to be widely distributed into body tissues. Benzodiazepines undergo biotransformation in the liver; however, it is interesting to note that the elimination half-life and body clearance of a particular compound often do not reflect the duration of action of the drug.

Benzodiazepines exert their pharmacologic effects by activating GABA(A) receptors in the brain.[180] Activation of the GABA(A)-benzodiazepine receptor complex can be blocked by the benzodiazepine antagonist, flumazenil. Tolerance to the depressant effects of benzodiazepines develops rapidly, but tolerance to the anxiolytic effects develops slowly and is limited. Nevertheless, benzodiazepines possess all characteristics of addictive substances, and a serious abstinence syndrome develops when the drug is discontinued abruptly after regular use.

Health Consequences

Benzodiazepines are potent anxiolytics, anticonvulsants, and muscle relaxants. They are used by adolescents to get high and counteract the effects of illicit stimulant drugs, such as cocaine or amphetamines. Drowsiness, ataxia, dizziness, and weakness are common adverse effects, even at therapeutic doses.[181] In addition, impairment of psychomotor performance and memory can occur with their use.

The salient feature of benzodiazepine overdose is sedation. Other effects include paresthesia, blurred vision, dysarthria, and nystagmus. There is little or no effect on blood pressure and respiratory status when benzodiazepines are used orally. Acute intoxication is more likely to occur when benzodiazepines are taken with alcohol or other depressants than when taken alone[179] not only because the effects are additive but also because alcohol increases the rate of absorption of benzodiazepines. Paradoxical reactions including agitation, although uncommon, occur. A field investigation of 66 adolescent users of flunitrazepam ("roches") in Texas found that almost all used other drugs, primarily alcohol and marijuana, and that many had experienced adverse consequences of benzodiazepine use, including amnesia, incoordination, motor vehicle crashes, sexual assault, and respiratory depression.[182] In addition, the study found that many subjects' descriptions of the tablets they took were consistent with benzodiazepines other than flunitrazepam. Thus, the investigators concluded that sedative-hypnotic abuse in Texas involved several different benzodiazepines.

Benzodiazepines with a long half-life, such as diazepam or flurazepam hydrochloride, tend to produce cumulative sedation; however, the cumulative sedation is offset partly by the development of tolerance. Physiologic dependence occurs, and an abstinence syndrome may begin as long as 5 to 8 days after the last dose of the longer half-life forms and continue for several weeks. For the benzodiazepines with a relatively short half-life (eg, oxazepam, lorazepam, alprazolam, or triazolam), withdrawal symptoms begin sooner. The mildest symptoms of withdrawal are insomnia, sensitivity to light and sound, and irritability. More severe symptoms may include tremulousness, diaphoresis, muscle twitching, tachycardia, systolic hypertension, and confusion, and seizures may occur.[183]

Benzodiazepines cross the placenta and accumulate in the fetus. There is some evidence that their use during the first trimester of pregnancy may result in increased risk of cleft lip and palate.

Laboratory Evaluation
Benzodiazepines can be detected in blood and urine (see Chapter 4).

Treatment Considerations
Treatment of overdose in a conscious patient consists of the administration of ipecac syrup to empty the stomach and activated charcoal followed by a cathartic, such as magnesium citrate. If the patient is comatose or the condition otherwise is compromised

severely, intubation, ventilation, and circulatory support may be necessary. Administration of flumazenil, the benzodiazepine antagonist, is not recommended, because mixed ingestion cannot be ruled out and there is a risk of precipitating seizures if a proseizure drug, such as a tricyclic antidepressant, also has been ingested.

The abstinence syndrome is treated by reinstituting a long-acting benzodiazepine, such as diazepam, and slowly tapering the dosage during a 1- to 2-week period.[184]

Inhalants

Epidemiology

Inhaling volatile gases, such as nitrous oxide or ether, for their mind-altering effects was popular among adults during the 19th century. However, abuse of inhalants by adolescents became a concern in the United States during the early 1960s with the epidemic of glue sniffing among children and young adolescents. Through the 1970s and 1980s, other volatile substances and aerosols came into widespread use as inhalants.

The *Monitoring the Future* studies of US high school students indicates a steady increase in prevalence of ever having used inhalants during the 1990s with a peak in 1995 and slight decrease in the following 2 years among older students.[7] Inhalants are more likely to be used by younger than older adolescents; prevalence of use within the past year by eighth, tenth, and twelfth graders in 1997 was 11.8%, 8.7%, and 6.7%, respectively, and the prevalence of use within the past 30 days was 5.6%, 3.0%, and 2.5%, respectively. Few adolescents report using inhalants daily; only 0.1% of twelfth graders reported daily use in 1997. Recent use (within the past 30 days) by twelfth graders was 2.2%; however, the prevalence was twice as high for eighth graders at 4.5% in 2000 (see Table 0.1, p ix).[1-3] The *National Household Survey on Drug Abuse* provides data on all adolescents 12 to 17 years of age, including school dropouts.[185] This survey documented the largest incidence rates for initiation of inhalant use among

14- and 15-year-olds. The overall prevalence rates for inhalant use during the years 1990 through 1995 were 6.6% for girls and 6.9% for boys and were highest among non-Hispanic whites and lowest among non-Hispanic blacks. Between 1990 and 1995, a significant increase was noted in the prevalence of adolescents who reported ever having used aerosol inhalants or having sniffed glue. The *Monitoring the Future* study reported the prevalence of twelfth graders who reported ever having used inhalants at a high of 18% in 1990, which decreased to 14.2% in 2000.[1-3]

Much of the inhalant use among young adolescents is experimental, and it often occurs as a group activity. Substances such as model glue, gasoline, spray paints, aerosols used as propellants for deodorants, cleaning fluids, fabric guard, and correction fluid are legal, inexpensive, and readily available. School authorities and parents are not likely to become suspicious when they encounter a 13-year-old with a can of deodorant. Gasoline sniffing has been reported as a recreational behavior since the early 1970s, especially among children in certain ethnic and sociocultural groups. Several reports from the United States, Canada, and Australia document a high prevalence of gasoline sniffing among native Indian or aboriginal children living in isolated areas.[186] A survey of almost 400 Eskimo children in grades 6 through 12 in western Alaska found the prevalence of ever having used inhalants was 48%; 6% of these children reported using inhalants during the past 30 days.[187] Gasoline was the preferred inhalant by 62% of users, and 22% preferred glue. In the Eskimo population, boys and girls were equally likely to be inhalant users, but boys were 5 times more likely to be heavy users than girls.[187]

The volatile nitrites, such as amyl, butyl, or isobutyl nitrite, became popular during the 1970s among male homosexuals who used them to enhance the sexual experience. Epidemiologic data specific to the adolescent population are rare in the literature, although 1.2% of twelfth graders in 1997 reported using nitrites within the past year.[7] In 1 study, a survey of 173 adolescents in a long-term drug treatment facility, 43% reported using isobutyl nitrite at least once, and 13% reported using it 10 or more times.[188]

A few of the adolescents had used the drug in conjunction with a sexual experience; for those who did, intercourse was heterosexual.

Pharmacology

Inhalation is accomplished in a variety of ways. The volatile substance may be poured or sprayed into a plastic bag and inhaled from the bag. Liquid hydrocarbons, such as solvents or cleaning fluids, can be inhaled from soaked rags placed over the mouth and nose. Butyl and isobutyl nitrite are sold in small glass bottles in "head shops" and pornography stores or by mail order and carry street names such as "rush," "locker room," "bullet," "quicksilver," and "thrust." The drugs may be inhaled directly from the bottle. The prescription variety of amyl nitrite ("poppers"), used as a vasodilator for the treatment of angina pectoris, comes in a small glass vial that is crushed (popped) before inhalation.

The chemicals in most inhalants are absorbed rapidly in the lungs and exert their CNS effects within seconds, producing an altered mental state for about 5 to 15 minutes. Tolerance often develops in long-term users, but withdrawal symptoms are rare.

Health Consequences

Toluene is the most common hydrocarbon found in paints, lacquer thinners, and household and model glues. Inhalation of toluene, as well as other hydrocarbons, has been associated with renal and hepatic damage, peripheral neuropathy, seizures, encephalopathy, and other CNS toxic effects.[170] Sudden death associated with glue sniffing and especially with inhalation of aerosols containing halogenated hydrocarbons (refrigerants) has been reported in a number of adolescents.[189] The deaths are thought to be attributable to cardiac arrhythmias resulting from sensitization of the heart to epinephrine. This mechanism is similar to that known to occur with halothane, a related chemical that is used as an anesthetic agent. Death often occurs while the intoxicated adolescent is running or is very agitated because of hallucinations and presumably experiencing an increased secretion of epinephrine.

Gasoline sniffing has been associated with ataxia, chorea, tremor, organic lead encephalopathy, hepatic damage, peripheral neuropathy, and myopathy.[186] Long-term gasoline abusers may suffer neuropsychologic and intellectual deficits secondary to lead poisoning.

Trichloromethane, tetraper chloroethylene, and trichloroethylene, found in fabric guard, spot remover, correction fluid, and some glues have been implicated in acute hepatic and renal toxic effects and also in sudden death attributable to cardiac arrhythmias. King et al[190] reported the sudden deaths of 4 adolescents immediately after inhaling the vapors from typewriter correction fluid. Toxicologic analysis revealed trichloromethane, trichloroethylene, or both in blood samples from all 4 patients. Ethanol was not detected in blood samples from any of the adolescents. Autopsy revealed no evidence of acute hepatic or renal damage. The cause of all 4 deaths was thought to be cardiac arrhythmia.

Inhaling amyl, butyl, or isobutyl nitrite has been reported to cause headaches, tachycardia, syncope, and hypotension attributable to the vasodilator effects.[191] Volatile nitrites also have been associated with increased intraocular pressure and with methemoglobinemia leading to cyanosis and hypoxia. People with glaucoma and with clinically significant anemia who use nitrites are at particular risk; however, few deaths have been reported.

Laboratory Evaluation

Specific testing for most inhalants is difficult because of their rapid elimination and volatility. Because of the frequency of hepatic, renal, and hematologic damage caused by inhalants, however, complete blood cell counts, coagulation studies, and hepatic and renal function tests should be performed on all inhalant abusers. For gasoline sniffers, blood lead concentration should be determined, because the blood lead level has been elevated in children who have only sniffed gasoline a few times.[186]

Treatment Considerations

Treatment should be similar to that offered to adolescents with other substance abuse problems and should include, for those who are deeply involved, consideration of residential or community-based drug-treatment programs and family involvement. Chelation therapy is effective for the toxic effects of tetraethyl lead resulting from gasoline inhalation.

Club Drugs

The National Institute on Drug Abuse has identified a pattern of drug use in all-night party and "rave" dance clubs and bars that causes significant morbidity and even mortality among youth. These drugs include stimulants, depressants, and hallucinogens. Some are of recent abuse (methamphetamine, MDMA, gammahydroxybutyrate [GHB], flunitrazepam, ketamine), and others represent drugs of long-standing abuse (marijuana, cocaine).[4] Several were reviewed earlier in this chapter. Consequences of using these drugs can be very serious and even fatal (Table 8.1).[4]

It is important to inform vulnerable youth about the dangers of these drugs as part of preventive counseling interventions among youth. The National Institute on Drug Abuse has launched a major initiative to warn the nation not to underestimate the harm of these drugs.[192] For periodic updates on club drugs, the health care professional can access the National Institute on Drug Abuse Web site at http://www.clubdrugs.org.

Conclusion

An understanding of the epidemiology, pharmacology, health consequences, laboratory evaluation, and treatment for abuse of specific drugs can aid the health care professional in prevention, assessment, and intervention. It will also be helpful to the health care professional to remain alert to emerging trends and patterns of specific drug consumption by youth at local and national levels to optimize the provision of health care for children and adolescents who are vulnerable to drug use and abuse.

table 8.1 Club Drugs[4]

MDMA ("ecstasy," "X," "XTC," "Adam")
A stimulant similar to methamphetamine, MDMA is usually taken orally as a tablet. It causes increased heart rate and blood pressure and may lead to an elevation of body temperature that causes kidney and cardiovascular failure. When combined with alcohol, MDMA can be extremely dangerous, sometimes fatal. Chronic abuse of MDMA may produce long-lasting neurotoxic effects in the brain.

GHB ("liquid ecstasy," "Georgia home boy," "G")
A clear odorless liquid, GHB is a CNS depressant and has been associated with poisonings, overdoses, and date rape. GHB overdose can lead rapidly to loss of consciousness, coma, and death. The purity and strength of individual doses of the drug can vary greatly, making overdoses likely.

Ketamine ("K," "special K," "vitamin K," "cat Valium")
Ketamine is a veterinary anesthetic that produces dissociative dream-like or hallucinatory effects. The drug is used as a liquid applied to marijuana or tobacco products or as a white powder that is snorted like cocaine. At high doses, ketamine produces delirium, amnesia, impaired motor function, and sometimes fatal respiratory effects.

Flunitrazepam (Rohypnol, "roofies," "rophie," "roche," "forget-me")
A benzodiazepine sedative similar to Valium (Roche Pharmaceuticals, Manati, Puerto Rico) and Xanax (Pharmacia & Upjohn, Bridgewater, NJ), flunitrazepam is not approved for prescription use in the United States. The drug is taken orally in tablet form or dissolved in beverages. Because the drug is odorless and tasteless and produces amnesia, it can be administered to a person without his or her knowledge and has been associated with date rape and other sexual assaults.

Methamphetamine ("meth," "speed," "ice," "glass," "crystal," "crank")
Methamphetamine, an odorless white crystalline powder, is a highly addictive stimulant that can be snorted, smoked, injected, or taken orally. The drug produces increased levels of activity, excited speech, and decreased appetite. Methamphetamine is a neurotoxin associated with long-lasting effects on the dopamine transporter system as well as with other dangerous health effects, including aggression, violence, memory loss, psychotic behavior, and cardiac damage.

LSD ("acid," "blotter," "cubes," "dots," "L," "sugar")
LSD is a powerful hallucinogen that is taken orally, usually on squares of blotter paper, sugar cubes, or pills that have absorbed the liquid drug. The drug produces profound abnormalities in sensory perception, including distortions of sound and sight, and emotional effects that create rapid mood swings ranging from intense fear to euphoria.

References

1. Johnston LD, O'Malley PM, Bachman JG. *National Survey Results on Drug Use from the Monitoring the Future Study, 1975-1998.* Volume I: Secondary School Students. Rockville, MD: National Institute on Drug Abuse; 1999. NIH Publication No. 99-4660

2. Johnston LD, O'Malley PM, Bachman JG. *The Monitoring the Future National Survey Results on Adolescent Drug Use: Overview of Key Findings, 1999.* Rockville, MD: National Institute on Drug Abuse; 2000. NIH Publication No. 00-4690

3. Johnston L, O'Malley P, Bachman J. "Ecstasy" use rises sharply among teens in 2000; use of many other drugs stays steady but significant declines are reported for some [press release]. Ann Arbor, MI: University of Michigan, News and Information Services; December 14, 2000

4. Leshner AI. A club drug alert. In: *NIDA Notes.* Rockville, MD: National Institute on Drug Abuse; 2000;14:3-5. NIH Publication No. 99-3478

5. Ray O. *Drugs, Society, and Human Behavior.* 3rd ed. St Louis, MO: CV Mosby Co; 1983

6. Kessler DA, Natanblut SL, Wilkenfeld JP, et al. Nicotine addiction: a pediatric disease. *J Pediatr.* 1997;130:518-524

7. Johnston LD, O'Malley PM, Bachman JG. *National Survey Results on Drug Use from the Monitoring the Future Study, 1975-1997.* Volume I: Secondary School Students. Rockville, MD: National Institute on Drug Abuse; 1998. NIH Publication No. 98-4345

8. Centers for Disease Control and Prevention. Tobacco use among high school students: United States, 1997. *MMWR Morb Mortal Wkly Rep.* 1998;47:229-233

9. Centers for Disease Control and Prevention. Selected cigarette smoking initiation and quitting behaviors among high school students: United States, 1997. *MMWR Morb Mortal Wkly Rep.* 1998;47:386-389

10. Greenlund KJ, Johnson CC, Webber LS, Berensen GS. Cigarette smoking attitudes and first use among third- through sixth-grade students: the Bogalusa Heart Study. *Am J Public Health.* 1997;87: 1345-1348

11. Mittelmark MB, Murray DM, Luepker RV, Pechacek TF, Pirie PL, Pallonen UE. Predicting experimentation with cigarettes: the childhood antecedents of smoking study (CASS). *Am J Public Health.* 1987;77:206-208

12. Young TL, Rogers KD. School performance characteristics preceding onset of smoking in high school students. *Am J Dis Child.* 1986;140:257-259

13. Benowitz NL. Drug therapy: pharmacologic aspects of cigarette smoking and nicotine addiction. *N Engl J Med.* 1988;319:1318-1330

14. Fielding JE. Smoking: health effects and control: I. *N Engl J Med.* 1985;313:491-498

15. Cornelius MD, Taylor PM, Geva D, Day NL. Prenatal tobacco and marijuana use among adolescents: effects on offspring gestational age, growth, and morphology. *Pediatrics.* 1995;95:738-743

16. Greenberg RA, Haley NJ, Etzel RA, Loda FA. Measuring the exposure of infants to tobacco smoke: nicotine and cotinine in urine and saliva. *N Engl J Med.* 1984;310:1075-1078

17. Tager IB, Munoz A, Rosner IB, Weiss ST, Carey V, Speizer FE. Effect of cigarette smoking on the pulmonary function of children and adolescents. *Am Rev Respir Dis.* 1985;131:752-759

18. Dwyer JH, Lippert P, Rieger-Ndakorerwa GE, Semmer NK. Some chronic disease risk factors and cigarette smoking in adolescents: the Berlin-Bremen study. *MMWR Morb Mortal Wkly Rep.* 1987;36(suppl 4):35S-40S

19. Craig WY, Palomaki GE, Johnson AM, Haddow JE. Cigarette smoking-associated changes in blood lipid levels in the 8- to 19-year-old-age group: a meta-analysis. *Pediatrics.* 1990;85:155-158

20. Jones CJ, Schiffman MH, Kurman R, Jacob P III, Benowitz NL. Elevated nicotine levels in cervical lavages from passive smokers. *Am J Public Health.* 1991;81:378-379

21. Perry C, Killen J, Telch M, Slinkard LA, Danaher BG. Modifying smoking behavior of teenagers: a school-based intervention. *Am J Public Health.* 1980;70:722-725

22. Schinke SP, Gilchrist LD, Snow WH. Skills intervention to prevent cigarette smoking among adolescents. *Am J Public Health.* 1985;75:665-667

23. Botvin GJ, Baker E, Dusenbury L, Botvin EM, Diaz T. Long-term follow-up results of a randomized drug abuse prevention trial in a white middle-class population. *JAMA.* 1995;273:1106-1112

24. *Clinical Practice Guideline Number 18: Smoking Cessation.* Rockville, MD: Agency for Health Care Policy and Research, US Dept of Health and Human Services; 1996. AHCPR Publication No. 96-0692

25. Perry CL, Silvis GL. Smoking prevention: behavioral prescriptions for the pediatrician. *Pediatrics.* 1987;79:790-799

26. American Academy of Pediatrics, Committee on Substance Abuse. Tobacco, alcohol, and other drugs: the role of the pediatrician in prevention and management of substance abuse. *Pediatrics.* 1998;101:125-128

27. Franzgrote M, Ellen JM, Millstein SG, Irwin CE Jr. Screening for adolescent smoking among primary care physicians in California. *Am J Public Health.* 1997;87:1341-1345

28. Sargent JD, Mott LA, Stevens M. Predictors of smoking cessation in adolescents. *Arch Pediatr Adolesc Med.* 1998;152:388-393.

29. Elders MJ, Perry CL, Eriksen MP, Giovino GA. The report of the Surgeon General: preventing tobacco use among young people. *Am J Public Health.* 1994;84:543-547

30. Smith TA, House RF Jr, Croghan IT, et al. Nicotine patch therapy in adolescent smokers. *Pediatrics.* 1996;98:659-667

31. Gostin LO, Arno PS, Brandt AM. FDA regulation of tobacco advertising and youth smoking: historical, social, and constitutional perspectives. *JAMA.* 1997;277:410-418

32. Pollan M. How pot has grown. *New York Times Magazine.* February 19, 1995:31-35

33. Hunt A, Jones RT. Tolerance and disposition of tetrahydrocannabinol in man. *J Pharmacol Exp Ther.* 1980;215:35-44

34. Alcohol, Drug Abuse, and Mental Health Administration. Cannabinoid receptor gene cloned. *JAMA.* 1990;264:1389

35. Axelrod J, Felder CC. Cannabinoid receptors and their endogenous agonist, anandamide. *Neurochem Res.* 1998;23:575-581

36. Adams IB, Martin BR. Cannabis: pharmacology and toxicology in animals and humans. *Addiction.* 1996;91:1585-1614

37. Tanda G, Pontieri FE, Di Chiara G. Cannabinoid and heroin activation of mesolimbic dopamine transmission by a common μ 1 opioid receptor mechanism. *Science.* 1997;276:2048-2050

38. Wickelgren I. Marijuana: harder than thought? *Science.* 1997;276: 1967-1968

39. Rodriguez de Fonseca F, Carrera MRA, Navarro M, et al. Activation of corticotropin releasing factor in the limbic system during cannabinoid withdrawal. *Science.* 1997;276:2050-2054

40. Cook SA, Lowe JA, Martin BR. CB1 receptor antagonist precipitates withdrawal in mice exposed to ä-9-tetrahydro-cannabinol. *J Pharmacol Exp Ther.* 1998;285:1150-1156

41. Selden BS, Clark RF, Curry SC. Marijuana. *Emerg Med Clin North Am.* 1990;8:527-539

42. Tashkin DP, Calvarese BM, Simmons MS, et al. Respiratory status of seventy-four habitual marijuana smokers. *Chest.* 1980;78:699-706

43. Wu T-C, Tashkin DP, Djahed B, Rose JE. Pulmonary hazards of smoking marijuana as compared with tobacco. *N Engl J Med.* 1988;318:347-351

44. Barsky SH, Roth MD, Kleerup EC, et al. Histopathologic and molecular alterations in bronchial epithelium in habitual smokers of marijuana, cocaine, and/or tobacco. *J Natl Cancer Inst.* 1998;90:1198-1205

45. Fligiel SE, Roth MD, Kleerup EC, et al. Tracheobronchial histopathology in habitual smokers of cocaine, marijuana, and/or tobacco. *Chest.* 1997;112:319-326

46. Matthias P, Tashkin DP, Marques-Magallanes JA, et al. Effects of varying marijuana potency on deposition of tar and d-9-THC in the lung during smoking. *Pharmacol Biochem Behav.* 1997;58:1145-1150

47. Hembree WC, Nahas GG, Zeidenberg P, et al. Changes in human spermatozoa associated with high dose marijuana smoking. In: Nahas GG, Paton WDM, eds. *Marijuana: Biological Effects, Analysis, Metabolism, Cellular Responses, Reproduction and Brain.* Oxford, England: Pergamon Press; 1979:424-439

48. Diamond F Jr, Ringenberg L, MacDonald, D, et al. Effects of drug and alcohol abuse upon pituitary-testicular function in adolescent males. *J Adolesc Health Care.* 1986;7:28-33

49. Shiono PH, Klebanoff MA, Nugent RP, et al. The impact of cocaine and marijuana use on low birth weight and preterm birth: a multicenter study. *Am J Obstet Gynecol.* 1995;172:19-27

50. Dreher MC, Nugent K, Hudgins R. Prenatal marijuana exposure and neonatal outcomes in Jamaica: an ethnographic study. *Pediatrics.* 1994;93:254-260

51. Asch RH, Smith CG, Siler-Khodr TM, Pauerstein CJ. Effects of d-9 THC during the follicular phase of the rhesus monkey (Macaca mulatta). *J Clin Endocrinol Metab.* 1981;52:50-55

52. Silber TJ, Iosefsohn M, Hicks JM, et al. Prevalence of PCP use among adolescent marijuana users. *J Pediatr.* 1988;112:827-829

53. Institute of Medicine, National Research Council, Division of Health Science Policy. Behavioral and psychosocial effects of marijuana use. In: Relman A, ed. *Marijuana and Health.* Washington, DC: National Academy Press; 1982:112-138

54. Milstein SL, MacCannell K, Karr G, et al. Marijuana produced impairments of coordination. *J Nerv Ment Dis.* 1975;161:26-31

55. Pope HG, Jacobs A, Mialet JP, et al. Evidence for a sex-specific residual effect of cannabis on visuospatial memory. *Psychother Psychosom.* 1997;66:179-184

56. Block RI, Farinpour R, Braverman K. Acute effects of marijuana on cognition: relationships to chronic effects and smoking techniques. *Pharmacol Biochem Behav.* 1992;43:907-917

57. Pope HG Jr, Gruber AJ, Yurgelun-Todd D. The residual neuropsychological effects of cannabis: the current status of research. *Drug Alcohol Depend.* 1995;38:25-34

58. Block RI, Ghoneim MM. Effects of chronic marijuana use on human cognition. *Psychopharmacology (Berl).* 1993;110:219-228

59. Pope HG Jr, Yurgelun-Todd D. The residual cognitive effects of heavy marijuana use in college students. *JAMA.* 1996;275:521-527

60. Schwartz RH, Gruenwald PJ, Klitzner M, Fedio P. Short-term memory impairment in cannabis-dependent adolescents. *Am J Dis Child.* 1989;143:1214-1219

61. Millman RB, Sbriglio R. Patterns of use and psychopathology in chronic marijuana users. *Psychiatr Clin North Am.* 1986;9:533-545

62. American Psychiatric Association. *Diagnostic and Statistical Manual of Mental Disorders, Third Edition, Revised (DSM-III-R)*. Washington, DC: American Psychiatric Association; 1989

63. Trosi A, Pasini A, Saracco M, Spalletta G. Psychiatric symptoms in male cannabis users not using other illicit drugs. *Addiction*. 1998;93:487-492

64. Weisbeck GA, Schuckit MA, Kalmijn JA, et al. An evaluation of the history of a marijuana withdrawal syndrome in a large population. *Addiction*. 1996;91:1469-1478

65. Duffy A, Milin R. Case study: withdrawal syndrome in adolescent chronic cannabis users. *J Am Acad Child Adolesc Psychiatr*. 1996;35:1618-1621

66. Crowley TJ, MacDonald MJ, Whitmore EA, Mikulich SK. Cannabis dependence, withdrawal, and reinforcing effects among adolescents with conduct symptoms and substance use disorders. *Drug Alcohol Depend*. 1998;50:27-37

67. Wechsler H, Isaac N. "Binge" drinkers at Massachusetts colleges. *JAMA*. 1992;267:2929-2931

68. Wechsler H, Moeykens B, Davenport A, Castillo S, Hansen J. The adverse impact of heavy episodic drinkers on other college students. *J Stud Alcohol*. 1995;56:628-634

69. Melzer-Lange MD. Violence and associated high-risk health behavior in adolescents. *Pediatr Clin North Am*. 1998;45:307-317

70. Caballeria J, Frezza M, Hernandez-Munoz R, DiPadova C, Korsten MA, Liebercs BE. Gastric origin of the first-pass metabolism of ethanol in humans: effect of gastrectomy. *Gastroenterology*. 1989;97:1205-1209

71. Frezza M, Di Padova C, Pozzato G, et al. High blood alcohol levels in women: the role of decreased gastric alcohol dehydrogenase activity and first-pass metabolism. *N Engl J Med*. 1990;322:95-99

72. Charness ME, Simon RP, Greenberg DA. Ethanol and the nervous system. *N Engl J Med*. 1989;321:442-454

73. Loiselle JM, Baker MD, Tempelton JM Jr, et al. Substance abuse in adolescent trauma. *Ann Emerg Med*. 1993;22:1530-1534

74. Jones NE, Pieper CF, Robertson LS. The effect of legal drinking age on fatal injuries of adolescents and young adults. *Am J Public Health*. 1992;82:112-115

75. Friedman IM. Alcohol and unnatural deaths in San Francisco youths. *Pediatrics*. 1985;79:191-193

76. Stephenson JN, Moberg P, Daniels BJ, Robertson JF. Treating the intoxicated adolescent: a need for comprehensive services. *JAMA*. 1984;252:1884-1888

77. King CA, Ghaziuddin N, McGovern L, et al. Predictors of comorbid alcohol and substance abuse in depressed adolescents. *J Am Acad Child Adolesc Psychiatry*. 1996;35:743-751

78. Donovan JE, Jessor R. Adolescent problem drinking. *J Stud Alcohol.* 1978;39:1506-1524
79. Ouelette EM, Rosett HL, Rosman NP, et al. Adverse effects on offspring of maternal alcohol use during pregnancy. *N Engl J Med.* 1977;297: 528-530
80. Streissguth AP, Aase JM, Clarren SK, et al. Fetal alcohol syndrome in adolescents and adults. *JAMA.* 1991;265:1961-1967
81. Centers for Disease Control and Prevention. Blood alcohol concentrations among young drivers: United States, 1982. *MMWR Morb Mortal Wkly Rep.* 1983;32:646-648
82. American Academy of Pediatrics, Committee on Substance Abuse. Alcohol use and abuse: a pediatric concern. *Pediatrics.* 1995;95: 439-442
83. Brown RT, Coupey SM. Illicit drugs of abuse. *Adolesc Med.* 1993;4: 321-340
84. Schwartz RH, Luxenberg MG, Hoffmann, NG. "Crack" use by American middle-class adolescent polydrug abusers. *J Pediatr.* 1991;118:150-155
85. Mofenson HC, Caraccio TR. Cocaine. *Pediatr Ann.* 1987;16:864-874
86. Hatsukami DK, Fischman MW. Crack cocaine and cocaine hydrochloride: are the differences myth or reality? *JAMA.* 1996;276:1580-1588
87. Farrar HC, Kearns GL. Cocaine: clinical pharmacology and toxicology. *J Pediatr.* 1989;115:665-675
88. Gawin FH, Ellinwood EH Jr. Cocaine and other stimulants: actions, abuse, and treatment. *N Engl J Med.* 1988;318:1173-1182
89. Koob GT, Vaccarino FJ, Amalric M, et al. Neural substrates for cocaine and opiate reinforcement. In: Fisher S, Raskin A, Uhlenhuth EM, eds. *Cocaine: Clinical and Behavioral Aspects.* New York, NY: Oxford University Press; 1987:80-108
90. Jones RT. Psychopharmacology of cocaine. In: Washton AM, Gold MS, eds. *Cocaine: A Clinician's Handbook.* New York, NY: Guilford Press; 1987:55-72
91. Isner JM, Estes M, Thompson PD, et al. Acute cardiac events temporally related to cocaine abuse. *N Engl J Med.* 1986;315:1438-1443
92. Marzuk PM, Tardiff K, Leon AC, et al. Ambient temperature and mortality from unintentional cocaine overdose. *JAMA.*1998;279: 1795-1800
93. Edlin BR, Irwin KL, Farque S. et al. Intersecting epidemics: crack cocaine use and HIV infection among inner-city young adults. *N Engl J Med.* 1994;331:1422-1427
94. Estroff TW. Medical and biological consequences of cocaine abuse. In: Washton AM, Gold MS, eds. *Cocaine: A Clinician's Handbook.* New York, NY: Guilford Press; 1987:23-32

95. Mayes LC, Granger RH, Bornstein MH, Zuckerman B. The problem of prenatal cocaine exposure. *JAMA.* 1992;267:406-408

96. King TA, Perlman JM, Laptook AR, et al. Neurologic manifestations of in utero cocaine exposure in near-term and term infants. *Pediatrics.* 1995;96:259-264

97. Mayes LC, Bornsetin MH, Chawarska MA, Granger RH. Information processing and developmental assessments in 3-month-old infants exposed prenatally to cocaine. *Pediatrics.* 1995;95:539-545

98. Chiriboga CA, Brust JCM, Bateman D, Hauser WA. Dose-response effect of fetal cocaine exposure on newborn neurologic function. *Pediatrics.* 1998;103:79-85

99. Morehouse ER. Treating adolescent cocaine abusers. In: Washton AM, Gold MS, eds. *Cocaine: A Clinician's Handbook.* New York, NY: Guilford Press; 1987:135-151

100. Kleber HD, Gawin FH. Pharmacological treatments of cocaine abuse. In: Washton AM, Gold MS, eds. *Cocaine: A Clinician's Handbook.* New York, NY: Guilford Press; 1987:118-134

101. Mendelson JH, Mello NK. Management of cocaine abuse and dependence. *N Engl J Med.* 1996;334:965-972

102. Pentel P. Toxicity of over-the-counter stimulants. *JAMA.*1984;252: 1898-1903

103. US Food and Drug Administration. FDA issues public health warning on phenylpropanolamine [press release]. Rockville, MD: Office of Public Affairs, US Food and Drug Administraion; November 6, 2000. Talk Paper T00-58. Available at: http://www.fda.gov/cder/drug/infopage/ppa/default.htm. Accessed March 14, 2001

104. Litovitz T. Amphetamines. In Haddad LM, Winchester JF, eds. *Clinical Management of Poisoning and Drug Overdose.* Philadelphia, PA: WB Saunders; 1983:469-475

105. Lan KC, Lin YF, Yu FC, et al. Clinical manifestations and prognostic features of acute methamphetamine intoxication. *J Formos Med Assoc.* 1998;97:528-533

106. El-Omar MM, Ray K, Geary R. Intracerebral hemorrhage in a young adult: consider amphetamine abuse. *Br J Clin Pract.* 1996;50:115-116

107. Forman HP, Levin S, Stewart B, et al. Cerebral vasculitis and hemor-rhage in an adolescent taking diet pills containing phenylpropanolamine: case report and review of literature. *Pediatrics.* 1989;83:737-741

108. Logan DK. Methamphetamine and driving impairment. *J Forensic Sci.* 1996;41:457-464

109. Cernerud L, Eriksson M, Jonsson M, et al. Amphetamine addiction during pregnancy: 14-year follow-up of growth and school performance. *Acta Paediatr.* 1996;85:204-208

110. Pelssinger MA. Prenatal exposure to amphetamines: risks and adverse outcomes in pregnancy. *Obstet Gynecol Clin North Am.* 1998;25:119-138

111. Stewart JL, Mecker JE. Fetal and infant deaths associated with maternal methamphetamine abuse. *J Anal Toxicol.* 1997;21:515-517

112. Schwartz RH. LSD: its rise, fall, and renewed popularity among high school students. *Pediatr Clin North Am.* 1995;42:403-413

113. Chilcoat HD, Schutz CG. Age-specific patterns of hallucinogen use in the U.S. population: an analysis using generalized additive models. *Drug Alcohol Depend.* 1996;43:143-153

114. Heym J, Jacobs BL. Serotonergic mechanisms of hallucinogenic drug effects. *Monogr Neural Sci.* 1987;13:55-81

115. Buckholtz NS, Zhou DF, Freedman DX, Potter WZ. Lysergic acid diethylamide (LSD) administration selectively downregulates serotonin 2 receptors in rat brain. *Neuropsychopharmacology.* 1990;3:137-148

116. Olney RK. Mescaline. *Tex Med.* 1972;68:80-82

117. Shervette RE, Schydlower M, Lampe RM, et al. Jimson "loco" weed abuse in adolescents. *Pediatrics.* 1979;63:520-523

118. Cohen S. The hallucinogens and the inhalants. *Psychiatr Clin North Am.* 1984;7:681-688

119. Beck JE, Gordon DV. Psilocybin mushrooms. *Pharm Chem Newslett.* 1982;4:1-4

120. Raff E, Halloran PF, Kjellstrand CM. Renal failure after eating "magic mushrooms." *CMAJ.* 1992;147:1339-1341

121. Abraham HD, Aldridge AM, Gogia P. The psychopharmacology of hallucinogens. *Neuropsychopharmacology.* 1996;14:285-298

122. Markel H, Lee A, Holmes RD, Domino EF. LSD flashback syndrome exacerbated by selective serotonin reuptake inhibitor antidepressants in adolescents. *J Pediatr.* 1994;125:817-819

123. Goldfrank L, Osborn H. Phencyclidine (angel dust). *Hosp Physician.* 1978;5:18-21

124. Hurlbut KM. Drug-induced psychoses. *Emerg Med Clin North Am.* 1991;9:31-52

125. Grove FE Jr. Painless self-injury after ingestion of "angel dust." *JAMA.* 1979;242:655

126. Welch MJ, Correa GA. PCP intoxication in young children and infants. *Clin Pediatr (Phila).* 1980;19:510-514

127. Strauss AA, Mondanlou HD, Bosu SK. Neonatal manifestations of maternal phencyclidine (PCP) abuse. *Pediatrics.* 1981;68:550-552

128. Aronow R, Done AK. Phencyclidine overdose: an emerging concept of management. *J Am Coll Emerg Phys.* 1978;7:56-59

129. Climko RP, Roehrich H, Sweeney DR, A-Razi J. Ecstasy: a review of MDMA and MDA. *Int J Psychiatry Med.* 1986-87;16:359-372

130. Cuomo MJ, Dyment PG, Gammino VM. Increasing use of ecstasy (MDMA) and other hallucinogens on a college campus. *J Am Coll Health*. 1994;41:271-274

131. Schwartz RH, Miller NS. MDMA (ecstasy) and the rave: a review. *Pediatrics*. 1997;100:705-708

132. Williams H, Dratcu L, Taylor R, et al. Saturday night fever: ecstasy related problems in a London accident and emergency department. *J Accid Emerg Med*. 1998;15:322-326

133. Sultana SR, Byrne DJ. Raver's hematuria. *J R Coll Surg Edinb*. 1996;41:419-420

134. Dowling GP, McDonough ET III, Bost RO. "Eve" and "ecstasy": a report of 5 deaths associated with the use of MDEA and MDMA. *JAMA*. 1987;257:1615-1617

135. Andreu V, Mas A, Bruguera M, et al. Ecstasy: a common cause of severe acute hepatotoxicity. *J Hepatol*. 1998;29:394-397

136. Brauer RB, Heidecke CD, Nathrath W, et al. Liver transplantation for the treatment of fulminant hepatic failure induced by the ingestion of ecstasy. *Transpl Int*. 1997;10:229-233

137. Parrot AC, Lees A, Garnham NJ, et al. Cognitive performance in recreational users of MDMA "ecstasy": evidence for memory deficits. *J Psychopharmacol (Oxf)*. 1998;12:79-83

138. Ricaurte GA, Forno LS, Wilson MA. 3,4-methylene dioxymethamphetamine selectively damages central serotonergic neurons in nonhuman primates. *JAMA*. 1988;260:51-55

139. American Medical Association Council on Scientific Affairs. Medical and nonmedical uses of anabolic-androgenic steroids. *JAMA*. 1990;264:2923-2927

140. Yesalis CE, Barsukiewicz CK, Kopstein AN, Bahrke MS. Trends in anabolic-androgenic steroid use among adolescents. *Arch Pediatr Adolesc Med*. 1997;151:1197-1206

141. Terney R, McLain LG. The use of anabolic steroids in high school students. *Am J Dis Child*. 1990;144:99-103

142. DuRant RH, Escobedo LG, Heath GW. Anabolic steroid use, strength training, and multiple drug use among adolescents in the United States. *Pediatrics*. 1995;96:23-28

143. Department of Health and Human Services Office of the Inspector General. *Adolescents and Steroids: A User Perspective*. Washington, DC: Department of Health and Human Services; 1990. Publication OEI-06-90-01081

144. Department of Health and Human Services, Office of the Inspector General. *Adolescent Steroid Use*. Washington, DC: Department of Health and Human Services; 1991. Publication No. OEI-06-90-01080

145. Tennant F, Black DL, Voy RO. Anabolic steroid dependence with opioid-type features. *N Engl J Med.* 1988;319:578

146. Fingerhood MI, Sullivan JT, Testa M, Jasinski DR. Abuse liability of testosterone. *J Psychopharmacol (Oxf).* 1997;11:59-63

147. Masonis AE, McCarthy MP. Direct interactions of androgenic/anabolic steroids with the peripheral benzodiazepine receptor in rat brain: implications for the psychological and physiological manifestations of androgenic/anabolic steroid abuse. *J Steroid Biochem Mol Biol.* 1996;58:551-555

148. Clark AS, Lindenfield RC, Gibbons CH. Anabolic-androgenic steroids and brain reward. *Pharmacol Biochem Behav.* 1996;53:741-745

149. Hallagan JB, Hallagan LF, Snyder MB. Anabolic-androgenic steroid use by athletes. *N Engl J Med.* 1989;321:1042-1045

150. Canadian Center for Drug-free Sport. The use of anabolic-androgenic steroids by Canadian students. *Clin J Sport Med.* 1996;6:9-14

151. Pope HG Jr, Katz DL. Psychiatric and medical effects of anabolic-androgenic steroid use: a controlled study of 160 athletes. *Arch Gen Psychiatry.* 1994;51:375-382

152. Tricker R, Casaburi R, Storer TW, et al. The effects of supraphysiological doses of testosterone on angry behavior in healthy eugonadal men: a clinical research center study. *J Clin Endocrinol Metab.* 1996;81:3754-3758

153. Middleman AB, Faulkner AH, Woods ER, et al. High-risk behaviors among high school students in Massachusetts who use anabolic steroids. *Pediatrics.* 1995;96:268-272

154. Meilman PW, Crace RK, Presley CA, Lyerla R. Beyond performance enhancement: polypharmacy among collegiate users of steroids. *Am J Coll Health.* 1995;44:98-104

155. Schanzer W, Delahaut P, Geyer H, et al. Long-term detection and identification of metandienone and stanozolol abuse in athletes by gas chromatography–high resolution mass spectrometry. *J Chromatogr B Biomed Appl.* 1996;6:93-108

156. Caitlin DH, Hatton CK, Starcevic SH. Issues in detecting abuse of xenobiotic anabolic steroids and testosterone by analysis of athletes' urine. *Clin Chem.* 1997;43:1280-1288

157. Goldberg L, Elliot D, Clarke GN, et al. Effects of a multi-dimensional anabolic steroid prevention intervention. *JAMA.* 1996;276:1555-1562

158. Goldberg L, Bents R, Bosworth, E, et al. Anabolic steroid education and adolescents: do scare tactics work? *Pediatrics.* 1991;87:283-286

159. Bruner AB, Fishman M. Adolescents and illicit drug use. *JAMA.* 1998;280:597-598

160. Ziporyn T. Growing industry and menace: makeshift laboratory's designer drugs. *JAMA.* 1986;256:3061-3063

161. Brittain JL. China white: the bogus drug. *J Toxicol Clin Toxicol.* 1982;19:1123-1126

162. Hibbs J, Perper J, Winek CL. An outbreak of designer drug–related deaths in Pennsylvania. *JAMA.* 1991;265:1011-1013

163. Ford M, Hoffman RS, Goldfrank LR. Opioids and designer drugs. *Emerg Med Clin North Am.* 1990;8:495-511

164. Easom JM, Lovejoy FH Jr. Opiates: In Haddad LM, Winchester JF, eds. *Clinical Management of Poisoning and Drug Overdose.* Philadelphia, PA: WB Saunders; 1983:424-433

165. Shesser R, Jotte R, Olshaker J. The contribution of impurities to the acute morbidity of illegal drug use. *Am J Emerg Med.* 1991;9:336-342

166. Centers for Disease Control and Prevention. Scopolamine poisoning among heroin users: New York City, Newark, Philadelphia, and Baltimore, 1995 and 1996. *MMWR Morb Mortal Wkly Rep.* 1996;45:457-460

167. Langston JW. Parkinson's disease: current view. *Am Fam Physician.* 1987;35:201-206

168. Widner H, Tetrud J, Rehncrona S, et al. Bilateral fetal mesencephalic grafting in 2 patients with parkinsonism induced by 1-methyl-4-phenyl-1,2,3,6-tetrahydropyridine (MPTP). *N Engl J Med.* 1992;327:1556-1563

169. Effective medical treatment of opiate addiction. National Consensus Development Panel on Effective Medical Treatment of Opiate Addiction. *JAMA.* 1998;280:1936-1943

170. Treatment of acute drug abuse reactions. *Med Lett Drugs Ther.* 1987;29:83-86

171. Yaster M, Kost-Byerly S, Berde C, Billet C. The management of opioid and benzodiazepine dependence in infants, children, and adolescents. *Pediatrics.* 1996;98:135-140

172. Coupey SM. Barbiturates. *Pediatr Rev.* 1997;18:260-265

173. Osborn H, Goldfrank LR. Sedative-hypnotic agents. In: Goldfrank LR, Flomenbaum NE, Lewin NA, Weisman RS, Howland MA, Hoffman RS, eds. *Toxicologic Emergencies.* 5th ed. Norwalk, CT: Appleton & Lange; 1994

174. Litovitz T. Methaqualone. In: Haddad LM, Winchester JF, eds. *Clinical Management of Poisoning and Drug Overdose.* Philadelphia, PA: WB Saunders; 1983:466-469

175. Reinisch JM, Sanders SA, Mortensen EL, Rubin DB. In utero exposure to phenobarbital and intelligence deficits in adult men. *JAMA.* 1995;274:1518-1525

176. Wesson DR, Smith DE, Seymour RB. Sedative-hypnotics and tricyclics. In: Lowinson JH, Ruiz P, Millman RB, Langrod JG, eds. *Substance Abuse: A Comprehensive Textbook.* 2nd ed. Baltimore, MD: Williams & Wilkins; 1992:271-279

177. Smith DE, Wesson DR. Phenobarbital technique for treatment of barbiturate dependence. *Arch Gen Psychiatry.* 1971;24:56-60
178. Rickert VI, Wiemann CM, Berenson AB. Prevalence, patterns, and correlates of voluntary flunitrazepam use. *Pediatrics.* 1999;103(1). URL: http://www.pediatrics.org/cgi/content/full/103/1/e6
179. Litovitz T. Benzodiazepines. In: Haddad LM, Winchester JF, eds. *Clinical Management of Poisoning and Drug Overdose.* Philadelphia, PA: WB Saunders Co; 1983:475-482
180. Pratt JA, Brett RR, Laurie DJ. Benzodiazepine dependence: from neural circuits to gene expression. *Pharmacol Biochem Behav.* 1998;59:925-934
181. Choice of benzodiazepines. *Med Lett Drugs Ther.* 1988;30:25-28
182. Calhoun SR, Wesson DR, Galloway GP, Smith DE. Abuse of flunitrazepam (Rohypnol) and other benzodiazepines in Austin and south Texas. *J Psychoactive Drugs.* 1996;28:183-189
183. Mellor CS, Jain VK. Diazepam withdrawal syndrome: its prolonged and changing nature. *Can Med Assoc J.* 1982;127:1093-1096
184. Higgitt AC, Lader MH, Fonagy P. Clinical management of benzo-diazepine dependence. *Br Med J (Clin Res Ed).* 1985;291:688-690
185. Neumark YD, Delva J, Anthony JC. The epidemiology of adolescent inhalant drug involvement. *Arch Pediatr Adolesc Med.* 1998;152: 781-786
186. Fortenberry JD. Gasoline sniffing. *Am J Med.* 1985;79:740-744
187. Zebrowski PL, Gregory RJ. Inhalant use patterns among Eskimo school children in western Alaska. *J Addict Dis.* 1996;15:67-77
188. Schwartz RH, Peary P. Abuse of isobutyl nitrite inhalation (Rush) by adolescents. *Clin Pediatr (Phila).* 1986;25:308-310
189. Bass M. Sudden sniffing death. *JAMA.* 1970;212:2075-2079
190. King GS, Smialek JE, Troutman WG. Sudden death in adolescents resulting from the inhalation of typewriter correction fluid. *JAMA.* 1985;253:1604-1606
191. Cohen S. The volatile nitrites. *JAMA.* 1979;241:2077-2078
192. National Institute on Drug Abuse. *Community Alert Bulletin.* Bethesda, MD: National Institute on Drug Abuse; 1999. NIH Publication No. 00-4723

Chapter 9

Tobacco Use and Abuse

Richard B. Heyman, MD, FAAP

Scope of the Problem

The early onset of tobacco use defines it as a pediatric disease,[1] because an estimated 6000 young people smoke their first cigarette each day.[2-4] Approximately 90% of all tobacco users begin before 19 years of age, at an average age of 12.5 years.[5] Each year more than 400 000 people die of tobacco-related illnesses in the United States,[1] including an estimated 3000 who die from lung cancer caused by environmental tobacco smoke (ETS).[6]

The *Monitoring the Future* study[7] suggests that, despite some recent progress made in decreasing youth smoking, more than one third of today's high school students are active smokers when they graduate. The cigarette smoking rate reached its peak among this age group in the mid 1990s. As of 1999, 17.5% of eighth graders identified themselves as current smokers, as did 25.7% of tenth graders and 36.5% of twelfth graders.

Smokeless tobacco (SLT) products are perceived by many young people as less dangerous, because they are unaware of SLT's intrinsic health hazards. A pouch of chewing tobacco consists of ground leaf and usually is chewed in golf ball-sized "wads." Cured ground tobacco is marketed as dry or moist snuff (usually in small tins), and those who "dip" place a pinch between the lower lip and cheek. Use of such products has remained steady for the last 5 years; 8.4%, 6.5%, and 4.5% of twelfth, tenth, and eighth graders, respectively, regularly use SLT.[7]

Many consider that the onset of tobacco use is a marker that predicts progression to the use of other drugs[8] and describe how it may help young people gradually move into the drug culture.[9] The availability of tobacco and society's "acceptance" of its use encourage young people to try it. By so doing, they learn how to acquire and use a drug and explore how a psychoactive drug works.

Furthermore, they learn to control their use to achieve the desired effect and build defenses against those who would criticize their use.[9] Young people readily identify that those who smoke are indeed more likely to use other drugs, including marijuana.[10] Therefore, the choice to use tobacco must be placed in perspective as a major risk behavior that may be part of a series of similar choices to pursue other risk behaviors.

Risk Factors for Initiation of Tobacco Use

Young people choose to initiate tobacco use for a wide variety of reasons, and insight into this issue may provide the health care professional with tools for prevention. The 1994 *Report of the Surgeon General*[2] identifies 4 basic categories of risk factors:

1. Environmental: availability, family use, social support for smoking and use of SLT, peer use, and exposure to the tobacco industry's advertising and promotion programs;
2. Sociodemographic: low socioeconomic status, limited parental education, and early stage of adolescent development (when most tobacco use begins);
3. Behavioral: low academic achievement, low aspiration for future success, lack of commitment to school and activities, and other risk behaviors (such as truancy, encounters with the juvenile justice system, rebelliousness); and
4. Personal: perceived value and functional meaning of tobacco use (what the cigarette or SLT does for the young person or the image obtained by using), psychologic sense of well-being, self-efficacy (one's assessment of how much control one has over one's activities), and knowledge of consequences.

Recent research suggests that advertising, promotion, and media exposure may have the strongest role in convincing young people to try tobacco products.[11] The portrayal of smoking as the norm and of smokers as sexy, independent, popular, successful, wealthy, thin, athletic, and rebellious is enticing to adolescents. Studies of brand preferences of young people reveal that the 3 most heavily advertised brands of cigarettes (Marlboro [Philip Morris USA,

New York, NY], Camel [RJ Reynolds Tobacco Holdings Inc, Winston-Salem, NC], and Newport [Lorillard Tobacco Co Inc, Greensboro, NC]) account for some 80% of cigarette sales to adolescents.[12] These 3 brands control less than a third of the adult market, suggesting that young people are more susceptible to the effects of advertising and make consumer choices more on the basis of image. Current antismoking campaigns sponsored by the tobacco industry that promote smoking as an adult habit and a choice to be made by those mature enough to make such a choice may be counterproductive, because young people may decide that smoking is a quick and easy way to "buy" the adult image.

Research in the area of risk behavior theory[13] suggests that the choice to use tobacco is but one of many behaviors subject to risk and protective factors. Tobacco use often is associated with illicit drug use, delinquency, running away, truancy, unhealthy lifestyle choices, and inability to hold a job. Tobacco use in the context of other risk behaviors identifies a young person who is willing to take chances, rebel against authority, and risk future good health.

Nicotine as the Reason for Tobacco Use

Young people begin to use tobacco for a variety of reasons, and most experiment with cigarettes; however, smoking as few as 3 cigarettes increases the likelihood of becoming a regular smoker.[14] Nearly half of high school students who smoke report they wish they could stop. Furthermore, most twelfth graders who smoke do not think they will be smoking 5 years after they graduate. Most assume they can quit smoking at will, yet surveys suggest that most will make a number of attempts to quit and that their success rate is no better than that of adult smokers.[2]

Nicotine is perhaps the most addictive of all substances. Its presence in tobacco products generally is accepted by researchers and the tobacco industry to be the reason people continue to use tobacco. Intake via the lungs in the volatile form is the most effective way to ingest the chemical, and the vaporization of nicotine from cigarettes represents an extremely efficient mechanism for its delivery. A puff on a cigarette delivers nicotine to the brain within 20 seconds, and the half-life of the chemical is 2 to 3 hours. A single cigarette can create detectable nicotine levels for 8 to 12 hours in most users. Regular users modulate their nicotine levels during the day, allow them to decrease through the night, and then need a quick morning dose to begin the process again.[14]

The biochemistry of nicotine is well understood. Structurally, the chemical resembles acetylcholine and is selectively bound to certain cholinergic receptors in the brain and other organs of the body. Activation of these cholinergic receptors enhances the release of a variety of neurotransmitters and hormones, including acetylcholine, vasopressin, epinephrine and norepinephrine, β-endorphin, and serotonin.

Research suggests that the release of specific neurotransmitters is responsible for many of the observed physiologic effects of nicotine. For example, dopamine release is associated with appetite suppression and a general sensation of pleasure, norepinephrine with arousal, acetylcholine with cognitive enhancement, vasopressin with improved memory, serotonin with a sense of mellowness, and β-endorphin with decrease of tension and anxiety. Other physiologic effects of nicotine include skeletal muscle relaxation, increased basal metabolism, acceleration of heart rate, generalized vasoconstriction, increased cardiac output and blood pressure, and changes in brain wave patterns.[15]

Discontinuation of tobacco use creates a syndrome of nicotine withdrawal that, in many aspects, reflects the obverse of the physiologic effects of the chemical. Symptoms may include restlessness, increased appetite, anxiety, impatience, irritability, difficulty concentrating, depression, loss of energy, digestive problems, sweating, headaches, insomnia, palpitations, tremors, and cigarette craving. Many of these symptoms are decreased dramatically with nicotine replacement therapy, giving further credence to the fact that tobacco use creates nicotine dependency.[16]

The actions and effects of nicotine meet the criteria for an addictive substance according to the *Diagnostic and Statistical Manual of Mental Disorders, Fourth Edition (DSM-IV)*.[17] These criteria include tolerance (need for increasing amounts to achieve the same effect); withdrawal (specific symptoms related to discontinuation of use); use in larger amounts over time than was intended; persistent efforts to cut down or discontinue use; increasing time spent using the substance to obtain the desired effects; effect on social, occupational, or recreational activities; and continued use despite physical or psychologic consequences of such use.

Toxic Effects of Tobacco

Thousands of compounds are released as tobacco burns. In addition to the pharmacologically active nicotine, other chemicals found in inhaled and sidestream cigarette smoke include carbon monoxide, cyanide, and a host of toxic hydrocarbons that represent products of combustion.[2] These compounds have well-documented effects on the smoker and the nonsmoker exposed to ETS. A variety of chemicals are released when SLT is used as well.

Effects on the Smoker

The main effect of tobacco smoke is on the respiratory tract. The various noxious chemicals found in smoke irritate and damage the cilia and mucous membranes with resultant increased phlegm production, decreased natural resistance to infectious agents, wheezing, and damage to alveolar air sacs. This irritation and damage results in a significantly increased incidence of chronic cough, increased nasal secretions, and upper respiratory and sinus infection. Long-term effects of cigarette smoking include the development of acute and chronic bronchitis and emphysema, abnormalities of blood lipids, and atherosclerotic cardiovascular disease. Cigarette smoking as a cause of lung cancer is well documented and is clearly subject to a dose-response effect[2] (see Chapter 8).

Effects on the Child or Adolescent Exposed to Cigarette Smoke

Children born to mothers who smoke during pregnancy are more likely to have low birth weight and underdeveloped lungs and respiratory distress. A number of epidemiologic studies indicate that prenatal and parental smoking are major risk factors for sudden infant death syndrome, the most common cause of death during the first year of life.[18] Children who grow up in homes with a parent who smokes may experience suboptimal lung development and are more likely to have repeated upper respiratory and ear infections. This risk has been demonstrated in a variety of prospective and retrospective studies and persists while controlling for a host of other variables. Exposure to ETS also increases the likelihood that a child will need tonsillectomy, adenoidectomy, and tympanostomy tube placement. The incidence of bronchitis and pneumonia is dramatically increased, and as many as 20% of hospitalizations for the treatment of lower respiratory tract illness in children are directly related to exposure to ETS.[19]

Young people with asthma suffer more exacerbations and hospitalizations if they are exposed to smoke in the home, and ETS may trigger the onset of the disease.[2] Exposure to ETS is associated with higher rates of school absenteeism and increased emergency department visits for treatment of respiratory ailments (see Chapter 8).

Effects of SLT

Because nicotine is absorbed readily through the oral mucous membranes, SLT is as addictive as smoked tobacco. In addition, the prolonged exposure of the sensitive buccal tissues to the moist tobacco causes an increased incidence of leukoplakia and various forms of oral cancer. Prolonged use of SLT can cause tooth discoloration and decay, gum recession, and consequent tooth loss. Chewing tobacco promotes excess salivation that necessitates frequent spitting—a social, health, and environmental drawback.[20]

Role of the Health Care Professional in Addressing Tobacco Use

Because nicotine is addictive and there are discouraging problems that face young people trying to quit tobacco use once the habit is established, it is clear that primary prevention is likely to be the most successful approach for dealing with tobacco use. There is a clear role for the health care professional in addressing this issue, and it should be placed on the anticipatory guidance and prevention agenda. The American Academy of Pediatrics,[6] the American

Medical Association,[21] and the Maternal and Child Health Bureau[22] have stressed the importance of tobacco prevention messages when providing routine health care to children and adolescents.

Perhaps the most important role for the health care professional is simply to raise the issue. Discussing sensitive topics with parents and patients can be difficult, and many health care professionals sidestep issues such as tobacco, alcohol, and other drug use when interviewing families. Parents and children expect to be asked about these sensitive topics,[23] and these issues can be handled effectively by most health care professionals. Raising an issue or discovering a problem does not mean that it must be "solved" at that visit. Simply discussing it may be therapeutic, and at the least, follow-up and referral can be arranged (see Chapter 2).

Tobacco Use Prevention and the Health Care Professional

Messages to prevent the use of tobacco fall into 3 general categories, which all may be valuable. Specifics should be individualized on the basis of age and developmental stage of the patient.

Factual Education

All children and adolescents should be given information about tobacco use. The dangers of tobacco—smoked and smokeless—should be stressed. Health effects should be pointed out as indicated.

Affective Education

Messages about self-esteem and self-image may help young people avoid problem behaviors, such as delinquency, lack of motivation, and beginning to use tobacco. Emphasizing responsibility to self, family, and community may elicit feelings of self-worth that decrease the likelihood of tobacco use. Better endurance for athletes, sexual attractiveness, and more money to spend on things desired rather than watching it "go up in smoke" make sense to young people, who may feel invincible when it comes to their health.

Social Influences Resistance

The misperception that most people use tobacco, the vulnerability to image advertising of tobacco products, and the desire to appear and act more like adult role models are, perhaps, the 3 most prominent reasons young people begin using tobacco. A critical aspect in the prevention of tobacco use is to break down these social influences by stressing that most people do not smoke; that smoking will not make one more glamorous, sexy, cool, independent, or macho; and that although smoking is portrayed as an adult habit, tobacco use does not make one an adult.

The National Cancer Institute's *How to Help Your Patients Stop Smoking: A Manual for Physicians*[24] organizes the physician's role into 5 basic categories, all conveniently beginning with the letter "A." Other health care professionals can use these guidelines as well.[3] The character of these activities may differ depending on the family situation.

Anticipate

The health care professional meeting prospective parents should stress the importance of a tobacco-free environment and mention the relationship of smoking to sudden infant death syndrome and a variety of childhood illnesses. Discussions about tobacco use should begin with the child and family at an early age as values and standards are developing. Age-appropriate messages should focus on health effects, dangers, obeying parents, and role models. Allowing children to have candy cigarettes should be discouraged. Older children showing signs of rebelliousness and other risk behaviors are at greater risk of beginning tobacco use and should receive a confidential discussion about its use. Prevention activities should begin during the early grades, and specific discussion of tobacco and its short-term effects should be part of every health maintenance visit beginning in elementary school.

Ask

Ask parents if they smoke and if their children are exposed to ETS at home or other locations. Ask children if they know about tobacco and its dangers, and ask older children and adolescents if they have friends who smoke or find themselves in places where others are smoking. Ask if anyone has ever offered them tobacco products and if they have tried smoking or chewing. Affix a prominent label or stamp to the chart of every tobacco-using patient, and discuss the issue at every visit. Even brief antismoking messages are effective prevention and cessation strategies.

Advise

Parents and children who smoke and use SLT should be given a "quit" message at every visit. Stress the relationship between recurrent childhood and chronic illnesses and exposure to ETS. Remind parents that they are the role models of acceptable behavior for their children and that children who choose to use tobacco products may be at risk of using other drugs of abuse.

Assist

All tobacco users should be offered help in quitting. Older children may begin to feel pressure to try tobacco and should be offered strategies to resist. Role-playing about how to say "no" and setting limits may be appropriate for parents, children, and adolescents. Specific strategies, including use of counseling and nicotine replacement therapy, are reviewed elsewhere in this chapter.

Arrange

Arrange follow-up for all smokers and users of SLT, at which time additional help can be offered and progress toward cessation can be monitored.

The Health Care Professional's Role in Tobacco Cessation Efforts

It is the responsibility of the health care professional to address the issue of tobacco cessation with parents and young people who smoke or use SLT. Surveys suggest that substantially more than half of all homes contain at least 1 smoker and that 90% of parents who smoke do not object to having this issue raised by their child's physician.[23] Studies confirm that as many as three fourths of all adolescent smokers have made at least 1 quit attempt,[2,10,25] which suggests that the average health care professional has many opportunities every day to influence adolescents to quit smoking.

Evidence-based research suggests that tobacco intervention programs for young people should follow the general guidelines of programs that have been successful with adults.[25] Motivating tobacco users to quit, especially young users, can be difficult. The concept of the "5 Rs" provides a useful strategy for addressing this issue with parents and young people who smoke or use SLT.[4,26,27]

Relevance

Provide information and motivation that is directly relevant to the user's situation. For example, pregnant mothers who smoke can be educated about the effects of tobacco on the fetus and newborn. Parents of young children who are experiencing ETS-related illness are especially good candidates for smoking cessation advice, because there may be profound economic and health implications. Young people may be particularly susceptible to issues such as exposing the tobacco industry's manipulation, the fact that most young people do not smoke, the annual cost of purchasing tobacco, and the fact that nicotine addiction robs them of true freedom.

Risks

The potential risks of tobacco use are known to most users, but highlighting the most personally significant risks may be useful. Young people think concretely and may relate best to consequences such as bad breath, stained fingers and teeth, smelly clothes, expense, and peer pressure.

Rewards

Young people may recognize the immediate benefits of cessation, including saving money, feeling better about oneself, better sports performance, freedom from addiction, and the end of parental pressure to quit.

Roadblocks

Smokers encounter a number of challenges in their attempts to quit tobacco use. Reassuring adolescent smokers about a number of issues can be most helpful. Weight gain is likely to be minimal and limited; friends who smoke are unlikely to be offended by a quit attempt; half of all people who have ever smoked have successfully quit; and life and good times will go on after stopping smoking.

Repetition

Regularly reviewing the motivation to quit may help the tobacco user feel more inclined to try.

Tobacco Cessation Therapy for Adolescents

The clinical guideline on smoking cessation published by the Agency for Healthcare Research and Quality suggests 3 general strategies for treating tobacco use in children and adolescents. The use of tobacco should be identified in the patient chart, and health care professionals should feel comfortable raising the issue and offering a brief message about not using tobacco or about cessation of use at every opportunity. Treatment strategies include the following[25]:

1. Provide social support. By communicating caring and concern, the health care professional can encourage the patient to talk about tobacco use and promote the motivation to quit. Identification of the 5 Rs can make this strategy particularly personal and effective for young people. Health care professionals should be aware of formal smoking cessation programs offered in their communities by agencies such as health maintenance organizations, the American Cancer Society, the American Heart Association, and the American Lung Association.

2. Offer problem-solving and skills training advice. Because so much use of tobacco by children and adolescents has a social origin, the health care professional can help young people identify specific situations in which they are likely to smoke or use SLT. Examples include times of stress, exposure to other smokers, getting into an argument, or being in a "trigger situation" in which tobacco use is a coping reflex. Learning to identify such situations is an important first step in the quitting process.

3. Provide pharmacologic therapy on a selective basis.[28] Nicotine transdermal systems (eg, NicoDerm CQ [SmithKline Beecham Consumer Healthcare, Pittsburgh, PA], Habitrol [Novartis Consumer Health, Summit, NJ], Nicotrol [McNeil Consumer Products, Fort Washington, PA]) and gum are available for

over-the-counter purchase. Studies suggest that nicotine replacement therapy can be effective in tobacco cessation programs for youth, and there is no reason the health care professional cannot prescribe nicotine replacement therapy for carefully selected patients. Although a detailed discussion of the use of patches and gum is beyond the scope of this guide, the following points are relevant:

a. Nicotine replacement increases the rate of smoking cessation for motivated patients. There is little statistical evidence for its efficacy in young people or use in light smokers (ie, those using fewer than 10 cigarettes per day).

b. Nicotine replacement therapy should generally not be used by those who continue to smoke or use SLT. Therefore, the motivation to quit should be explored carefully and documented before nicotine replacement therapy is instituted, especially for young people for whom tobacco use has significant social and psychologic implications.

c. Studies suggest that the nicotine patch provides more uniform and predictable blood nicotine levels and is probably the most useful form of nicotine replacement therapy. Many clinicians supplement the baseline nicotine level provided by the patch by encouraging the concomitant use of nicotine gum or spray to control sudden urges to smoke.

d. Treatment for 8 weeks has been shown to be as effective as longer treatment. Most nicotine patches are marketed in several strengths. Package inserts give detailed instructions that can be modified based on the user's previous attempts to quit, experience with nicotine replacement therapy, and the level of use and addiction. In general, the higher dose patches are used for 1 month, followed by gradual tapering to lower strengths. Careful follow-up visits are indicated to monitor progress and provide ongoing support.

e. Other medications, including bupropion hydrochloride, clonidine hydrochloride, and nortriptyline hydrochloride, may be effective second-line pharmacologic choices when nicotine replacement is deemed inappropriate or ineffective.

Conclusion

The choice to use tobacco is commonly the first of a series of bad choices young people make as they enter adolescence. Tobacco use should be viewed as an important risk behavior that may serve as a marker for current and future risk behaviors. Health care professionals should be aware of the various factors that govern a young person's decision to use tobacco and should consider instituting the following policies into their practice:

1. Identify prominently the charts of all patients and parents who use tobacco.
2. Talk about tobacco-related issues at every health maintenance visit and use episodic illness related to tobacco use as an opportunity to discuss cessation with parents and young users.
3. Recognize the dangers associated with tobacco use and exposure to ETS and review these problems with families in which there is a tobacco user.
4. Be prepared to discuss cessation techniques with parents and young people, and help identify factors that might provide the motivation to quit.

References

1. Kessler DA, Natanblut SL, Wilkenfeld JP, et al. Nicotine addiction: a pediatric disease. *J Pediatr.* 1997;130:518-524
2. Centers for Disease Control and Prevention, National Center for Chronic Disease Prevention and Health Promotion, Office on Smoking and Health. *Preventing Tobacco Use Among Young People: A Report of the Surgeon General.* Washington, DC: Government Printing Office; 1994
3. Epps RP, Manley MW, Glynn TJ. Tobacco use among adolescents. Strategies for prevention. *Pediatr Clin North Am.* 1995;42:389-402
4. American Academy of Pediatrics, Committee on Substance Abuse. Tobacco's toll: implications for the pediatrician. *Pediatrics.* 2001;107:794-798
5. Heyman RB. Tobacco: prevention and cessation strategies. In: *Adolescent Health Update.* Vol. 9. Elk Grove Village, IL: American Academy of Pediatrics; 1997:1-8
6. American Academy of Pediatrics, Committee on Substance Abuse. Tobacco-free environment: an imperative for the health of children and adolescents. *Pediatrics.* 1994;93:866-888

7. Johnston LD, Bachman JG, O'Malley PM. *The Monitoring the Future National Survey Results on Adolescent Drug Use: Overview of Key Findings, 1999.* Rockville, MD: National Institute on Drug Abuse; 2000. NIH Publication No. 00-4690

8. Yamaguchi K, Kandel DB. Patterns of drug use from adolescence to young adulthood, III: predictors of progression. *Am J Public Health.* 1984;74:673-681

9. Slade J. Adolescent nicotine use and dependence. *Adolesc Med.* 1993;4:305-320

10. Columbia University, Center on Addiction and Substance Abuse. *CASA National Survey of American Attitudes on Substance Abuse.* New York, NY: Center on Addiction and Substance Abuse; 1995

11. Evans N, Farkas A, Gilpin E, Berry C, Pierce JP. Influence of tobacco marketing and exposure to smokers on adolescent susceptibility to smoking. *J Natl Cancer Inst.* 1995;87:20;1538-1545

12. Pierce JP, Gilpin E, Burns DM, et al. Does tobacco advertising target young people to start smoking? Evidence from California. *JAMA.* 1991;266:3154-3158

13. Jessor R. Risk behavior in adolescence: a psychosocial framework for understanding and action. *J Adolesc Health.* 1991;12:597-605

14. Institute of Medicine, Committee on Preventing Nicotine Addiction in Children and Youths. *Growing Up Tobacco Free: Preventing Nicotine Addiction in Children and Youths.* Lynch BS, Bonnie RJ, eds. Washington, DC: National Academy Press; 1994

15. Centers for Disease Control and Prevention. *The Health Consequences of Smoking: Nicotine Addiction: A Report of the Surgeon General, 1988.* Rockville, MD: US Dept of Health and Human Services; 1988. DHHS Publication No. CDC 88-8406

16. Gritz ER, Carr CR, Marcus AC. The tobacco withdrawal syndrome in unaided quitters. *Br J Addict.* 1991;86:1, 57-69

17. American Psychiatric Association. *Diagnostic and Statistical Manual of Mental Disorders, Fourth Edition (DSM-IV).* Washington, DC. American Psychiatric Association; 1994

18. Schoendorf KC, Kiely JL. Relationship of sudden infant death syndrome to maternal smoking during and after pregnancy. *Pediatrics.* 1992;90:905-908

19. DiFranza JR, Lew RA. Morbidity and mortality in children associated with the use of tobacco products by other people. *Pediatrics.* 1996;97:560-568

20. US Department of Health and Human Services, Public Health Service: *The Health Consequences of Using Smokeless Tobacco: A Report to the Advisory Committee to the Surgeon General.* Bethesda, MD: US Department of Health and Human Services; 1986. NIH Publication No. 86-2874

21. Levenberg PB, Elster AB. *Guidelines for Adolescent Preventive Services (GAPS)*. Chicago, IL: American Medical Association; 1995

22. Green M, ed. *Bright Futures: Guidelines for Health Supervision of Infants, Children and Adolescents*. Arlington, VA: National Center for Education in Maternal and Child Health; 1994

23. Burns D, ed. *Tobacco and the Clinician: Interventions for Medical and Dental Practice*. Bethesda, MD: US Department of Health and Human Services; 1994. NIH Publication No. 94-3693

24. Glynn TJ, Manley MW. *How to Help Your Patients Stop Smoking*. Bethesda, MD: US Department of Health and Human Services, National Cancer Institute; 1991. NIH Publication No. 92-3064

25. Fiore MC, Bailey WC, Cohen SJ, et al. *Treating Tobacco Use and Dependence*. Clinical Practice Guideline. Rockville, MD: Agency for Healthcare Research and Quality; 2000. AHRQ Publication No. 00-0032

26. Agency for Health Care Policy and Research. *Smoking Cessation Clinical Practice Guidelines*. Rockville, MD: Agency for Health Care Policy and Research; 1996. AHCPR Publication No. 96-0692

27. Fiore MC, Bailey WC, Cohen SJ, et al. *Treating Tobacco Use and Dependence. Quick Reference Guide for Clinicians*. Rockville, MD: US Department of Health and Human Services, Public Health Service. October 2000.

28. Centers for Disease Control and Prevention, National Center for Chronic Disease Prevention and Health Promotion, Office on Smoking and Health. *Reducing Tobacco Use: A Report of the Surgeon General*. Atlanta, GA: Centers for Disease Control and Prevention; 2000

Chapter 10

Perinatal Exposure to Maternal Substances of Abuse: Effect on the Developing Child

Ira J. Chasnoff, MD, FAAP

Although substance abuse is not a new phenomenon, it was not until the early 1970s that the modern description of fetal alcohol syndrome[1] turned clinicians' attention to the use of recreational drugs during pregnancy. This description was soon followed by the description of neonatal abstinence syndrome in newborns undergoing withdrawal attributable to their mothers' use of opiates, especially heroin, during pregnancy.[2] The emergence of cocaine in the 1980s as a drug of choice among large portions of the population of the United States marked a new era in perinatal medicine, because this was a drug that was viewed as safe and nonaddictive and did not need to be injected, all of which made it attractive to women. Data from the National Institute on Drug Abuse suggest that more than 1 million children per year are exposed to alcohol, tobacco, or illicit substances during gestation.[3]

The effect of this prenatal exposure to alcohol, cocaine, marijuana, and other drugs on pregnancy and the neonate has been described in a variety of studies, and exploration is beginning of the long-term implications of prenatal substance exposure for the child. Woven throughout this research is the realization that multiple factors mediate the effect of prenatal substance exposure on the child's neurologic and behavioral development. This chapter attempts to provide an overview of the effect of prenatal substance exposure on the developing child and to describe the role of the primary health care provider in identifying and providing services to the child exposed prenatally to maternal substances of abuse.

Perinatal Complications of Maternal Substance Abuse

In pregnancies affected by prenatal substance abuse, the use of a number of substances produces many of the same problems. Because the most common form of drug use in this country is "polydrug" use, this section discusses the implications of prenatal substance abuse in the context of polydrug use.

Spontaneous Abortion

Women who smoke tobacco have been shown to have higher rates of spontaneous abortion than those who do not smoke.[4] The only illicit drug perhaps associated with early spontaneous abortion is cocaine,[5,6] but it is difficult to differentiate cocaine's role from that of tobacco, which commonly is used in addition to cocaine. Nicotine and cocaine produce vasospasm and fetal hypoxia that could explain the resultant pregnancy loss. One study of 299 women whose test results were positive for cocaine, amphetamines, or opiates found a significant increase in the rate of spontaneous abortion compared with control subjects. However, this difference did not persist when nulliparas were excluded or when the study group was separated by drug.[7]

Abruptio Placentae

One of the complications first noted in the early studies of cocaine use during pregnancy was abruptio placentae.[5,8-10] The earliest clinical report of cocaine use during pregnancy focused on abruptio placentae,[8] and the first controlled study, published in 1985, also found an increased rate of abruption among the women who used cocaine during pregnancy.[5] The risk of abruption seems to be attributable to the damage caused by cocaine to the placental vasculature, even if the woman used cocaine only the during first trimester of pregnancy.[11] Although the risk of abruption also is increased in pregnancies complicated by opiate use, the abruption is most closely associated with sudden cessation of the opiate use by the addict.[12]

Intrauterine Growth Retardation

Intrauterine growth retardation has been documented in association with the use of alcohol,[13] heroin,[14] tobacco,[15] marijuana,[16] and cocaine[17-19] during pregnancy. The common denominator among all of these drugs is the inadequate nutrition and prenatal care that often occur among the population that uses drugs. Beyond the nutritional, environmental, and social confounding elements, however, studies consistently have documented intrauterine growth retardation attributable to prenatal substance exposure.

Preterm Labor

Multiple factors are associated with preterm labor, many of which are present in the woman who abuses substances, for example, lack of prenatal care, inadequate nutrition, and tobacco smoking. Heavy marijuana use also may be associated with preterm delivery.[20] In addition, women abusing substances are likely to have a history of preterm delivery, which is a risk factor for preterm labor in the current pregnancy. However, even when controlling for a preterm delivery history, a significantly shorter gestational age is found among neonates born to women who use cocaine.[7] The uterine irritability and smooth muscle contractions induced by cocaine use seem to have a significant role in increasing the risk of preterm labor and delivery.

Congenital Anomalies

Alcohol seems to be the substance of abuse most closely related to dysmorphic changes in the fetus, affecting facial structure, the cardiovascular system, and the genitourinary system.[13,21] Several reports of maternal cocaine use suggested the possibility of genitourinary tract malformations,[5] and findings were corroborated by data from published studies using rats.[22] These reports were followed by reports of cardiac, intestinal, and central nervous system (CNS) anomalies[9,23] as well as limb-reduction anomalies.[23,24] The mechanism through which these anomalies arise seems to be an interruption of the intrauterine blood supply with subsequent disruption or destruction of structures that previously had formed normally from an embryologic standpoint. This interruption of blood flow most likely is related to the pharmacologic effects of cocaine: hemorrhage accompanying a rapid rise in systemic and cerebral blood pressure; hemorrhage accompanying hypoperfusion; and hypoxia secondary to uterine, placental, embryonic, or fetal vasoconstriction.

CNS Lesions

One of the early case reports of an infant exposed to cocaine in utero was a child who suffered an intrauterine cerebral infarction.[25] Also reported is an increased incidence of intracerebral hemorrhage in children born to women who were using cocaine or amphetamine.[26] Of 32 exposed neonates, 7% had intraventricular hemorrhage, 13% had subarachnoid hemorrhage, 10% had ventricular dilatation indicative of cerebral atrophy, 13% had white matter density indicative of hemorrhage, 10% had white matter cavitation, and 3% had cerebral infarction. The patterns of effects also emphasize the vascular disruption caused by cocaine at varying times during gestation.

Apnea and Sudden Infant Death Syndrome (SIDS)

It has been well documented that children exposed in utero to heroin or tobacco are at increased risk of SIDS.[27,28] Apnea and abnormalities of respiratory patterns during sleep have been documented in cocaine-exposed infants.[29] In addition, several investigators have studied the risk of SIDS among cocaine-exposed infants,[29,30] but the level of risk has not been determined clearly. A systematic study of infants exposed prenatally to cocaine did not document an increased rate of SIDS.[31] Rather, the authors believed that the associated polydrug use and environmental factors led to any increase in the SIDS rate among this population. Environmental or accidental exposure to cocaine also could result in illness or death of a child and could be mistakenly diagnosed as SIDS.[32] Whatever the cause or mechanism, biologic or environmental, health care professionals should recognize that substance-exposed infants are at risk of SIDS.

Neonatal Neurobehavioral Deficiencies

Neurobehavioral changes found in neonates exposed to marijuana, alcohol, cocaine, and tobacco usually do not reflect a process of neonatal withdrawal from the drug, as has been found specifically with heroin, but rather reflect neurotoxic effects.[5,11,33] Thus, the patterns of behavior in the neonate can be quite varied. Overall, substance-exposed infants can be classified as fragile infants who may have a low threshold for overstimulation and require a great deal of assistance from the parent to maintain control of their hyperexcitable nervous systems. This fragility is seen clearly in the infants' responses to many of the items on the Neonatal Behavioral Assessment Scale,[34] although the severity of the response deficiencies and the rate of recovery of the infant during the first few months of life varies substantially from infant to infant. The key neurobehavioral areas affected by intrauterine substance exposure seem to be motor behavior (reflexes, motor control, coordination of motor activities), state control (the infant's ability to move appropriately through the various states of arousal in response to the demands of the environment), and orientation (the infant's ability to interact actively with the outside world by attending to and responding to visual and auditory stimuli).[5,11,35-37] In most instances, these deficiencies in neurobehavioral functioning do not need to be treated pharmacologically but rather through structured interventions that assist the infant to regulate neurobehavioral functions.

Because there is so much variability in the behavior changes that occur as a result of intrauterine substance exposure, it sometimes is difficult in the hospital nursery to determine the difficulties the child may be experiencing. Careful tracking by nursing personnel and formal evaluation of the infant by a trained specialist can help facilitate the child's neurobehavioral recovery. There rarely is a need to use medications, such as phenobarbital or paregoric, to quiet the infant or improve neurobehavioral functioning.

Long-term Outcome of Substance-Exposed Infants

Little information about the long-term implications for intrauterine substance exposure exists. The transience and chaos of the lifestyle of many of the families enmeshed in substance abuse make it extremely difficult to evaluate the effects of tobacco, alcohol, or illicit drugs on the cognitive and behavioral development of the exposed child. A study of 3-month-old infants who had been exposed prenatally to cocaine found that such exposure affected arousal and attention regulation rather than early cognitive processes.[38] Tobacco smoking by the pregnant woman was related to inadequate language development and cognitive functioning in the child at 3 and 4 years of age; alcohol exposure was related to decreased cognitive abilities at 3 years of age, and marijuana exposure was associated at 4 years of age, with lower scores in the verbal and memory domains.[39] In a separate study, alcohol consumption during pregnancy by white, middle class women had a negative effect on the intelligence quotient scores of their children at 4 years of age. This relationship held after controlling for various prenatal and postnatal confounding variables.[21]

Several studies have found that prenatal cocaine exposure does not have a direct effect on cognitive development of the child at school age, but environmental factors have a role in predicting global developmental scores.[40-42] Ornoy et al[43] studied 2 groups of children born to heroin-dependent mothers; 1 group was adopted and the other group was raised by the birth parent or parents. Ornoy et al[43] concluded that the developmental delays and behavioral problems demonstrated by the heroin-exposed infants resulted from environmental deprivation and the addiction of 1 or both birth parents in the home in which the children were raised.

In a prospective study of 4- to 6-year-old children exposed prenatally to cocaine and other drugs, it was found that prenatal cocaine or polydrug exposure did not have a direct effect on global cognitive functioning but a strong indirect effect as mediated through the home environment.[44] However, prenatal exposure to cocaine and other drugs had a significant direct effect on the child's behavior at 4 to 6 years of age; prenatally exposed children showed higher rates of impulsive behavior, aggressive behavior, attention problems, thought problems, and distractibility. The self-regulatory difficulties interfered with school achievement and success and occurred independent of the home environment.

Loss of behavioral control or withdrawal in children with self-regulatory problems may be triggered by a number of environmental situations and stimuli. Anything that increases the inconsistency and decreases the predictability of a child's environment (eg, multiple caregivers, multiple placements in foster care, or continued substance abuse by a parent) likely will exacerbate the self-regulatory difficulties of the children with problems and create such difficulties in children who previously had no difficulties with self-regulation. The children then have erratic and difficult-to-control behavior when faced with transitions or changes in their lives. New demands placed on the child, as in the classroom situation, exacerbate the difficulties.

The overall outcomes of children exposed prenatally to maternal substances of abuse in utero can be positive if other major risk factors in their lives are addressed and interventions to correct the other factors are undertaken. Unfortunately, the child who is exposed prenatally has a host of environmental risk factors that can impede developmental progress, and the emotional, behavioral, and learning problems likely will occur more often and be more severe in the children who do not receive the interventions they need. The role of the health care professional is the early identification of the children, for there is not a child who cannot be helped through thoughtful nurturing intervention.

Issues in Child Welfare

Several studies of physically abused children have shown that among the abusers, there is a high rate of substance abuse. In New York City, it was estimated that 50% of all child abuse and neglect cases involved drug abuse, and if alcohol was included, substance abuse was involved in 64% of child abuse cases.[45]

Infants removed from their homes because of substance abuse problems in the family represent a large proportion of the recent influx into the already burdened child welfare system, and drug and alcohol abuse are among the most commonly named factors cited as contributing to the increase in child maltreatment.[46]

In 1990, the Inspector General's survey reported that 30% to 50% of drug-exposed infants are placed in foster care.[47] In 1991, 55% of the very young children placed in foster care were estimated to have been exposed to cocaine or cocaine derivatives. Another 11% were estimated to have been exposed prenatally to alcohol and other drugs.[48] By 1990, the influx of drug-exposed infants into a system that already had a short supply of foster homes had stretched the foster care system to its breaking point.[49]

Nationally, studies reveal that children placed in foster care because of parental substance abuse, compared with children placed for other reasons, are separated from their mothers earlier, stay in out-of-home placements longer, experience more changes in placement, are less likely to return home, and have lower rates of adoption. This is particularly true for children of color.[50]

Role of the Primary Care Physician

The central responsibility of the primary care physician is the early identification of the high-risk pregnant woman and her infant so that timely interventions can be initiated that will protect the child and enhance the child's ultimate medical, developmental, and behavioral outcomes. Guidelines for the identification and evaluation of infants exposed prenatally to maternal substances of abuse must be kept general because of the rapidly changing body of knowledge in the field. However, some recommendations for the primary care physician are as follows:

1. Elicit a complete maternal substance use history for ever neonate. Every health care professional should be able to obtain a lifestyle and substance abuse history in a nonthreatening, nonjudgmental manner. With clinical skill, the substance abuse history takes a relatively short time to obtain and will not be perceived as inappropriate or intrusive by most patients. Several screening instruments are available that can guide the health care professional in eliciting an appropriate and correct history (see Chapter 3).

2. Obtain a urine screen for substances of abuse for any neonate in whom there are indications. Most states do not require written consent to obtain a urine toxicology screen for a neonate, but the laws in each state and the guidelines for the hospital should

be reviewed. In any case, from a clinical perspective, a parent always should be informed of any test that will be ordered for the neonate. If the urine toxicology screen result is positive or if the screen result is negative but there is still strong evidence or suspicion of maternal drug use, continue with the following steps.

3. If the mother has not had a screen for hepatitis B or C, syphilis, or human immunodeficiency virus (HIV) during the third trimester of pregnancy, perform these screening tests on the neonate. Specific state or hospital guidelines should be consulted about the need to obtain parental consent before obtaining an HIV screen on the neonate.[51,52]

4. If growth retardation or microcephaly is present, consider screening for other causes, such as toxoplasmosis or cytomegalovirus.

5. Universal screening of exposed infants by using renal or cranial ultrasonography or electroencephalography is not indicated unless clinical evaluation warrants such testing. Careful neurologic examination and close observation of urinary output and evaluation for renal masses during the physical examination will aid in this decision.

6. Instruct the parents in neonatal and infant cardiopulmonary resuscitation. Evaluation by pneumogram and home apnea monitors do not successfully decrease chances for the occurrence of SIDS.[53]

7. Counsel the mother against breastfeeding, because substances of abuse cross readily into breast milk and can have a significant effect on the infant.[54]

8. Refer the mother to social services for evaluation of the home and initiation of drug treatment.

9. Refer the family to governmental child protection services if mandated by the state or if there are indications of potential endangerment of the child.

10. Track infant growth and development closely to ensure that early interventions are initiated as needed. Regular formal neurodevelopmental evaluation will be necessary if screening reveals delays or difficulties in psychomotor, cognitive, or behavioral development.

Conclusion

The health care professional often must serve as the advocate for the family and child. The hysteria of the media that has accompanied the recognition of large numbers of substance-exposed children has resulted in increasingly punitive measures against mothers and families. In turn, the pendulum has recently begun to swing in the opposite direction, with reports in the press that the problems purported to be displayed by cocaine-exposed infants are a myth.[55] The truth lies somewhere in between. Children exposed to drugs, especially cocaine, in utero are not permanently damaged infants as inferred by many articles in the lay press,[56] but they are also not free from risk. The skill and clinical perceptions of a concerned and well-trained health care professional are needed to discern children in need and to provide and manage their care, helping them to reach their full potential.

References

1. Jones KL, Smith DW, Ulleland CN, et al. Pattern of malformation in offspring of chronic alcoholic mothers. *Lancet.* 1973;1:1267-1271
2. Finnegan LP, Connaughton JF, Kron RE, et al. Neonatal abstinence syndrome: assessment and management. In: Harbison RD, ed. *Perinatal Addiction.* New York, NY: Spectrum Publications; 1975:141-158
3. National Institute on Drug Abuse. *National Pregnancy and Health Survey.* Rockville, MD: National Institute on Drug Abuse; 1994
4. US Department of Health, Education, and Welfare. *Health Consequences of Smoking for Women: A Report of the Surgeon General.* Washington, DC: US Department of Health, Education, and Welfare; 1980. NIH Publication No. 0-326-003
5. Chasnoff IJ, Burns WJ, Schnoll SH, et al. Cocaine use in pregnancy. *N Engl J Med.* 1985;313:666-669
6. Frank DA, Zuckerman BS, Amaro H, et al. Cocaine use during pregnancy: prevalence and correlates. *Pediatrics.* 1988;82:888-895

7. Gillogley KM, Evans AT, Hansen R, et al. The perinatal impact of maternal substance abuse detected by universal intrapartum screening. *Am J Obstet Gynecol.* 1990;163:1535-1541

8. Acker D, Sachs BP, Tracey KJ, et al. Abruptio placentae associated with cocaine use. *Am J Obstet Gynecol.* 1983;146:220-221

9. Bingol N, Fuchs M, Diaz V, et al. Teratogenicity of cocaine in humans. *J Pediatr.* 1987;110:93-96

10. MacGregor SN, Keith LG, Chasnoff IJ, et al. Cocaine use during pregnancy: adverse perinatal outcome. *Am J Obstet Gynecol.* 1987;157:696-690

11. Chasnoff IJ, Griffith DR, MacGregor S, et al. Temporal patterns of cocaine use in pregnancy. *JAMA.* 1989;261:1741-1744

12. Zuspan FP, Gumpel JA, Mejia-Zelaya A, et al. Fetal stress from methadone withdrawal. *Am J Obstet Gynecol.* 1973;122:43-46

13. Oulellette EM, Rosett HL, Rosman NP, et al. Adverse effects on offspring of maternal alcohol abuse during pregnancy. *N Engl J Med.* 1977;297:528-531

14. Naeye RL, Blanc W, Leblanc W, et al. Fetal complications of maternal heroin addiction: abnormal growth, infections and episodes of stress. *J Pediatr.* 1973;83:1055-1061

15. Butler NR, Godstein H, Ross EM. Cigarette smoking in pregnancy: its influence on birth weight and prenatal mortality. *Br Med J.* 1972;2:127-130

16. Hatch EE, Bracken MB. Effect of marijuana use in pregnancy on fetal growth. *Am J Epidemiol.* 1986;124:986-988

17. Chouteau M, Namerow PB, Leppert P. The effect of cocaine abuse on birth weight and gestational age. *Obstet Gynecol.* 1988;72:351-354

18. Neerhof MG, MacGregor SN, Retzky SS, et al. Cocaine abuse during pregnancy: peripartum prevalence and perinatal outcome. *Am J Obstet Gynecol.* 1989;161:688-690

19. Ryan L, Ehrlich S, Finnegan L. Cocaine abuse in pregnancy: effects on the fetus and newborn. *Neurotoxicol Teratol.* 1987;9:295-299

20. Fried PA, Watkinson B, Willan A. Marijuana use during pregnancy and decreased length of gestation. *Am J Obstet Gynecol.* 1984;150:23-27

21. Streissguth A, Sampson P, Barr H. Neurobehavioral dose-response effects of prenatal alcohol exposure in humans from infancy to adulthood. *Ann N Y Acad Sci.* 1989;562:145-158

22. Fantel AG, Macphail BJ. The teratogenicity of cocaine. *Teratology.* 1982;26:17-19

23. Chasnoff IJ, Chisum GM, Kaplan WE. Maternal cocaine use and genitourinary tract malformations. *Teratology.* 1988;37:201-204

24. Hoyme HE, Jones KL, Dixon SD, et al. Prenatal cocaine exposure and fetal vascular disruption. *Pediatrics.* 1990;85:743-746

25. Chasnoff IJ, Bussey ME, Savich R, et al. Perinatal cerebral infarction and maternal cocaine use. *J Pediatr.* 1986;108:456-458

26. Dixon SD, Bejar R. Brain lesions in cocaine and methamphetamine exposed neonates [abstract]. *Pediatr Res.* 1988;23:405

27. Rajegowda BK, Kandall SR, Falciglia H. Sudden unexpected death in infants of narcotic-dependent mothers. *Early Hum Dev.* 1978;2/3:219-225

28. Haglund B, Cnattingius S. Cigarette smoking as a risk factor for sudden infant death syndrome: a population-based study. *Am J Public Health.* 1990;80:29-32

29. Chasnoff IJ, Hunt CE, Kletter R, et al. Prenatal cocaine exposure is associated with respiratory pattern abnormalities. *Am J Dis Child.* 1989;143:583-587

30. Durand DJ, Espinoza AM, Nickerson BG. Association between prenatal cocaine exposure and sudden infant death syndrome. *J Pediatr.* 1990;117:909-911

31. Bauchner H, Zuckerman B, McClain M, et al. Risk of sudden infant death syndrome among infants with in-utero exposure to cocaine. *J Pediatr.* 1988;13:831-834

32. Rivkin M, Gilmore HE. Generalized seizures due to environmentally acquired cocaine. *Pediatrics.* 1989;84:1100-1101

33. Chasnoff IJ, Griffith DR, Freier C, et al. Cocaine/polydrug use in pregnancy: two-year follow-up. *Pediatrics.* 1992;89:284-289

34. Brazelton TB. *Neonatal Behavioral Assessment Scale.* Philadelphia, PA: Spastics International; 1984

35. Griffith DR. The effects of perinatal cocaine exposure on infant neurobehavior and early maternal-infant interactions. In: Chasnoff IJ, ed. *Drug Use in Pregnancy: Mother and Child.* Boston, MA: MTP Press; 1988:105-113

36. Lester BM, Corwin MJ, Sepkoski C, et al. Neurobehavioral syndromes in cocaine-exposed newborn infants. *Child Dev.* 1991;62:694-705

37. Singer LT, Garber R, Kliegman R. Neurobehavioral sequelae of fetal cocaine exposure. *J Pediatr.* 1991;119:667-672

38. Mayes LC, Bornstein MH, Chawarska K, et al. Information processing and developmental assessments in 3-month-old infants exposed prenatally to cocaine. *Pediatrics.* 1995;95:539-545

39. Fried AP, Watkinson B. 36- and 48-month neurobehavioral follow-up of children prenatally exposed to marijuana, cigarettes, and alcohol. *Dev Behav Pediatr.* 1990;11:49-58

40. Azuma SD, Chasnoff IJ. Outcome of children prenatally exposed to cocaine and other drugs: a path analysis of three-year data. *Pediatrics.* 1993;92:396-402

41. Hurt H, Brodsky NL, Betancourt L, et al. Cocaine-exposed children: follow-up through 30 months. *J Substance Abuse.* 1995;7:267-280

42. Nulman I, Rovet J, Altmann D, et al. Neurodevelopment of adopted children exposed in utero to cocaine. *J Dev Behav Pediatr.* 1995;16: 418-424

43. Ornoy A, Michilevskaya V, Lukashov I, et al. The developmental outcome of children born to heroin-dependent mothers, raised at home or adopted. *Can Med Assoc J.* 1994;151:1591-1597

44. Chasnoff IJ, Anson A, Hatcher R, Stenson H, Iaukea K, Randolph LA, et al. Prenatal exposure to cocaine and other drugs: outcome at four to six years. *Ann N Y Acad Sci.* 1998;846:314-328

45. Marriott M. Child abuse cases swamping New York City's family court. *New York Times.* 1987;15:17

46. Herskowitz J, Seck M, Fogg C. *Substance Abuse and Family Violence: Identification of Drug and Alcohol Usage During Child Abuse Investigations.* Boston, MA: Massachusetts Department of Social Services; 1989

47. US Office of the Inspector General. *Crack Babies.* Washington, DC: US Department of Health and Human Services; 1990

48. US General Accounting Office. *Foster Care: Parental Drug Abuse Has Alarming Impact on Young Children.* Washington, DC: US General Accounting Office; 1994. GAO/HEHS Publication No. 94-89

49. *The Enemy Within: Crack-Cocaine and the American Family.* Washington, DC: US House of Representatives, Committee on Ways and Means, Subcommittee on Human Resources; 1990

50. *Hearings Before the Senate Subcommittee on Children, Families, Drugs & Alcoholism,* 101st Cong, Second Sess (1990) (testimony of Douglas J. Besharov)

51. American Academy of Pediatrics. Human immunodeficiency virus infection. In: Pickering LK, ed. *2000 Red Book: Report of the Committee on Infectious Diseases.* 25th ed. Elk Grove Village, IL: American Academy of Pediatrics; 2000:325-349

52. Mofenson LM, and the Committee on Pediatric AIDS. Technical report: perinatal human immunodeficiency virus testing and prevention of transmission. *Pediatrics.* 2000;106:1476-1477

53. American Academy of Pediatrics, Task Force on Infant Sleep Position and Sudden Infant Death Syndrome. Changing concepts of sudden infant death syndrome: implications for infant sleeping environment and sleep position. *Pediatrics.* 2000;105:650-659

54. American Academy of Pediatrics. Transfer of drugs and other chemicals into human milk. In: Kleinman RE, ed. *Pediatric Nutrition Handbook.* 4th ed. Elk Grove Village, IL: American Academy of Pediatrics; 1998:633-641

55. Goodman E. Debunking myth about "crack kids." *The Atlanta Constitution.* January 28, 1992:A-9

56. Hopkins E. Childhood's end. *Rolling Stone.* 1990;589:66-72, 108-110

Chapter 11

Assessment, Diagnosis, and Treatment of the Adolescent With a Dual Diagnosis

Marie Armentano, MD, and Michael S. Jellinek, MD, FAAP

Many adolescents receiving treatment for substance abuse have other psychiatric diagnoses. Awareness of the most likely disorders and formulation of an integrated treatment plan are important. This chapter reviews what is known about comorbidity and offers guidelines for management and consultation.

Adolescents who manifest other psychiatric diagnoses in addition to substance abuse have elicited increasing concern.[1-19] In this chapter, the terms "dual diagnosis" and "comorbidity" are used as general terms to refer to patients who meet the criteria for a psychoactive substance use disorder and for another psychiatric diagnosis on axis I or II using the *Diagnostic and Statistical Manual of Mental Disorders, Third Edition Revised (DSM-III-R),*[20] the *DSM, Fourth Edition (DSM-IV),*[21] and *Diagnostic and Statistical Manual for Primary Care (DSM-PC), Child and Adolescent Version.*[22] The term "substance abuse" is used as a generic term that includes substance dependence. Adolescents who initially seek or are referred for treatment of substance abuse may be different from those who seek or are referred for psychiatric treatment[23,24]; this chapter focuses on adolescents whose initial treatment was for diagnosed substance use disorders.

According to Bukstein and Kaminer,[25] issues of nosology in adolescent substance abuse continue to be problematic despite the advent of *DSM-IV* and *DSM-PC* criteria.[22] The criteria that have been developed have not been validated with adolescents. There may be some discontinuities between adolescent and adult populations.[25,26] When diagnostic criteria are based on problem behaviors, it is often unclear whether the behaviors are attributable to substance use or a coexisting or preexisting problem. Although

craving and loss of control are included in the criteria, no studies
have established whether these criteria are present in adolescents.[25]
Nosology is only the best attempt to make sense of reality; therefore, an imperfect system designed for adults is used to make
substance abuse diagnoses in adolescents.[25-28]

Dual diagnosis issues as well were studied initially in adults,[29-34]
leaving the health care professional to extrapolate from this research
to the adolescent population. More recently,[5-9,11-17,35-45] adolescent
clinical and community populations have been studied. For adults
and adolescents, some of the methodologic questions are the same.
The course and treatment of the same 2 disorders may vary depending on which one is primary or, in other words, which disorder pre-
ceded the other[30] and on their relative severity.[23,24,32,45-47] It is
unhelpful to assume that all patients with dual diagnoses are the
same and require the same treatment.[45] Although a high prevalence
of comorbidity has been reported among adolescent patients with
drug use disorders,[11,13,14,47-54] it is unclear how many exhibit psychiatric symptoms secondary to the substance use disorder and how
many have a primary or coexisting psychiatric diagnosis. Miller
and Fine[30] argue that methodologic considerations, including the
length of abstinence required before the diagnosis is made, the
population sampled, and the perspective of the examiner affect
prevalence rates for psychiatric disorders in persons who abuse
substances and account for the variability. They see the prevalence
rates for psychiatric disorders as artificially elevated by the tendency to make a diagnosis before abatement of some of the psychiatric
symptomatology secondary to substance use.

Despite the controversy about the degree of comorbidity, primary
care physicians need to treat the patients they encounter. Some of
the patients will have a psychiatric diagnosis, and the treatment
provided may need modification. Health care professionals will
serve these patients well if they:

1. Conduct a comprehensive evaluation of each patient that
   includes a mental status examination and an inquiry into
   other psychiatric symptomatology and obtain information
   from multiple sources.

2. Have a high index of suspicion for psychiatric comorbidity in adolescents whose conditions do not respond to treatment or who are presenting problems in treatment.
3. Individualize treatment to accommodate other psychiatric diagnoses.
4. Know when to consult a psychiatrist or another specialist.

Health care professionals should know the kinds of comorbidity they are likely to encounter in practice. Large-scale population studies, until recently, did not focus on adolescents. The *National Institute of Mental Health Epidemiological Catchment Area Study*[35] attempted to estimate the true prevalence rates of alcohol and other drug use disorders and mental disorders in an adult community and institutional sample of more than 20 000 subjects standardized to the US Census. Of the total, 37% of persons with alcohol use disorders had another mental disorder, with the highest prevalence for affective, anxiety, and antisocial personality disorders. More than 50% of those with drug use disorders other than alcohol abuse had a comorbid mental disorder; 28% had anxiety disorders, 26% had affective disorders, 18% had antisocial personality disorder, and 7% had schizophrenia. This study verified the widely held impression that comorbidity rates are much higher among clinical and institutional populations than in the general population.

Until very recently, studies involving adolescents were smaller and involved clinical populations. Stowell and Estroff[15] studied 226 adolescents receiving inpatient treatment in private psychiatric hospitals for a primary substance use disorder. Psychiatric diagnoses were made 4 weeks into treatment by using a semistructured diagnostic interview. Of the total, 82% of the patients met *DSM-III-R* criteria for an axis I psychiatric disorder, 61% had mood disorders, 54% had conduct disorders, 43% had anxiety disorders, and 16% had substance-induced organic disorders. Three quarters of the patients (74%) had 2 or more psychiatric disorders. Westermeyer et al[16] studied 100 adolescents 12 to 20 years of age who sought care at 2 university-based outpatient substance abuse treatment programs and found much comorbidity and multiple diagnoses. Of the adolescents, 22 had eating disorders, 8 had conduct disorders, 7 had major depressive disorder, 6 had minor depressive disorder, 5 had bipolar disorder, 5 had schizophrenia, and 4 had anxiety disorders. Three had another psychotic disorder, 3 had an organic mental disorder, and 2 had attention-deficit/hyperactivity disorder (ADHD). The distribution of diagnoses as a function of age showed that older adolescents had increased eating disorder diagnoses and depressive symptoms.[16]

Several recent population studies have included adolescents. Giaconia et al[37] also studied the issue of age in a predominantly white, working class community sample of 386 eighteen-year-olds. They compared adolescents who had met the criteria for 1 of 6 psychiatric diagnoses, including substance abuse, before and after they were 14 years of age. Adolescents with early onset of any psychiatric disorder were 6 times as likely to have 1 and 12 times as likely to have 2 additional disorders by 18 years of age than those with later onset psychiatric disorder.[37] This would imply that the health care professional's index of suspicion for dual diagnosis must be particularly high for younger patients with substance use disorders. Burke et al[35] studied data from the *National Institute of Mental Health Epidemiological Catchment Area Study* to determine hazard rates for the development of disorders and concluded that the peak age range for the onset of depressive disorders in females and for the onset of substance use disorders and bipolar disorders in both sexes was 15 to 19 years.

The *National Comorbidity Study* included a large noninstitutional sample of persons 15 to 24 years of age, although adolescents were not studied separately from young adults.[41] Compared with older adults, 15- to 24-year-olds had the highest prevalence of 3 or more disorders occurring together and of any disorders, including substance use disorders. The *Methods for the Epidemiology of Child and Adolescent Mental Disorders Study* obtained data for 401 subjects 14 to 17 years of age.[39] Adolescents with substance use disorders had much higher rates of mood and conduct disorder than did those without substance use disorders.

Major Diagnostic Categories

Depressive Disorder

Much has been written about the interplay between depression and substance abuse.[5,17,19,32-34,36,38,40,42,47,48] The emerging concept is that in adolescents[5,13,25,36,47,48] and adults,[32-34] 2 groups exhibit significant depressive symptoms—those with a substance-induced mood disorder and those with primary depressive disorders.[21] The chief symptom of depression consists of a disturbance of mood usually characterized as sadness or feeling "down in the dumps" and a loss of interest or pleasure. Adolescents may report or exhibit irritability instead of sadness. In addition, depression is characterized by guilt, hopelessness, sleep disturbances, appetite disturbances, loss of the ability to concentrate, diminution of energy, and thoughts of death or suicide. To meet the criteria, the patient must exhibit or experience depressed mood most of the day, every day, for 2 weeks.[21] Patients with a substance-induced mood disorder exhibit the same depressive symptoms.

Schuckit[32-34] and Miller[29] stress the importance of distinguishing the 2 disorders. Studies of adults who abused substances showed that the substance-induced mood disorder dissipated with abstinence from substance use, but the primary depressive disorder did not, and if left untreated, could interfere with treatment and recovery.[29,30,32,34] Deykin et al[36] interviewed 223 adolescents in residential treatment for substance abuse and found that almost 25% met the *DSM-III-R* criteria for depression. Of these, 8% met the criteria for a primary depression; the other 16% had a secondary mood disorder. Bukstein et al[5] studied adolescent inpatients on a dual diagnosis unit and reported that almost 31% had a comorbid major depression, with secondary depressive disorder much more common than primary depressive disorder. Unlike findings reported for adults, Bukstein et al[5] found that the secondary depression did not remit with abstinence from substance use. This finding, if replicated, would argue for more vigorous treatment of depressive syndromes in adolescents.

During the mental status examination, depressed adolescents may seem taciturn and show poor eye contact and a sad-looking face. They may be poorly groomed or drably dressed and may become tearful during the interview. Often they deny feelings of sadness, although their demeanor states it eloquently. Depression interferes with treatment because of the lack of concentration, motivation, and hope and the tendency toward isolation. Kempton et al[50] found cognitive distortions, including magnification (all-or-nothing thinking) and personalizing, to be particularly prominent among adolescents with the multiple diagnoses of conduct disorder, depressive disorder, and substance abuse. A depressed adolescent may benefit from a specific cognitive intervention for depression.[27,55]

If the adolescent has a depressive disorder that predates the substance abuse, has a family history of depression, and has a mood disorder that interferes with treatment several weeks into abstinence from substance use despite cognitive interventions, pharmacotherapy is indicated. Serotoninergic agents, such as fluoxetine hydrochloride, have a relatively safe profile for adverse effects and may be most appropriate, considering reports that young substance abusers have a preexisting serotonin deficit.[7,12] It would be advisable before prescribing medication to determine whether the patient is abstinent from substance use, whether the abstinence is secure, and whether supports are in place or the patient is in a secure drug-free environment; and whether the patient will adhere to a medication regimen or has a family to help with adherence to the medication regimen. Study of the referral and prescribing practices of primary care physicians has shown a tendency to underdiagnose and undertreat depression.[49,56] If there are doubts about the diagnosis of depression or about how to treat, a consultation with a psychiatrist experienced in treating adolescents with addictions is indicated. When the primary care physician is concerned about possible suicidal behavior, consultation should be sought without delay.[3,38,40]

Bipolar Disorder

In bipolar disorder, which often begins during late adolescence,[6,37,51] the initial symptoms of mania include a persistent elevated, expansive, or irritable mood lasting at least 1 week accompanied by grandiosity or inflated self-esteem, decreased need for sleep, pressured speech, racing thoughts, increased purposeful activity, and excessive involvement in pleasurable activities, such as spending money, sexual indiscretions, or substance abuse.[21] Wilens et al[51] have found an increased risk of substance use disorders in adolescents with bipolar disorder. Children in whom bipolar disorder was diagnosed and treated appropriately at a younger age had a lower risk of substance abuse. Some patients use substances, particularly alcohol, to calm themselves during a manic phase. Clearly, some of these symptoms also are seen with substance intoxication. If a patient exhibits these symptoms after a period of abstinence, the diagnosis of bipolar disorder should be considered. Bipolar disorders are treated with mood stabilizers, the most common of which is lithium carbonate.[10] Valproic acid, carbamazepine, and other anticonvulsants also are used.[27,46] Before treating for bipolar disorder, a psychiatric consultation should be obtained.

Anxiety Disorders and Post-traumatic Stress Disorder

Anxiety disorders include generalized anxiety disorder, panic disorder, obsessive-compulsive disorder, and post-traumatic stress disorder.[21] Anxiety disorders often are not detected or treated, especially when present with depression or psychoactive substance use disorders.[6,52] Sometimes a closer examination of patients who resist attending self-help meetings may reveal a social phobia or agoraphobia. Panic attacks are periods of intense discomfort that develop abruptly and reach a peak within 10 minutes. Symptoms include palpitations, sweating, trembling, sensations of shortness of breath or choking, chest discomfort, nausea, dizziness, and fear of losing control or of dying. Because some of these symptoms also might be seen in substance intoxication or withdrawal, it is important to establish abstinence before making a diagnosis. Patients with a social phobia may isolate themselves in an inpatient unit or in a group. A careful interview in which anxiety symptoms and family history of anxiety disorders are pursued may be quite revealing. Behavioral treatment, including relaxation training, often is helpful for anxiety disorders.[27] The issue of pharmacotherapy is controversial. Many argue that the use of benzodiazepines is contraindicated in anyone with a history of substance abuse. Buspirone hydrochloride and serotonin reuptake inhibitors have been recommended as nonaddictive antianxiety agents. Clinical experience and anecdotal reports suggest that for many, buspirone is ineffective. Often when treating patients who insist that only benzodiazepines are effective, it is unclear whether the statement represents drug-seeking behavior or a bona fide observation. If abstinence has been established, adequate trials of behavioral or cognitive therapy[27] and alternative medications have failed, and the patient adheres to the treatment and medication regimen, the judicious use of a long-acting benzodiazepine, such as clonazepam, may be justified.

In clinical reports on adolescents, the incidence of severe trauma and symptoms of post-traumatic stress disorder are surprisingly high.[8,39,52-54] An adolescent who has been acting out and abusing substances may not have dealt with previous trauma, such as physical and sexual abuse and exposure to violence, or with the trauma that may be incurred when abusing substances.[53] Symptoms and memories of trauma may manifest themselves only during abstinence. Symptoms of post-traumatic stress disorder can be divided into 3 groups.[21] The first group involves reexperiencing the trauma through intrusive thoughts, dreams, or flashbacks, which make the person feel as if the event is reoccurring. Second, the patient has a numbing of general responsiveness and avoids thinking about the trauma. Third, there are symptoms of increased arousal, including difficulty sleeping, irritability, hypervigilance, and an exaggerated startle response. Trauma and the symptoms associated with trauma should be considered and inquired about to ensure adequate treatment of adolescents who abuse substances. Care should be taken to acknowledge the trauma without arousing anxiety that will interfere with abstinence and substance abuse treatment. Groups that support self-care and a first-things-first attitude may be the best approach; the patient needs to learn to stay safe, and treatment for substance abuse is a most important aspect of safety. The patient can be counseled that recovery is a process and must be taken in stages and that some of the effects of the trauma can be dealt with later, when the patient's abstinence and safety are better established. When trauma is suspected, the health care professional should obtain mental health consultation if there are questions about diagnosis or management.

Organic Mental Disorders

The abuse of substances, including alcohol, marijuana, cocaine, hallucinogens, and inhalants, is associated in some patients with acute and residual cognitive damage.[15,21,50] Acute symptoms may include impaired concentration and receptive and expressive language abilities as well as irritability. Long-term interference with memory and other executive functions occurs. The possibility of substance-induced dementia should be considered in adolescents who have difficulty coping with the cognitive and organizational demands of a structured and supportive program. Some adolescents will be able to use the program if instructions are simplified and if they comprehend information accurately. There may be rapid improvement in cognitive functioning, but the cognitive functioning of some patients continues to improve for as long as a year or more after cessation of the chemical assault to the brain. Some may be left with residual impairment. Adolescents and their families should be informed about the cognitive consequences of their substance use in a way that does not engender despair but clearly warns against further abuse. The presence of cognitive deficits, if they persist, should be considered in rehabilitation, educational, and vocational planning for the adolescent. Adolescents need neuropsychologic evaluation and follow-up.

Schizophrenia

Patients who simultaneously meet the criteria for schizophrenia and a substance abuse diagnosis are less likely to receive treatment in a substance abuse unit than in a psychiatric unit.[23,24] Because the late adolescent years are a time when many schizophrenic disorders begin and the use of substances may precipitate an incipient psychosis, patients with this disorder may seek treatment during early stages of schizophrenia.[14,30,31] Characteristic symptoms are hallucinations that are more often auditory, delusions, disorganized speech, grossly disorganized or catatonic behavior, and negative symptoms, including affective flattening, impoverished speech, or avolition.[20] Therefore, for patients with bizarre manifestations that seem grossly different from the rest of the treatment population, the diagnosis of schizophrenia should be considered. Increasingly, younger schizophrenic patients abuse substances,[57-59] some in an attempt to manage or deny their symptoms. Their abuse of substances often interferes with treatment of their psychotic disorder. These patients are best managed in special dual diagnosis programs for psychotic patients in whom psychosis and substance abuse are addressed in a parallel manner.[23,24,31,43,49,54,57,58]

Attention-Deficit/Hyperactivity Disorder

Many involved in the treatment of adolescents who abuse substances have noted the large numbers of adolescents who also have ADHD.[4,7,18,19,44,46,60,61] Bukstein and colleagues[4] postulate that there is no direct connection but that both are often comorbid with conduct disorder. Crowley and Riggs[7] noted comorbidity with affective, anxiety, and antisocial disorders in the patients and their families. The symptoms of ADHD include inattention, such as failure to listen, difficulty with organization, the tendency to lose objects, or easy distractibility; and hyperactivity and impulsivity, such as fidgeting, restlessness, and the tendency to interrupt.[21,59] These symptoms must be present in more than 1 setting, and it may be helpful to use rating scales to establish the diagnosis and monitor progress. Treatment should include behavioral and educational intervention. Pharmacotherapy for adolescents has been controversial, particularly because some have argued that the use of stimulants might predispose adolescents to abuse other substances. Riggs et al[61] have reported some success with the use of bupropion hydrochloride. Wilens et al[18] suggest that successful treatment with stimulants of adolescents who have ADHD may actually lower the probability of developing a substance use disorder. Because the successful treatment of substance abuse involves teaching patients to plan and to delay impulses, the effective treatment of ADHD is necessary in an integrated plan.

Conduct Disorders and Antisocial Personality Disorders

Particularly in males, conduct disorder and antisocial personality disorder are the most common comorbid diagnoses with substance abuse.[7,14-17,19,32,39,46-48] The characteristic symptom of antisocial personality disorder is a pervasive pattern of disregarding and violating the rights of others, and the disorder may include deceitfulness, impulsivity, failure to conform to rules or the law, aggressiveness, and irresponsibility.[21] Conduct disorder has similar criteria but includes manifestations that are likely to be seen in younger persons, such as cruelty to animals, running away, truancy, and vandalism. Many who have studied adolescent substance abuse have commented that it usually occurs as part of a constellation of problem behaviors.[7,9,39,44,62] Cloninger[62] presented an interesting scheme of hereditary factors on 3 axes that may account for many psychiatric diagnoses and their interrelationships. The 3 axes are reward-dependence, harm-avoidance, and novelty seeking. On the basis of these axes, Cloninger[62] distinguished type 1 and type 2 alcoholic patients. Type 2 alcoholic patients score low on reward-dependence and harm-avoidance and high on novelty seeking. Younger alcoholic patients with antisocial personality fit the type 2 classification. The higher prevalence of antisocial personality and conduct disorder among younger alcoholic patients may explain why many health care professionals find adolescent substance abusers more difficult to treat. Horowitz et al[12] consider many young patients who abuse substances to have a combination of characteristics, including increased hostility, depression, and suicidal ideation, that suggest an underlying, perhaps neurochemically determined difficulty with self-regulation and aggression. Adolescents with conduct disorders and antisocial personality disorder need a strong behavioral program with clear limits. If there is a comorbid disorder, such as a mood or attention disorder, that can be treated successfully, adolescents are more likely to do well.[7,18,61]

Borderline and Narcissistic Personality Disorders

In addition to psychiatric diagnoses on axis I, the personality disorders described on axis II of *DSM-IV* are relevant during the treatment of adolescents who abuse substances.[21,63-65] Personality disorders are enduring patterns of inner experience and behavior that affect cognition, interpersonal behavior, emotional response, and impulse control. Personality factors often make an adolescent difficult to treat. Borderline personality disorder is marked by impulsivity and instability of interpersonal relationships that affect self-image. A marked sensitivity and wish to avoid abandonment, chronic feelings of emptiness, inappropriate and intense anger, and suicidal or self-mutilating behavior are characteristic of borderline personality disorder. In a treatment setting, the patient with borderline personality disorder can wreak havoc because of the severe regression often manifested and the divisiveness they often cause among staff. Narcissistic personality disorder is characterized by a pervasive pattern of grandiosity, a need for admiration, and a lack of empathy. The patient feels unique and entitled to special treatment. A patient with narcissistic personality disorder may have difficulty participating in groups or seeing other people in ways other than as need gratifiers.

Both of these personality disorders can present challenges to the health care professional and staff in the treatment setting. Powerful and negative feelings, conscious and unconscious,[47] can be aroused easily by patients who are manipulative and full of rage, who feel entitled, and whose behavior saps the emotional strength of the staff and health care professional.[63] If the treatment of a patient requires a great amount of emotional energy, personality issues likely are involved. It is essential to be aware of the effect that such patients exert to take care of the health care professional, the staff in the treatment setting, and the patient. Expert psychiatric consultation can be very helpful in these situations.

Eating Disorders

As the incidence of eating disorders and substance abuse have increased in our adolescent population,[16,66-68] it is not uncommon to find them together; one quarter of all patients with an eating disorder have a history of substance abuse or are currently abusing substances.[66] Anorexia nervosa, which involves weight restriction and increased activity, distorted body image, and intense fear of losing control and becoming fat,[21] is not as prevalent as bulimia in the general population and among persons who abuse substances.[68] Bulimia involves recurrent episodes of binge eating, sometimes accompanied by compensatory measures, such as vomiting or laxative abuse, and a preoccupation with food and weight. Of all eating disorders, 90% to 95% occur in females.[66] Although anorexic patients have a characteristic emaciated appearance, bulimic patients can be any weight. Patients who consistently spend time in the bathroom after meals may be purging. Persons with an eating disorder may abuse amphetamines to lose weight. Katz[66] postulates that the proneness to substance abuse in bulimic patients may be attributable to borderline personality features.

Conclusion

An awareness of the prevalence and manifestations of psychiatric diagnoses is essential for the quality treatment of adolescents who abuse substances. An ongoing relationship with a psychiatrist who can be available for consultation as needed is helpful. The primary care physician and the psychiatrist should keep up to date on psychopharmacologic interventions.[69,70] Careful observation, history taking, and appropriate consultation result in better detection and treatment of comorbid disorders and, ultimately, of the initial substance abuse problem.

References

1. American Academy of Pediatrics, Committee on Substance Abuse. Indications for management and referral of patients involved in substance abuse. *Pediatrics.* 2000; 106:143-148

2. Armentano M. Assessment, diagnosis, and treatment of the dually diagnosed adolescent. *Pediatr Clin North Am.* 1995;42:479-490

3. Bukstein OG, Brent DA, Perper JA, et al. Risk factors for completed suicide among adolescents with a lifetime history of substance abuse: a case-control study. *Acta Psychiatr Scand.* 1993;88:403-408

4. Bukstein OG, Brent DA, Kaminer Y. Comorbidity of substance abuse and other psychiatric disorders in adolescents. *Am J Psychiatry.* 1989;146:1131-1141

5. Bukstein OG, Glancy LJ, Kaminer Y. Patterns of affective comorbidity in a clinical population of dually diagnosed adolescent substance abusers. *J Am Acad Child Adolesc Psychiatry.* 1992;31:1041-1045

6. Burke JD Jr, Burke KC, Rae DS. Increased rates of drug abuse and dependence after onset of mood or anxiety disorders in adolescence. *Hosp Community Psychiatry.* 1994;45:451-455

7. Crowley TJ, Riggs PD. Adolescent substance use disorder with conduct disorder and comorbid conditions. In: Rahdert E, Czechowicz D, eds. *Adolescent Drug Abuse: Clinical Assessment and Therapeutic Interventions.* Bethesda, MD: National Institute on Drug Abuse; 1995:49-111

8. Deykin EY, Buka SL. Prevalence and risk factors for posttraumatic stress disorder among chemically dependent adolescents. *Am J Psychiatr.* 1997;154:752-757

9. Fergusson DM, Horwood LJ, Lynskey MT. Prevalence and comorbidity of DSM-III-R diagnoses in a birth cohort of 15 year olds. *J Am Acad Child Adolesc Psychiatry.* 1993;32:1127-1134

10. Geller B, Cooper TB, Sun K, Frazier J, Williams M, Heath J. Double-blind and placebo-controlled study of lithium for adolescent bipolar disorders with secondary substance dependency. *J Am Acad Child Adolesc Psychiatr.* 1998;37:171-178

11. Grilo CM, Becker DF, Walker ML, Levy KN, Edell WS, McGlashan TH. Psychiatric comorbidity in adolescent inpatients with substance use disorders. *J Am Acad Child Adolesc Psychiatry.* 1995;34:1085-1091

12. Horowitz HA, Overton WF, Rosenstein D, Steidl JH. Comorbid adolescent substance abuse: a maladaptive pattern of self-regulation. *Adolesc Psychiatry.* 1992;18:465-483

13. Hovens JG, Cantwell DP, Kiriakos R. Psychiatric comorbidity in hospitalized adolescent substance abusers. *J Am Acad Child Adolesc Psychiatry.* 1994;33:476-483

14. Kaminer Y, Tarter RE, Bukstein OG, Kabene M. Comparison between treatment completers and noncompleters among dually diagnosed substance-abusing adolescents. *J Am Acad Child Adolesc Psychiatry.* 1992;31:1046-1049

15. Stowell JA, Estroff TW. Psychiatric disorders in substance-abusing adolescent inpatients: a pilot study. *J Am Acad Child Adolesc Psychiatry.* 1992;31:1036-1040

16. Westermeyer J, Specker S, Neider J, Lingenfelter MA. Substance abuse and associated psychiatric disorder among 100 adolescents. *J Addict Dis.* 1994;13:67-89

17. Wilcox JA, Yates WR. Gender and psychiatric comorbidity in substance-abusing individuals. *Am J Addict.* 1993;2:202-206

18. Wilens TE, Biederman J, Spencer TJ. Attention deficit hyperactivity disorder and psychoactive substance use disorders. *Child Adolesc Psychiatr Clin North Am.* 1996;5:73-91

19. American Psychiatric Association. *Diagnostic and Statistical Manual of Mental Disorders, Third Edition (DSM-III).* Washington, DC: American Psychiatric Association; 1983

20. American Psychiatric Association. *Diagnostic and Statistical Manual of Mental Disorders, Third Edition Revised (DSM-III-R).* Washington, DC: American Psychiatric Association; 1987

21. American Psychiatric Association. *Diagnostic and Statistical Manual of Mental Disorders, Fourth Edition (DSM-IV).* Washington, DC: American Psychiatric Association; 1994

22. American Academy of Pediatrics. *The Classification of Child and Adolescent Mental Diagnoses in Primary Care: Diagnostic and Statistical Manual of Mental Disorders for Primary Care (DSM-PC) Child and Adolescent Version.* Wolraich MI, Felice ME, Drotar D, eds. Elk Grove Village, IL: American Academy of Pediatrics; 1996

23. Caton CL, Gralnick A, Bender S, Simon R. Young chronic patients and substance abuse. *Hosp Community Psychiatry.* 1989;40:1037-1040

24. Ries R, Mullen M, Cox G. Symptom severity and utilization of treatment resources among dually diagnosed inpatients. *Hosp Commun Psychiatry.* 1994;45:562-568

25. Bukstein O, Kaminer Y. The nosology of adolescent substance abuse. *Am J Addict.* 1994;3:1-13

26. Clark DB, Kirisci L, Tarter RE. Adolescent versus adult onset and the development of substance abuse disorders in males. *Drug Alcohol Depend.* 1998;49:115-121

27. Kaminer Y. *Adolescent Substance Abuse: A Comprehensive Guide to Theory and Practice.* New York, NY: Plenum Medical Book Co; 1994

28. Weinberg NZ, Rahdert E, Colliver JD, Glantz MD. Adolescent substance abuse: a review of the past 10 years. *J Am Acad Child Adolesc Psychiatry.* 1998;37:252-261

29. Miller NS. Comorbidity of psychiatric and alcohol/drug disorders: interactions and independent status. *J Addict Dis.* 1993;12:5-16

30. Miller NS, Fine J. Current epidemiology of comorbidity of psychiatric and addictive disorders. *Psychiatr Clin North Am.* 1993;16:1-10

31. Ries RK. Clinical treatment matching models for dually diagnosed patients. *Psychiatr Clin North Am.* 1993;16:167-175

32. Schuckit MA. The clinical implications of primary diagnostic groups among alcoholics. *Arch Gen Psychiatry.* 1985;42:1043-1049

33. Schuckit MA. Genetic and clinical implications of alcoholism and affective disorder. *Am J Psychiatry.* 1986;143:140-147

34. Schuckit MA. Alcohol and depression: a clinical perspective. *Acta Psychiatr Scand Suppl.* 1994;377:28-32

35. Burke KC, Burke JD Jr, Regier DA, Rae DS. Age at onset of selected mental disorders in five community populations. *Arch Gen Psychiatry.* 1990;47:511-518

36. Deykin EY, Buka SL, Zeena TH. Depressive illness among chemically dependent adolescents. *Am J Psychiatry.* 1992;149:1341-1347

37. Giaconia RM, Reinherz HZ, Silverman AB, Pakiz B, Frost AK, Cohen E. Ages of onset of psychiatric disorders in a community population of older adolescents. *J Am Acad Child Adolesc Psychiatry.* 1994;33:706-717

38. Flory M. Psychiatric diagnosis in child and adolescent suicide. *Arch Gen Psychiatry.* 1996;53:339-348

39. Kandel DB, Johnson JG, Bird HR, et al. Psychiatric comorbidity among adolescents with substance use disorders: findings from the MECA study. *J Am Child Adolesc Psychiatry.* 1999;36:693-699

40. Kandel DB, Raveis VH, Davies M. Suicidal ideation in adolescence: depression, substance use, and other risk factors. *J Youth Adolesc.* 1991;20:289-309

41. Kessler RC, Nelson CB, McGonagle KA, Edlund MJ, Frank RG, Leaf PJ. The epidemiology of co-occurring addictive and mental disorders: implications for prevention and service utilization. *Am J Orthopsychiatry.* 1996;66:17-31

42. Lewisohn PM, Hops H, Roberts RE, Seeley JR, Andrews JA. Adolescent psychopathology I: prevalence and incidence of depression and other DSM-III-R disorders in high school students. *J Abnormal Psychol.* 1993;102:133-144

43. Mason SE, Siris SG. Dual diagnosis: the case for case management. *Am J Addict.* 1992;1:77-82

44. Morrison MA, Smith DE, Wilford BB, Ehrlich P, Seymour RB. At war in the fields of play: current perspectives on the nature and treatment of adolescent chemical dependency. *J Psychoactive Drugs.* 1993;25: 321-330

45. Weiss RD, Mirin SM, Frances RJ. Alcohol and drug abuse: the myth of the typical dual diagnosis patient. *Hosp Community Psychiatry.* 1992;43:107-108

46. American Academy of Child and Adolescent Psychiatry. Practice parameters for the assessment and treatment of children and adolescents with substance abuse disorders. *J Am Acad Child Adolesc Psychiatry.* 1997;36(10 suppl):140S-156S

47. King CA, Ghaziuddin N, McGovern L, Brand E, Hill E, Naylor M. Predictors of comorbid alcohol and substance abuse in depressed adolescents. *J Am Acad Child Adolesc Psychiatry.* 1996;35:743-751

48. Rao U, Ryan ND, Dahl RE, et al. Factors associated with the development of substance use disorder in depressed adolescents. *J Am Acad Child Adolesc Psychiatry.* 1999;38:1109-1117

49. Costello EJ, Costello AJ, Edelbrock C, et al. Psychiatric disorders in pediatric primary care: prevalence and risk factors. *Arch Gen Psychiatry.* 1988;45:1107-1116

50. Kempton T, van Hasselt VB, Bukstein OG, Null JA. Cognitive distortions and psychiatric diagnosis in dually diagnosed adolescents. *J Am Acad Child Adolesc Psychiatry.* 1994;33:217-222

51. Wilens TE, Biederman J, Millstein RB, Wozniak J, Hahesy AL, Spencer TJ. Risk for substance use disorders in youths with child- and adolescent-onset bipolar disorder. *J Am Acad Child Adolesc Psychiatry.* 1999;46:618-320

52. Clark DB, Bukstein O, Smith MG, Kaczynski NA, Mezzich AC, Donovan JE. Identifying anxiety disorders in adolescents hospitalized for alcohol abuse and dependence. *Psychiatr Serv.* 1995;46:618-620

53. Clark DB, Lesnick L, Hegedus AM. Traumas and other adverse life events in adolescents with alcohol use and dependence. *J Am Acad Child Adolesc Psychiatry.* 1997;36:1744-1751

54. Van Hasselt VB, Ammerman RT, Glancy LJ, Bukstein OG. Maltreatment in psychiatrically hospitalized dually diagnosed adolescent substance abusers. *J Am Acad Child Adolesc Psychiatry.* 1992;31:868-874

55. Beck AT, Rush AJ, Shaw BF, Emery G. *Cognitive Therapy of Depression.* New York, NY: Guilford Press; 1979

56. Olfson M, Klerman GL. The treatment of depression: prescribing practices of primary care physicians and psychiatrists. *J Fam Pract.* 1992;35:627-635

57. Buckley PF. Substance abuse in schizophrenia: a review. *J Clin Psychiatry.* 1999;59(suppl 3):26-30

58. Minkoff K. An integrated treatment model for dual diagnosis of psychosis and addiction. *Hosp Community Psychiatry.* 1989;40: 1031-1036

59. Ries RK. The dually diagnosed patient with psychotic symptoms. *J Addict Dis.* 1993;12:103-122

60. American Academy of Pediatrics, Committee on Quality Improvement, Subcommittee on Attention-Deficit/Hyperactivity Disorder. Diagnosis and evaluation of the child with attention-deficit/hyperactivity disorder. *Pediatrics.* 2000;105:1158-1170

61. Riggs PD, Mikulich SC, Pottle LC. An open trial of bupropion for ADHD in adolescents with substance use disorder and conduct disorder. *J Am Acad Child Adolesc Psychiatry.* 1998;37:1271-1278

62. Cloninger CR. Neurogenetic adaptive mechanisms in alcoholism. *Science.* 1987;236:410-416

63. Groves JE. Taking care of the hateful patient. *N Engl J Med.* 1978;298:883-887

64. Jellinek MS, Ablon S. Character disorders in adolescence. In: Friedman SB, Fisher M, Schonberg SK, Alderman EM. *Comprehensive Adolescent Health Care.* 2nd ed. New York, NY: Mosby Year-Book; 1995:911-920

65. Myers WC, Burket RC, Otto TA. Conduct disorders and personality disorders in hospitalized adolescents. *J Clin Psychiatry.* 1993;54:21-26

66. Katz JL. Eating disorders: a primer for the substance abuse specialist, I: clinical features. *J Subst Abuse Treat.* 1990;7:143-149

67. Ross HE, Ivis F. Binge eating and substance abuse among male and female adolescents. *Int J Eat Disord.* 1999;26:245-260

68. Westermeyer J, Specker S. Social resources and social function in comorbid eating and substance disorder: a matched-pairs study. *Am J Addict.* 1999;8:332-336

69. Kaminer Y. Pharmacotherapy for adolescents with psychoactive substance use disorders. In: Rahdert E, Czechowicz D, eds. *Adolescent Drug Abuse: Clinical Assessment and Therapeutic Interventions.* Bethesda, MD: National Institute on Drug Abuse; 1995:49-111

70. Sohlkhah R, Wilens TE. Pharmacotherapy of adolescent alcohol and other drug use. *Alcohol Health Res World.* 1998;22:122-125

Appendix 1

Self-help and Advocacy Group Resources*

National Clearinghouse for Alcohol and Drug Information (NCADI)
The NCADI has trained information specialists available 24 hours a day.

PO Box 2345
Rockville, MD 20847-2345
Toll Free: 800/729-6686
Local Call: 301/468-2600
Hablamos Espanol: 877/767-8432
TDD: 800/478-4889
Fax: 301/468-6433
Internet: http://www.health.org/Index.htm

National Federation of Parents for Drug-Free Youth (NFP)
Activities include Project Graduation and Safe Homes.

8730 Georgia Avenue, #200
Silver Spring, MD 20910
Telephone: 301/585-5437

Parent Resources and Information for Drug Education (PRIDE)
Information and referral resource for parents and others. PRIDE is the largest and oldest organization in the nation devoted to drug- and violence-free youth.

Robert Woodruff Building
Volunteer Service Center, Suite 1012
100 Edgewood Avenue NE
Atlanta, GA 30303
Telephone: 800/241-9746
Internet: http://www.prideusa.org

---

*This listing does not indicate AAP endorsement of program efficacy or approach.

Alcoholics Anonymous (AA)

Grand Central Station
PO Box 459
New York, NY 10163
Telephone: 212/870-3400
Internet: http://www.alcoholics-anonymous.org/

Narcotics Anonymous (NA)

Narcotics Anonymous is a national network of more than 2000
regional groups that is patterned closely after Alcoholics Anonymous (AA). NA groups are conducted by recovered drug
addicts who follow the AA program to aid in rehabilitation.
NA publishes a variety of helpful materials for its members,
including a directory of group meetings.

World Service Office – Los Angeles
PO Box 9999
Van Nuys, CA 91409
Telephone: 818/773-9999
Fax: 818/700-0700
Internet: http://www.na.org

World Service Office – Europe
48 Rue de lt/Zomerstraat
B-1050 Brussels, Belgium
Telephone: 32-2-646-6012
Fax: 32-2-649-9239

Mothers Against Drunk Driving (MADD)

Membership is open to youth, senior citizens, individuals,
families, organizations and businesses, injured victims, and
families of victims who want to stop drunk driving, support the
victims of this violent crime, and prevent underage drinking.

National Headquarters
Victim Assistance and Book Orders
511 East John Carpenter Freeway, Suite 700
Irving, TX 75062
Telephone: 214/744-6233

Parent Teacher Association (PTA)

The National PTA is the nation's largest and oldest child advocacy volunteer association.

300 North Wabash Avenue, Suite 2100
Chicago, IL 60611
Telephone: 800/307-4782
Fax: 312/670-6783
E-mail: info@pta.org
Internet: http://www.pta.org
(Some information on the PTA Web site is available in English and Spanish)

Washington, DC Office
1090 Vermont Avenue NW, Suite 1200
Washington, DC 20005-4905
Telephone: 202/289-6790
Fax: 202/289-6791
Internet: http://www.pta.org/programs/dcoffice.htm

Families Anonymous (FA)

Self-help group patterned after AA.

PO Box 528
Van Nuys, CA 91408
Telephone: 818/989-7841

Adult Children of Alcoholics (ACOA)

Addresses the trauma of growing up in an alcoholic family.

PO Box 880517
San Francisco, CA 94188
Telephone: 415/931-2262

National Association for Children of Alcoholics (NACOA)

11426 Rockville Pike, Suite 100
Rockville, MD 20852
Telephone: 888/554-2627
E-mail: nacoa@erols.com
Internet: http://www.health.org/nacoa

Students Against Driving Drunk (SADD)
Chapters in high schools and colleges. Weekend hotline service to provide safe rides.

PO Box 800
Marlboro, MA 01752
Telephone: 617/481-3568

---

*This listing does not indicate AAP endorsement of program efficacy or approach.

Appendix 2

Medical and Medical Specialty Organizations

American Academy of Pediatrics (AAP)

Through AAP committees and scientific meetings on substance abuse and its Department of Education, many resources are available, including the annual and spring meetings, this guide, and hands-on programs offered by state chapters. The official journal of the AAP is *Pediatrics*. For more information about the wide range of educational materials on substance abuse available, contact the Department of Education.

141 Northwest Point Boulevard
Elk Grove Village, IL 60007
Telephone: 800/433-9016
Fax: 847/434-8000
E-mail: kidsdocs@aap.org
Internet: http://www.aap.org

American Society of Addiction Medicine (ASAM)

Holds an annual meeting devoted to adolescent and young adult addiction medicine. The *Journal of Addictive Diseases* is the official publication of the ASAM.

740 Buckingham Drive
Redland, CA 92374
Telephone: 714/427-5128
Internet: http://www.asam.org

Association for Medical Education and Research in Substance Abuse (AMERSA)

Continuing education programs are offered. *Substance Abuse* is the official journal of AMERSA.

125 Whipple Street
Third Floor, Suite 300
Providence, RI 02908
Telephone: 401/349-0000
Fax: 877/418-8769
Internet: http://www.amersa.org

American Medical Association (AMA)

Offers a great variety of continuing medical education materials and conferences. *Profiles of Adolescent Health,* Volumes I and II, are an excellent general reference, and the official journal is the *Journal of the American Medical Association (JAMA).* A directory of continuing medical education offerings is available.

515 North State Street
Chicago, IL 60610
Toll Free: 800/262-2350
Local Call: 312/751-6000

American Academy of Child and Adolescent Psychiatry

428 East Preston Street
Baltimore, MD 21202
Telephone: 800/638-6423

American Academy of Family Physicians

1740 West 92nd Street
Kansas City, MO 64114
Toll Free: 800/274-2237
Local Call: 816/333-9700

Society for Adolescent Medicine

1916 Copper Oaks Circle
Blue Springs, MO 64015
Telephone: 816/224-8010
E-mail: sam@adolescenthealth.org
Internet: http://www.adolescenthealth.org

Society for General Internal Medicine (SGIM)

c/o Judy Ann Bigby, MD
Division of General Medicine
Brigham and Women's Hospital
77 Francis Street, Boston, MA 02115
Telephone: 617/732-7063

Society of Teachers of Family Medicine

Publishes the *Family Medicine Curriculum Guide to Substance Abuse.*

8880 Ward Parkway
PO Box 8729
Kansas City, MO 64114
Telephone: 800/274-2237

Appendix 3

Additional Resources

National Institute on Drug Abuse (NIDA)

Visit NIDA's home page on the World Wide Web at http://www.nida.nih.gov. To learn more about prevention research, click on the Division of Epidemiology and Prevention Research. For information on community-based data from the Community Epidemiology Work Group, click on CEWG. For PREVLINE information from the National Clearinghouse for Alcohol and Drug Information home page, go to http://www.health.org.

NIDA
US Department of Health and Human Services
5600 Fishers Lane
Rockville, MD 20857
Telephone: 301/443-4060

For NIDA publications and prevention materials:
National Clearinghouse for Alcohol and Drug Information (NCADI)

PO Box 2345
Rockville, MD 20847-2345
Telephone: 800/729-6686

New NIDA materials on prevention:
All new publications are announced in *NIDA Notes,* NIDA's newsletter to the field. To get on the mailing list, write to:

Subscription Department, *NIDA Notes*
c/o ROW Sciences, Inc.
1700 Research Boulevard, Suite 400
Rockville, MD 20850
Fax: 301/294-5401

National Institute on Alcohol Abuse and Alcoholism (NIAAA)

Visit NIAAA's home page on the World Wide Web at http://www.niaaa.nih.gov. Full texts of many NIAAA publications are available as well as program announcements identifying research priorities and NIAAA's online bibliographic database, which contains approximately 100 000 records.

Join Together

A national resource center for communities working to prevent alcohol and other drug abuse across the nation.

441 Stewart Street, 7th Floor
Boston, MA 02116
Telephone: 617/437-1500
Internet: http://www.jointogether.org

National Council on Alcoholism and Drug Dependence (NCADD)

Provides educational materials on alcohol abuse and alcoholism as well as phone numbers of local NCADD affiliates who can provide information on local treatment resources.

12 West 21st Street
New York, NY 10010
Telephone: 800/NCA-CALL
Internet: http://www.ncadd.org

National Institute on Alcohol Abuse and Alcoholism (NIAAA) Scientific Communications Branch

Makes available free informational materials on many aspects of alcohol use, alcohol abuse, and alcoholism.

6000 Executive Boulevard, Suite 409
Bethesda, MD 20892-7003
Telephone: 301/443-3860
Internet: http://www.niaaa.nih.gov

Center for Substance Abuse Treatment (CSAT)

CSAT, a part of the Substance Abuse and Mental Health Services Administration, is responsible for supporting treatment services through block grants and developing knowledge about effective drug treatment, disseminating the findings to the field, and promoting their adoption. CSAT also operates the National Treatment Referral 24-hour Hotline (800/662-HELP) which offers information and referral to people seeking treatment programs and other assistance. CSAT publications are available through the National Clearinghouse on Alcohol and Drug Information (800/729-6686). Additional information about CSAT can be found on their Web site at http://www.samhsa.gov/csat.

National Network of Tobacco Prevention and Control Contacts

National Cancer Institute

Office of Cancer Communications
Building 31, Room 10A24
Bethesda, MD 20892
Telephone: 800/4-CANCER

Office on Smoking and Health

National Center for Chronic Disease Prevention
and Health Promotion
Centers for Disease Control and Prevention
Mail Stop K-50
4770 Buford Highway, NE
Atlanta, GA 30341-3742
Telephone: 770/488-5705

If there is any difficulty reaching any of the state contacts listed below, please contact the Office on Smoking and Health at 770/488-5705.

Alabama
Mobile County Health Department
Bureau of Health Promotion Administrative Services
PO Box 2867
Mobile, AL 36652
Telephone: 334/690-8186
Fax: 334/432-7443

Federal Express Address:
251 North Bayou Street
Mobile, AL 36603

Alaska
Manager, Health Promotion Program
Division of Public Health
Department of Health and Social Services
PO Box 110614
Juneau, AK 99811-0614
Telephone: 907/465-3140
Fax: 907/465-2770

Federal Express Address:
333 Willoughby Street, Room 713
Juneau, AK 99801

Arkansas
Director, Office of Tobacco Control and Prevention
4815 West Markham Street
Little Rock, AR 72205
Telephone: 501/661-2783
Fax: 501/661-2082

Arizona
Program Director, Tobacco Use Prevention and Control Program
Office of Health Promotion and Education
1400 West Washington Street
Phoenix, AZ 85007
Telephone: 602/542-7234
Fax: 602/542-0141

California
California Department of Health Services
744 P Street
PO Box 942732
Sacramento, CA 94234-7320
Telephone: 916/322-4787
Fax: 916/327-5424

Colorado
ASSIST Project Manager
Colorado Department of Health
4300 Cherry Creek Drive South
Denver, CO 80222-1530
Telephone: 303/692-2515
Fax: 303/782-0095

Connecticut
Health Program Supervisor
Department of Public Health and Addiction Services
150 Washington Street
Hartford, CT 06106
Telephone: 203/566-6618
Fax: 203/566-1217

Delaware
Prevention Coordinator
Department of Health and Social Services
PO Box 637
Dover, DE 19903
Telephone: 302/739-4724
Fax: 302/739-6617

Federal Express Address:
Jessie Cooper Building
Federal and Water Streets
Dover, DE 19901

District of Columbia
Public Health Educator
Department of Human Services
2nd Floor
800 Ninth Street, SW
Washington, DC 20024
Telephone: 202/645-5556
Fax: 202/645-0526

Florida
Program Administration
HRS Health Promotion and Wellness
Building 2-HSH, Room 321
1317 Winewood Boulevard
Tallahassee, FL 32399-0700
Telephone: 904/487-3220
Fax: 904/488-6495

Georgia
Tobacco Prevention Program Manager
Department of Human Resources
Tobacco Prevention Education Program
2 Peachtree Street, 6th Floor
Atlanta, GA 30303
Telephone: 404/657-2570
Fax: 404/657-6631

Guam
Health Educator Administrator
Department of Public Health and Social Services
PO Box 2816
Agana, Guam 96910
Telephone: 671/734-7129
Fax: 671/734-5910

Hawaii
Department of Health
952 North King Street, Bay 06
Honolulu, HI 96817
Telephone: 808/832-5951
Fax: 808/832-5955

Idaho
Health Promotion Coordinator
Idaho Department of Health and Welfare
PO Box 83728
450 West State Street
Boise, ID 83720-0036
Telephone: 208/334-4936
Fax: 208/334-6573

Illinois
Chief Public Health Educator
Illinois Department of Public Health
Division of Health Promotion
535 West Jefferson Street
Springfield, IL 62761
Telephone: 217/785-2060
Fax: 217/782-1235

Indiana
Director, ASSIST Project
Division of Health Education
Indiana Department of Health
1330 West Michigan Street
PO Box 1964
Indianapolis, IN 46206-1964
Telephone: 317/633-0267
Fax: 317/633-0776

Iowa
Director, Division of Substance Abuse and Health Promotion
Iowa Department of Public Health
Lucas State Office Building
Des Moines, IA 50319-0075
Telephone: 515/281-7248
Fax: 515/281-4535

Kansas
Office of Chronic Disease and Health Promotion
Kansas Department of Health and Environment
900 Southwest Jackson Street
Topeka, KS 66612-1290
Telephone: 913/296-1233
Fax: 913/296-8059

Kentucky
Tobacco Control Coordinator
Kentucky Department for Health Services
275 East Main Street
Frankfort, KY 40621
Telephone: 502/564-7243
Fax: 502/564-6533

Louisiana
Chronic Disease Control Program
Louisiana Department of Health and Hospitals
325 Loyola Avenue, Room 414
New Orleans, LA 70112
Telephone: 504/568-7210
Fax: 504/568-2543

Maine
ASSIST Project
Division of Health Promotion and Education
Maine Department of Human Services
151 Capitol Street
State House Station 11
Augusta, ME 04333
Telephone: 207/287-5180
Fax: 207/287-4631

Mariana Islands
Psychiatric Clinical Coordinator
Department of Public Health and Environmental Services
PO Box 409 CK
Saipan, MP 96950
Telephone: 670/234-8950, ext 2500
Fax: 670/234-8930

Marshall Islands
Director of Human Services
Alcohol and Substance Abuse
Ministry of Health and Environment
PO Box 16
Majuro, Republic of the Marshall Islands 96960
Telephone: 011-692-625-3249
Fax: 011-692-625-3432

Maryland
Division of Health Education
Department of Health and Mental Hygiene
201 W Preston Street
Baltimore, MD 21201
Telephone: 410/225-1362
Fax: 410/333-7903

Massachusetts
Office for Nonsmoking and Health
Massachusetts Department of Public Health
250 Washington Street, 4th Floor
Boston, MA 02111
Telephone: 617/624-5900
Fax: 617/624-5922

Michigan
ASSIST Project Director
Chief, Tobacco Section
Michigan Department of Public Health
3423 N Logan Street
PO Box 30195 – CHP
Lansing, MI 48909
Telephone: 517/335-8380
Fax: 517/335-9648

Federal Express Address:
Drop PO Box

Micronesia
Secretary, Department of Health
FSM National Government
Palikir Station, PS 70
Palikir, Pohnpei FSM 96941
Telephone: 011-691-320-2619
Fax: 011-691-5263/2785

Minnesota
ASSIST Project Manager
Minnesota Department of Health
717 Delaware Street, SE
PO Box 9441
Minneapolis, MN 55440-9441
Telephone: 612/623-5623
Fax: 612/623-5775

Mississippi
Coordinator
Tobacco Prevention
Mississippi State Department of Health
PO Box 1700
Jackson, MS 39215-1700
Telephone: 601/960-7828
Fax: 601/354-6278

Federal Express Address:
2423 N State Street
Jackson, MS 39216

Missouri
Project Manager, ASSIST
Tobacco Control Coordinator
Missouri Department of Health
101 Park DeVille Drive
Columbia, MO 65203
Telephone: 314/876-3260
Fax: 573/446-8777

Montana
Health Services Manager
Department of Health and Environmental Sciences
1400 Broadway
Cogswell Bldg, Rm C314
Helena, MT 59620
Telephone: 406/444-4488
Fax: 406/444-2606

Nebraska
Health Promotion and Education
Nebraska Department of Health
301 Centennial Mall South
PO Box 95007
Lincoln, NE 68509-5007
Telephone: 402/471-2101
Fax: 402/471-6446

Federal Express Address:
Drop PO Box

Nevada
Tobacco Control Coordinator
Nevada Department of Human Resources
505 E King St, Rm 304
Carson City, NV 89710
Telephone: 702/687-4800
Fax: 702/687-4988

New Hampshire
Bureau of Health Promotion
New Hampshire Division of Public Health Services
Health and Welfare Building
6 Hazen Drive
Concord, NH 03301-6527
Telephone: 603/271-6892
Fax: 603/271-6116

New Jersey
Coordinator
ASSIST Project—Tobacco Program
New Jersey Department of Health
CN 362, 129 Hanover Street
Trenton, NJ 08625-0369
Telephone: 609/984-1310
Fax: 609/292-3816

New Mexico
Program Manager
Tobacco Use Prevention/ASSIST
2329 Wisconsin, NE, Suite A
Albuquerque, NM 87110
Telephone: 505/841-8335
Fax: 505/841-8333

New York
Program Manager
Tobacco Control Program, ASSIST Project
New York State Department of Health
Corning Tower Building
Empire State Plaza, Room 515
Albany, NY 12237-0620
Telephone: 518/474-1515
Fax: 518/473-2853

North Carolina
Manager
Division of Adult Health, ASSIST Project
North Carolina Department of Environment, Health,
   and Natural Resources
PO Box 27687
Raleigh, NC 27611-7687
Telephone: 919/733-1676
Fax: 919/733-0488

Federal Express Address:
1330 St. Mary's Street
Raleigh, NC 27611-7687

North Dakota
Coordinator
Tobacco Prevention and Control Program
600 E Boulevard Ave, Judicial Wing, 2nd Floor
Bismarck, ND 58505-0200
Telephone: 701/328-3138
Fax: 701/328-1412

Ohio
Chief
Bureau of Chronic Diseases, Prevention Branch
Ohio Department of Health
246 N High Street
PO Box 118
Columbus, OH 43266-0118
Telephone: 614/466-2144
Fax: 614/644-7740

Federal Express Address:
Drop PO Box

Oklahoma
Health Information Section
Oklahoma State Department of Health
1000 NE 10th Street
Oklahoma City, OK 73117-1299
Telephone: 405/271-5601
Fax: 405/271-2865

Oregon
Chronic Disease
Oregon Department of Human Resources
800 NE Oregon Street
Portland, OR 97232
Telephone: 503/731-4025
Fax: 503/731-4082

Pennsylvania

Director
Tobacco and Control Program
Pennsylvania Department of Health
PO Box 90, Room 1003
Harrisburg, PA 17108
Telephone: 717/783-5900
Fax: 717/783-5498

Federal Express Address:
Tobacco Control Program
Health and Welfare Building, Room 1003
Commonwealth Avenue and Forster Street
Harrisburg, PA 17120

Palau

Minister of Health
Ministry of Health
PO Box 6027
Koror, Republic of Palau 96940
Telephone: 011-680-488-2813
Fax: 011-680-488-1725

Puerto Rico

SAMPSF, Preventive Medicine
Puerto Rico Department of Health
PO Box 70184
San Juan, PR 00936
Telephone: 809/274-5645
Fax: 809/274-7863

Rhode Island

ASSIST Project
Rhode Island Department of Health
Cannon Building, 3 Capitol Hill, Room 103
Providence, RI 02908-5097
Telephone: 401/277-3329
Fax: 401/861-5751

Samoa

Associate Director, Public Health Nursing
Department of Health
Pago Pago, American Samoa 96799
Telephone: 011-684-4606/5318
Fax: 011-684-633-5379

South Carolina

ASSIST Project, Center for Health Promotion
South Carolina Department of Health and
    Environmental Control
2600 Bull Street
Columbia, SC 29201
Telephone: 803/734-4446
Fax: 803/253-4001

South Dakota

South Dakota Department of Human Services
Division of Alcohol and Drugs
3800 E Highway 34; Hillsview Plaza
Pierre, SD 57501
Telephone: 605/773-3123
Fax: 605/773-5483

Tennessee

Tennessee Department of Health
Health Promotion/Disease Control
Tennessee Tower Building, 13th Floor
312 8th Avenue, N
Nashville, TN 37247-5201
Telephone: 615/741-7366
Fax: 615/432-8478

Texas
Office of Smoking and Health
Texas Department of Health
1100 W 49th Street
Austin, TX 78756-3199
Telephone: 512/458-7402
Fax: 512/458-7618

Utah
Statewide Risk Reduction
Utah Department of Health
288 N 1460, W
Salt Lake City, UT 84116-0660
Telephone: 801/538-6270
Fax: 801/538-6036

Vermont
Tobacco Control Coordinator
Health Promotion/Epidemiology Division
Vermont Department of Health
PO Box 70
Burlington, VT 05402
Telephone: 802/865-7783
Fax: 802/863-7425

Virgin Islands
Virgin Islands Department of Social and Health Services
Charles Harword Complex, Room E-25
Christiansted, St Croix, VI 00820
Telephone: 809/774-7700
Fax: 809/774-4701

Virginia
Virginia Department of Health
1500 E Main Street
PO Box 2448, Suite 245
Richmond, VA 23218-2448
Telephone: 804/786-3551
Fax: 804/371-6152

Washington
ASSIST Project, Heart Disease and Cancer Prevention
Department of Social and Health Services
Airdustrial Park 10, PO Box 4783
Olympia, WA 98504-7835
Telephone: 206/586-6082
Fax: 206/664-8779

Federal Express Address:
Drop PO Box

West Virginia
Program Manager
ASSIST Project
West Virginia Department of Health and Human Resources
1411 Virginia Street, E
Charleston, WV 25301
Telephone: 304/558-0644
Fax: 304/558-1553

Wisconsin
ASSIST Project
Wisconsin Division of Health
1400 E Washington Avenue, Room 240
Madison, WI 53703-3041
Telephone: 608/266-8322
Fax: 608/266-8925

Wyoming
Program Manager
Health Risk Reduction
Wyoming Department of Health
Hathaway Building, 4th Floor
Cheyenne, WY 82002
Telephone: 307/777-5949
Fax: 307/777-5402

Astho Headquarters
Director, Tobacco Control Projects
415 Second Street, NE
Suite 200
Washington, DC 20002
Telephone: 202/546-5400
Fax: 202/544-9349

Index

* Page numbers with *f* indicate figures; page numbers with *t* indicate tables; page numbers with *n* indicate footnotes.

A

Abortion, 178, 294
 amphetamine use and, 294
 cocaine use and, 219–20, 294
 opiate use and, 247
 spontaneous, 219, 294
 tobacco use and, 294
Abruptio placentae, 219, 294
Abscesses, heroin and, 247
Abstinence philosophy, 138
Abstinence syndrome
 anticipation of, 255
 neonatal, 248, 293
 opiate, 247, 248, 249
 sedative-hypnotic, 254, 255
 tranquilizers, 259
 treatment of, 249, 255, 259
Acceptance of responsibility, 90–91
Acetaldehyde, 210
Acetylcholine, 227
Acetylprocaine, 245
Achenbach Child Behavior
 Checklist, 77
Acid, 226, 264*t*
Acidification of urine, 234
Action stage, 89, 92
Acute renal failure, MDMA as cause
 of, 236
Acute transient toxic psychosis, 234
Adam, 264*t*
Addiction
 to cocaine, 218, 222–23
 to opiates, 248
 stage change models of, 89–91

Addiction medicine
 patient-treatment matching in, 127
 use of formal assessment
  instruments in, 43
Adolescent Alcohol Prevention
 Trial, 154
*Adolescent Assessment/Referral System
 (AARS) Manual*, 78–79, 81, 82
Adolescent CAGE, 70–71
Adolescent Diagnostic Interview
 (ADI), 83
Adolescents. *See also* Minors
 alcohol use by, 208–9, 211–13
 amphetamine use by, 221–22, 223–25
 cocaine use by, 215–16, 217–20
 confidentiality of information
  disclosed by, 48–51
 constitutional protections for female,
  178
 designer hallucinogen use by, 234–37
 dual diagnosis in, diagnosis,
  assessment, and treatment
  of, 206, 307–19
 fluctuations in prevalence of
  substance use among, 11
 inhalant use by, 259–62
 interviewing for substance abuse,
  51–52
 legal and ethical considerations in
  care of, 179–82
 LSD use by, 226–27, 229–30
 marijuana use by, 199, 201–6
 obtaining sensitive information from,
  66–67

opiate use by, 243–44, 246–48
PCP use by, 231, 232–33
placement criteria, 130–36*t*
populations of, with heightened
    vulnerability to substance
    abuse, 44–45
resistance to consulting with
    psychiatrist/psychologist, 32
sedative-hypnotic use by, 251–52,
    253–54
substance abuse in, viii, 2, 3, 4*f*
    categorizing dimensions of, 85
    counseling strategies for, 91–92,
        93*t*, 94–98
    stages of, 124*t*
    testing for, 26*t*
tobacco cessation therapy for,
    287–88
tobacco use by, 192–94, 196,
    277–78, 281–82
tranquilizer use by, 256, 257–58
Adolescents Training and Learning
    to Avoid Steroids (ATLAS)
    program, 242
Adolescent Substance Abuse Subtle
    Screening Inventory (SASSI),
    75–76
Adult Children of Alcoholics (ACOA),
    139, 327
Adversarial relationship, 126
Adverse consequences, 90
    associated with the abuse, 63, 64*t*
Advertisements
    development of counter-, 165–66
    tobacco products in, 198, 278–79
Advocacy roles and opportunities of
    primary care physicians, 37–38
Affective disorders, 309
Affective education, 165, 168–69
    promoting personal growth
        through, 147

Age-appropriate psychosocial function-
    ing, inquiry into, 24
Agency for Healthcare Research and
    Quality, 287
Age of initiation of alcohol use, and
    use of other drugs, 2–3
Aggressive behavior as risk factor in
    substance abuse, 5, 6
Agoraphobia, 313
AIDS, 183, 186, 244. *See also* Human
    immunodeficiency virus (HIV)
    infection
Air bags, 167*n*
Al-Anon, 137, 139
Alateen, 139, 215
Alcohol, 208–15
    Adolescent Alcohol Prevention Trial
        in preventing use of, 154
    age of initiation of, 2–3
    benzodiazepine use and, 257–58
    decrease in adolescent use of, viii
    drinking and driving prevention
        program for, 167–68
    epidemiology, 208–9
    as gateway drug, 125
    health consequences, 211–13
    intoxication, 214
    intrauterine growth retardation and,
        294–95
    laboratory evaluation of, 214
    legal and ethical issues in use of,
        176–77
    marijuana use and, 212
    motor vehicle crashes and, viii, 2, 9,
        211
    neonatal neurobehavioral deficien
        cies and, 296–97
    pharmacology of, 209–11
    prenatal exposure to, 213, 293
    prevalance of use, ix
    problem strategies and, 167–68

steroid use and, 242
treatment of intoxication, 214–15
withdrawal syndrome, 210–11
Alcoholic parents, children of, 209
Alcoholics Anonymous (AA), 137, 139, 215, 326
Alcoholism, 209
in adolescents, 214
complications of chronic, 212
family history of, and risk of, 5
link between genetics and, 5
Alternative highs, providing, 147–49
Amenorrhea, heroin use and, 247
American Academy of Child and Adolescent Psychiatry, 330
American Academy of Family Physicians, 330
American Academy of Pediatrics (AAP), 282, 329
Model Act of, 185
policy statement on laboratory testing for drugs of abuse, 24
American Cancer Society, 287
American Heart Association, 287
American Lung Association, 287
American Medical Association (AMA), 282–83, 330
American Society of Addiction Medicine (ASAM), 129, 329
γ-Aminobutyric acid (GABA), 210
Amobarbital sodium, 251
Amotivational syndrome, marijuana and, 205–6
Amphetamine look-alikes, 222, 223
Amphetamines, 27, 144, 215, 221–26
benzodiazepines in counteracting effects of, 257
central nervous system lesions and, 296
distinguishing psychosis from schizophrenia and use of, 225

epidemiology, 221–22
health consequences, 223–25
immunoassay tests for, 107t
laboratory evaluation, 225
pharmacology, 222–23
prenatal exposure to, 225
prevalance of use, ix
spontaneous abortion and, 294
steroid use and, 240, 242
street names for, 221
treatment considerations, 225–26
Amphetamine with isomers, 222
Amyl nitrite, 260, 262
Anabolic-androgenic steroids, 237–43
epidemiology, 237–39
health consequences, 240–42
laboratory evaluation, 242
pharmacology, 239–40
prevalance of use, ix
tests for, 106
treatment, 242
Anemias, anabolic-androgenic steroids in, 237
Angel dust, 226, 231
Angel mist, 231
Anorexia nervosa, 319
cocaine and, 219
Anovulatory cycles, heroin use and, 247
Anticholinergic hallucinogens, 228–29, 230
treatment of, 230
Anticipatory guidance
for adolescents, 22–23, 27–28
for alcohol use, 214
group encounters in accomplishing, 36
for parents, 23
for tobacco use, 282–83
Anticonvulsants for bipolar disorder, 313
Antihistamines, in triggering flash-backs, 230

Antismoking campaigns, 279
Antisocial personality disorders, 309,
    317–18
Anxiety disorders, 309, 313–15
    substance abuse risk in, 45
Anxiety relief, substance use for, 61
Apnea, 296
    PCP as cause of, 233
*ASAM Patient Placement Criteria for
    the Treatment of Substance-
    Related Disorders, Second
    Edition-Revised,* 129
Aspiration pneumonia
    alcohol intoxication and, 212
    sedative-hypnotic drugs in, 253
Association of Medical Educators and
    Researchers in Substance Abuse
    (AMERSA), 330
Associative processes abstraction, effect
    of marijuana on, 204
Asthma
    marijuana use and, 202
    smoking and, 195
Atherogenesis, 240
Atropine, 227
Atropine poisoning, 230
Attention deficit/hyperactivity disorder
    (ADHD), 310, 316–17
    amphetamines for, 221
    as risk factor in substance abuse,
    6, 45
Attention tasks, residual effects of
    marijuana on, 205
Auditory-verbal memory, effect of
    marijuana on, 205

B
BAM, 221
Barbiturates, 144, 210, 251. *See also*
    Sedative-hypnotics
    immunoassay tests for, 107*t*
    prevalance of use, ix
Behavior
    aggressive, as risk factor in
        substance abuse, 5
    alcohol use, and genetics, 5
    cocaine use and, 218, 219
    defensive, in substance abuse
        interviews, 51
    deviant, in obtaining drugs, 62
    disruptive, substance abuse and, 35
    enabling, 125–26
    marijuana use and, 203, 205–6
    steroid use and, 241–42
Behavioral treatment for anxiety
    disorders, 314
Bennie, 221
Benzodiazepines, 210, 256
    for agitation in PCP use, 234
    binding sites for, 240
    immunoassay tests for, 107*t*
    screening for, 116
    for treating LSD intoxication, 230
Beta-galactosidase, 114
Binge drinking, 208, 242
Bipolar disorder, 310, 313
    substance abuse risk in, 45
Bisexual adolescents, vulnerability to
    substance abuse, 44
Black beauties, 221
Black market, 238
Blood alcohol levels, 212, 214
Blood assays
    for amphetamines, 225
    for cocaine, 220
Blotter acid, 228, 264*t*
Blue heavens, 251

Boldenone undecylenate, 239
Borderline personality disorders, 318–19
Brachial plexitis, heroin and, 247
Brazelton Neonatal Assessment Scale, 203
Breakaway road sign posts, 167*n*
Breastfeeding, maternal substances of abuse and, 301
Bronchial epithelium, adverse effects of marijuana and tobacco on, 202
Bronchitis
    marijuana use and, 202
    smoking as cause of, 195, 281
Bronchoconstriction, marijuana use and, 202
Bronchodilation, 201–2
Brown v The Board of Education, 177
Bulimia, 319
    substance abuse risk in, 45
Bullet, 261
Bupropion hydrochloride
    for anxiety disorders, 314
    for attention deficit/hyperactivity disorder (ADHD), 316–17
    in smoking cessation, 198, 288
Butyl nitrite, 261, 262

C
Caffeine, 222
CAGE
    adolescent, 70–71
    adult, 70
CAGE-AA (CAGE Adapted for Adolescents), 71
Cancer, smoking as risk factor for, 196
Cannabinoid antagonist, 201
Cannabinoid receptor, 200–201
Cannabinoids, 200
    detection of, in urine, 207
    immunoassay tests for, 107*t*

Cannabis-dependence disorder, 206
Cannabis indica, 199
Cannabis sativa, 199
    x *indica,* 199
Capillary column, 116
Carbamazepine, for bipolar disorder, 313
Carbon monoxide
    marijuana use and, 202
    smoking and, 194, 196
Carboxyhemoglobin, 194, 196
Carcinogens, 194–95
Cardiac arrhythmias
    inhalants as cause of, 261, 262
    PCP as cause of, 233
Cardiopulmonary arrest, opiate use and, 248
Cardiovascular disease, advances in preventing, 1
Cardiovascular effects of marijuana, 201
Carey v Population Services International, 178
Cat Valium, 264*t*
Cellulitis, heroin and, 247
Center for Substance Abuse Treatment (CSAT), 129, 335
    adolescent placement criteria, 129, 130–36*t*
Central nervous system
    anomalies in, 295
    effects of cocaine on, 217
    lesions in, 296
    nicotine and, 194
    opiates and, 246
Cervical cancer, smoking and, 196
Chain of custody, 110
    documentation of, 109–10
Channel One, 163
Checkup visits, providing anticipatory guidance in, 23

Chelation therapy, 263
Chemical Dependency Assessment
	Scale, 77
Chewing tobacco, 191–92, 277
Child Behavior Checklist, 82
*Childhood Antecedents of Smoking
	Study,* 193–94
Children
	of alcoholic parents, 209
	effects of cigarette smoke on, 195,
		281–82
	testing for drugs of abuse in, 26*t*
Child welfare, substance abuse and,
	299–300
Chlorpromazine, 255
	for amphetamines overdose, 225–26
Chromosome breakage, 230
Chronic alcoholism, 212
Chronic diseases, vulnerability to
	substance abuse and, 44
Chronic hypoxia, 195
Cirrhosis of the liver, chronic
	alcoholism and, 212
Citizen-parent action groups, advocacy
	roles and opportunities in, 38
*Classification of Child and Adolescent
	Mental Diagnoses in Primary
	Care: Diagnostic and Statistical
	Manual for Primary Care (DSM-
	PC), Child and Adolescent
	Version,* 86–87, 87, 307
Cleft lip and palate, benzodiazepines as
	cause of, 258
Client Personal History Questionnaire,
	81
Clinical information, synthesizing,
	85–91
Clinical interviews. *See* Interviews
Clinical screening for substance abuse,
	44–45, 55. *See also* Interviews;
	Questionnaires

counseling strategies in, 91–92, 93*t*,
	94–98
formal assessment instruments in,
	66–68
formal diagnostic classification
	system, 86–88
interviews in, 54*t*, 63–66
stage change models of addiction,
	89–91
synthesizing clinical information in,
	85–91
tiered system approaches in, 76–82
Clitoral hypertrophy, steroid use and,
	241
Cloned-enzyme donor immunoassay
	(CEDIA), 114
Clonidine hydrochloride
	for opiate withdrawal, 250
	for smoking cessation, 288
Club drugs, 191, 226, 232, 235, 256,
	263, 264*t*
Cocaine, 215–21, 293
	in abruptio placentae, 294
	adolescent use of, 3
	apnea and, 296
	benzodiazepines in counteracting
		effects of, 257
	central nervous system lesions
		and, 296
	congenital anomalies and, 295
	epidemiology, 215–16
	health consequences, 217–20
	immunoassay tests for, 107*t*
	intrauterine growth retardation
		and, 294–95
	laboratory evaluation, 220
	mixing heroin with, 216
	neonatal neurobehavioral
		deficiencies and, 296–97
	neonates exposed to, 220
	pharmacology, 216–17

prenatal exposure to, 293
preterm labor and, 295
prevalance of use, ix
spontaneous abortion and, 294
steroid use and, 242
sudden infant death syndrome
(SIDS) and, 296
switch to amphetamines from, 222
treatment considerations, 220–21
Codeine, 243
Cognitive task performance in MDMA
users, 237
College of American Pathologists in
accrediting forensic laboratories,
105
Color tests, 113
Coma
alcohol intoxication and, 212
PCP as cause of, 233
Community
alcohol abuse programs in, 215
prevention programs focused on,
161–65, 169
role of primary care physicians in,
36, 37–38
Comorbidity, 206, 241, 307
antisocial personality disorders and,
317–18
anxiety disorders and, 45, 313–15
attention-deficit/hyperactivity
disorder and, 6, 45, 316–17
bipolar disorders and, 45, 310, 313
borderline personality disorders
and, 318–19
conduct disorders and, 45, 212,
310, 317–18
depressive disorders and, 45, 212,
311–12
eating disorders and, 45, 219, 310,
319
marijuana use and, 206

narcissistic personality disorders
and, 318–19
organic mental disorders and, 315
post-traumatic stress disorders and,
313–15
schizophrenia and, 225, 315–16
substance abuse and, 307–19
Competence enhancement approaches
to prevention, 155–57
Comprehensive Assessment Battery
(CAB), 81
Computer-assisted technology for
identification of sensitive health
issues, 67
Conduct disorders, 310, 317–18
substance abuse risk in, 45, 212
Confidentiality
in counseling, 28
of information disclosed by
adolescent, 29, 48–51, 183–88
in providing family support in
substance abuse, 33
Confirmation testing
gas chromatography in, 116
gas chromatography/mass
spectrometry in, 116–17, 237
high-performance liquid
chromatography in, 117
of immunoassay results, 106, 108
necessity of, 106, 108
specificity of, 109
Congenital abnormalities, 295–96
See also Pregnancy
relationship of cocaine to, 219–20
Consultation, role of primary care
physicians in, 32–33
Contemplation stage, 89, 90, 92
Contextual factors in substance abuse,
9–10
Continued substance use, 87, 88
Continuing care, 139
Contract for Life, 167

Controlled Substances Act
  Schedule I of, 234–35
  Schedule II of, 221, 251
  Schedule III of, 238
Cooperative consultation process, 166
Coordination, effect of marijuana on
    performance of tasks related
    to, 203–4
Coronary artery disease, smoking and
    risk of, 196
Cortinarius species mushrooms,
    hallucinogens in, 229
Cotinine, 195, 196
Counseling strategies for adolescents
    with substance abuse, 91–92,
    93*t*, 94–98
Counteradvertising programs, 165–66
Crack, 215, 216–17
CRAFFT mnemonic tool, 68–69
Crank, 221, 264*t*
Crash, 218
Cross-reactivity, 115–16
Crystal, 264*t*
Cubes, 264*t*
Cystic fibrosis, vulnerability to
    substance abuse and, 44
Cytomegalovirus, screening of mother
    for, 301

D
Darvon, 243
Date rape drug, 256
Death. *See* Mortality
Decerebrate rigidity, PCP as cause
    of, 233
Defensive behaviors, in substance
    abuse interviews, 51
Dehydrogenase, 209–10
Delirium tremens, 210–11, 254
Demerol, 243

Dependence
  on alcohol, 220
  on benzodiazepines, 258
  on cocaine, 218, 222–23
  on sedative-hypnotics, 220
Depression, 310, 311–12
  alcohol use and, 212
  amphetamine use and, 224–25
  steroid use and, 241
  substance abuse risk in, 45, 311
Designer drugs, 226, 244, 246–47
  steroid use and, 242
Designer euphoriants, 27
Designer opiates, 246–47–248
Detailed clinical interview, 67
Determination or preparation stage,
    89, 92
Deterrence-based programs, 161–62
Detoxification
  heroin and, 245
  methadone in, 249–50
Deviant behavior in obtaining drugs,
    62
Dextroamphetamine sulfate, 222–23
Diabetes mellitus, vulnerability to
    substance abuse and, 44
Diacetylmorphine, 245
*Diagnostic and Statistical Manual
    of Mental Disorders, Fourth
    Edition (DSM-IV)*, 87, 126
  addictive substances in, 280–81
  categories in, 88
  comorbid psychiatric disorders in,
    206, 307, 309
  criteria in, 86
  depression in, 311
  steroid use in, 241
  substance abuse in, 127*t*
  substance dependence in, 88, 128*t*
  substance-induced disorders in, 87
  substance use disorders in, 86, 87

Diagnostic Interview Schedule for
    Children (DISC), 82
Diagnostic testing, 26*t*
Diazepam, 256
    for agitation in PCP use, 234
Dilaudid, 243
2,5-Dimethoxy-4-methylamphetamine
    (DOM, STP), 227
Diphenoxylate hydrochloride, 243
Disruptive behaviors, substance abuse
    and, 35
Disulfiram for alcoholism, 214
Divorce of parents, substance abuse
    and, 7
Doctors Ought to Care, drug
    prevention programs of, 165
Dolophine, 243
Dopamine, 201
Dots, 264*t*
Downers, 251
Drinking and driving prevention
    program, 167–68
Driving ability, effect of methampheta-
    mine on, 224
Drug abuse. *See* Substance abuse
Drug and Alcohol Problem
    Quickscreen (DAP), 68
Drug dependence, lifetime prevalence
    of, 3
Drug-free rock concerts, 148
Drug-free therapeutic communities,
    250
Drug information education, 146–47
Drug resistance skills, 150, 157–58
Drug testing, 26*t*
    for amphetamines, 225
    for barbiturates, 254
    for cocaine, 220
    color or spot tests in, 113
    confirmation techniques in, 116–17
    in diagnosing substance abuse, 24
    diagnostic testing in, 26*t*

immunoassays in, 107*t*, 113–16
for inhalants, 262
involuntary testing in, 26*t*
for marijuana, 207
for maternal substances of abuse,
    300–301
for MDMA, 237
necessity of confirmation, 106, 108
for opiates, 248
for PCP, 234
scientific issues in, 105–6, 107*t*,
    108–12, 111*t*
    broadness of screen, 108
    confirmation of immunoassay
        results, 106, 108
    documentation of chain of
        custody, 109–10
    sensitivity of screening
        procedure, 108–9
    specificity of confirmatory
        procedure, 109
    urine testing in, 110–12
    variety of drugs being assayed,
        106, 107*t*
sensitivity of, 107*t*, 108–9
standards for, 118
for steroids, 242
thin-layer chromatography in, 113
voluntary screening in, 26*t*
Drug Use Screening Inventory (DUSI),
    76, 77–78
    diagnostic evaluation, 77–78
    screening assessment, 77
Dual diagnosis, 307
    assessment, diagnosis, and treat-
        ment of adolescents with,
        307–19
Dysphoric reactions of marijuana, 203

E

Eating disorders, 310, 319
    anorexia nervosa, 219, 319
    bulimia, 45, 319
Ecstasy, 27, 145, 188, 226, 227, 234,
    235, 263, 264*t*
Education
    affective, 147, 165, 168–69, 283
    effect of substance abuse on, 2
    factual, 283
    normative, 150, 157–58
    parent programs in, 159–60
    in preventing substance abuse, 36,
        146–47
Elephant (monkey) tranquilizer, 231
Emergency doctrine, 182
Emergency treatment of child, 181
Emphysema, smoking as cause of,
    195, 281
Enabling behavior, 125–26
Endocarditis
    cocaine and, 219
    heroin and, 247
Environmental tobacco smoke (ETS),
    277, 281, 282
Enzyme immunoassay in detecting
    cocaine, 220
Enzyme-linked immunosorbent assays
    (ELISA), 115
Enzyme-multiplied immunoassay
    technique (EMIT), 114
    in detecting marijuana, 207
Ephedrine, 222
    immunoassays for, 115
Erythroxylon coca, 215
Ethanol, 209–11
    spot tests for, 113
Ethchlorvynol, spot tests for, 113
Ether, 259
Ethical considerations. *See* Legal and
    ethical considerations
Exploratory issues, 58

F

F-40s, 251
False-negative test results, 106
False-positive test results, 108
Families Anonymous (FA), 327
Family
    alcohol use in, 209, 212
    drug use as problem in, 33–34
    dynamics theories of, 159
    as factor in substance abuse, 6–8
    prevention programs focused on,
        159–61, 169
    role of primary care physicians in
        providing support for, 33–36
Family and Educational Rights Privacy
    Act (1974), 185
Family court, 175–77
    establishment of, 177
    referral to, 176–77
Family Court Act (1899), 175–76
Fenfluramine hydrochloride, 223
Fentanyl citrate, 243
Fertility, effect of marijuana on, 202
Fetal abnormalities, barbiturates in, 254
Fetal alcohol syndrome, 213, 293
Fetal hypoxia, 294
Fetus, effect of smoking on, 195
"First-pass" metabolism, 209
Flame ionization, 116
Flashbacks, 229, 230
Flumazenil, 257, 259
Flunitrazepam, 256, 263, 264*t*
Fluorescence polarization immunoassay
    (FPIA), 115
Fluoxetine hydrochloride, 312
Follow-up, 139
    referral versus, 125–26
Food and Drug Administration (FDA)
    advisory on removing phenyl-
        propanolamine from drug
        products, 222
    regulations on tobacco, 198

Forced multiple-choice answers in getting formal substance use history, 60
Forensic laboratories, accreditation of, 105
Forget-me, 264*t*
Forget pill, 256
Formal assessment instruments, 66–68, 72–73
Formal diagnostic classification systems, 86–88
Formal substance use history, elements of, 59–62, 59*t*
Fourteenth Amendment, 177
Fourth Amendment right to protection against unreasonable searches, 178
Freebase, 216

G

"G," 264*t*
GABA(A)-benzodiazepine receptor complex, activation of, 257
Gammahydroxybutyrate (GHB), 263
Gas chromatography, 116
Gas chromatography/mass spectrometry (GC/MS), 105, 115, 116–17
confirmation by, 106
in detecting anabolic-androgenic steroids, 242
methods of, 105
in testing for MDMA, 237
Gasoline sniffing, 260, 262
Gastric lavage in treating lysergic acid diethylamide (LSD) intoxication, 230
Gastrointestinal bleeding, alcohol intoxication and, 212
Gateway drugs, 125
Gault, In re, 177
Genetics, link between alcohol use behaviors and, 5

Georgia home boy, 264*t*
GHB, 264*t*
Glass, 264*t*
Glucose-6-phosphate dehydrogenase [G6PD], 114
Glue sniffing, 259, 261
Glutaraldehyde, potential for interference with testing, 112
Group encounters in anticipatory guidance, 36
Growth hormone therapy, anabolic-androgenic steroids in testing, 237
Growth retardation, screening of mother for, 301
Gynecomastia, steroid use and, 241

H

Habilitation deficits, 159
Habitrol, 198
for tobacco cessation, 287
Hair, for drug testing, 110, 111*t*, 220
Hallucinations, amphetamine use and, 225
Hallucinogens. *See also* Lysergic acid diethylamide (LSD); MDMA (3,4-Methylenedioxymethamphetamine) ("ecstasy"); PCP
adverse psychologic effects of, 229
prevalance of use, ix
steroid use and, 242
Halogenated hydrocarbons, 261
Haloperidol, for treating LSD intoxication, 230
Halothane, 261
Hate crimes, vulnerability to substance abuse and, 44
HEADSS exam, 24
Health care professional. *See also* Primary care physicians
development of therapeutic alliance between adolescent and, 46

risk and protective factors and their implications for preventive interventions for, 1–12
in tobacco cessation efforts, 282–87
Health issues, computer-assisted technology for identification of sensitive, 67
Health maintenance visits, role of primary care physicians in providing anticipatory guidance in, 22–23
Hearing impairments, vulnerability to substance abuse and, 44–45
Heart disease, smoking and, 195
Hemodialysis, in treating barbiturate abuse, 255
Hemoperfusion, in treating barbiturate abuse, 255
Hepatic function, steroid use and, 240
Hepatitis
cocaine use and, 219
heroin use and, 247
steroids use and, 240
Hepatitis B, screening of mother for, 301
Hepatitis C, screening of mother for, 301
Hepatotoxic effects of MDMA, 236
Herbal ecstasy, 235
Heroin, 27, 188, 243, 244, 245–46
apnea and, 296
intrauterine growth retardation and, 294–95
mixing with cocaine, 216
prevalance of use, ix
sudden infant death syndrome (SIDS) and, 296
High-performance liquid chromatography (HPLC), 117
with diode array detector, 117

High-resolution mass spectrometry, in detecting anabolic-androgenic steroids, 242
Hirsutism, steroid use and, 241
Hog, 231
Homosexual adolescents
inhalant use by, 260
vulnerability to substance abuse, 44
Human immunodeficiency virus (HIV) infection, 2, 137. *See also* AIDS
amphetamine use and risk of, 224
cocaine use and risk of, 219
heroin use and risk of, 247
opiate use and, 248
screening of mother for, 301
steroid use and, 240–41
substance abuse risk in adolescents, 45
Hydrochloride, 243
immunoassays for, 115
Hydrocodone, immunoassays for, 115
Hydromorphone hydrochloride, 243
immunoassays for, 115
Hyperreflexia, PCP and, 233
Hypertension, PCP and, 233
Hyperthermia
MDMA use and, 236
sedative-hypnotic drugs in, 253
Hypnotics. *See* Sedative-hypnotics
Hypoglycemia, alcohol and, 214
Hypogonadism, anabolic-androgenic steroids in treating, 237
Hypomania, steroid use and, 241
Hypothermia, sedative-hypnotic drugs in, 253
Hypoxia, chronic, 195

I

Ice, 221, 264*t*
  prevalence of use, 222
Immunoassays, 107*t*, 113–16
  advantages and disadvantages, 115–16
  cloned-enzyme donor, 114, 115
  enzyme-linked, 115–16
  enzyme-multiplied, 114, 115
  fluorescence polarization, 115
  kinetic interaction of microparticles in solution, 114, 115
  radioimmunoassay, 114–15
  sensitivity of, 107*t*, 108–9
In-depth interview, 56
Indicated prevention approaches, 146
Individual factors in substance abuse, 5–6
Information disclosed by adolescent, confidentiality of, 48–51
Inhalants, 259–63
  epidemiology, 259–61
  as gateway drugs, 125
  health consequences, 261–62
  laboratory evaluation, 262
  pharmacology, 261
  prevalance of use, ix
  steroid use and, 242
  treatment considerations, 262–63
Insomnia
  cocaine use and, 219
  marijuana use and, 206
International Classification of Diseases, Ninth Edition, Clinical Modification (ICD-9-CM) codes, 86, 88
Intervention, role of primary care physicians in, 30*t*, 31, 34–36
Interviews, 43–98. *See also* Questionnaires
  clinical screening by, 55, 63–66

confidentiality of information disclosed by adolescent in, 48–51
  context of, 44–45, 45*t*
  detailed clinical, 67
  diagnosing substance abuse in, 24
  face-to-face, 67
  focused questions in, 63, 64*t*
  formal assessment instruments in, 66–68
  general techniques in, 46–48, 47*t*
  in-depth, 56
  mid-range evaluation in, 55–56
  psychosocial assessment in, 53, 54*t*, 55–56
  screening by, 63–66
  specialized evaluation in, 56
  strategies for, 51–52
  substance use history in, 56–63, 59*t*
Intoxicated adolescent, arrival at health care visit, 52
Intracerebral hemorrhage, amphetamines in, 224
Intracranial abscesses, heroin and, 247
Intrauterine growth retardation, 294–95
Involuntary testing, 26*t*
Isobutyl nitrite, 260, 261, 262

J

Jehovah's Witness, children of, 179
Jimsonweed, 227, 228–29
Juvenile delinquent, 176
Juvenile justice system, 177, 188

K

"K," 264*t*
Ketamine hydrochloride, 232, 263, 264*t*
  tests for, 106
Kinetic interaction of microparticles in solution, 114

L

"L," 264*t*

Lactose, 245

Learning
  alcohol use and, 212
  marijuana use and, 204, 205
  substance abuse and, 8–9

Legal and ethical considerations,
    175–89
  abortion, 178
  alcohol use, viii, 2, 9, 176–77,
      208, 211
  black market, 238
  confidentiality, 28, 29, 33,
      48–51, 183–88
  emergency doctrine, 181, 182
  juvenile justice system, 177
  mandatory reporting regulations,
      183
  medical care for adolescents,
      179–82
  parental consent, 175, 179,
      181–82, 184, 186, 187
  parens patriae doctrine, 187
  physician liability, 182
  physician-patient relationship,
      187
  police power, 187–88
  rights of minors, 49, 178, 180–82,
      184
  Schedule I drugs, 234–35
  Schedule II drugs, 221, 251
  Schedule III drugs, 238

Lethargy, PCP as cause of, 233

Life Skills Training (LST), 157–59,
    166

Limb-reduction anomalies, 295

Liquid chromatography/mass
    spectrometry, 117

Liquid ecstasy, 264*t*

Lithium carbonate, for bipolar
    disorder, 313

Local governments, advocacy roles
    and opportunities in, 38

Locker room, 261

Lomotil, 243

"Ludes," 251

Lumbosacral plexitis, heroin and, 247

Lung cancer, smoking as cause of,
    195, 277, 281

Lysergic acid diethylamide (LSD), ix,
    226–30, 264*t*
  epidemiology, 226–27
  flashback syndrome, 230
  health consequences, 229–30
  pharmacology, 227–29
  tests for, 106
  treatment considerations, 230

M

Ma huang, 222

Mainlining, 245

Maintenance stage, 89

Male pattern baldness, steroid use
    and, 241

Managed care, 129

Mandatory reporting regulations, 183

Mania, steroid use and, 241

Mannitol, 245

Marijuana, 199–207
  adolescent use of, 3
  alcohol use and, 212
  decrease in adolescent use of, viii
  epidemiology, 199
  health consequences, 201–6
  intrauterine growth retardation and,
      294–95
  laboratory evaluation, 207
  mixture of PCP with, 203
  neonatal neurobehavioral
      deficiencies and, 296–97
  pharmacology, 199–201
  prenatal exposure to, 293
  preterm labor and, 295

prevalance of use, ix
steroid use and, 242
treatment considerations, 207
trends in use of, 10f
in triggering flashbacks, 230
Mass spectrometry, 116
Maternal and Child Health Bureau,
 283
Maternal drug withdrawal, 247–48
Maternal substances of abuse, perinatal
 exposure to, 5, 293–302
MDEA, 236
MDMA (3,4-Methylenedioxymeth-
 amphetamine) ("ecstasy"), 27,
 145, 226, 227, 235, 263, 264t
 prevalance of use, ix
Media
 counteradvertising programs in,
 165–66
 portrayal of substance abuse in,
 166–67
 regulations on tobacco advertisements, 198
Medical complications, from substance
 abuse, 31
Medical history. *See also* Substance
 use history
 inclusion of questions on drug use
 in, 44
Medical organizations, 329–50
 advocacy roles and opportunities
 in, 37–38
Memory
 marijuana use and, 204, 205
 MDMA use and, 237
Mental disorders. *See also*
 Comorbidity
 identification of preexisting or
 coexisting, 29
Meperidine hydrochloride, 243, 246
Mescaline, 226, 227, 228, 229, 231
Meth, 264t

Methadone, 243, 245–46
 in detoxification, 249–50
 immunoassay tests for, 107t
Methadone maintenance, for opiate
 addiction, 248, 250
Methamphetamine hydrochloride, 223
Methamphetamines, 215, 221, 224,
 263, 264t
 prenatal exposure to, 225
 prevalance of use, ix
Methandrostenolone, 239
Methaqualone, 251, 252, 253, 256
 immunoassay tests for, 107t
 overdose with, 253
 treatment of intoxication, 255
Methemoglobinemia, inhalant use
 and, 262
Methenolone, 239
Methohexital sodium, 252
1-Methyl-4-phenyl-1,2,3,6-tetrahy-
 dropyridine (MPTP), 247
1-Methyl-4-phenyl-4-propionoxyp-
 iperidine, 246
3,4-Methylenedioxymethamphetamine
 (MDMA) ("ecstasy"). *See*
 MDMA (3,4-Methylenedioxy-
 methamphetamine) ("ecstasy")
2-Methylfentanyl ("China white"), 244
3-Methylfentanyl ("China white"), 244
Methylphenidate, 222
Mexican Valium, 256
Mexican yellows, 251
Microcephaly, screening of mother
 for, 301
Middle-ear effusions, smoking and,
 195
Mid-range evaluation, 55–56
 instruments for, 82–84
Minors. *See also* Adolescents
 emancipated, 180–81
 mature, 178, 180–81

right to outpatient counseling for drug and alcohol abuse, 49
right to privacy, 178
right to secure medical care for sexually transmitted diseases (STDs), 181–82
Miosis
opiate overdose and, 246
sedative-hypnotic drugs in, 253
Model Act of the American Academy of Pediatrics, 185
Mollies, 221
Monitoring the Future studies
inhalant use in, 259, 260
MDMA use in, 235
steroid use in, 238
tobacco use in, 277
Mood-altering effects of cocaine, 217
Mood stabilizers, for bipolar disorder, 313
Morphine, 243, 244
Mortality
amphetamine use and, 224
club drugs and, 263
cocaine use and, 218–19
inhalant use and, 261, 262
MDMA use and, 236
tobacco use and, 195
Mothers Against Drunk Driving (MADD), 326
Motor coordination, effect of alcohol on, 211
Motor vehicle crashes
alcohol-related, viii, 2, 9, 211, 213
drinking and driving prevention programs and, 167–68
methamphetamine and, 224
Muscle rigidity, PCP as cause of, 233

N
Nail, for drug testing, 111*t*
Naltrexone, 250
Nandrolone decanoate (Deca-Durabolin), 239
Narcissistic personality disorders, 318–19
Narcotics Anonymous (NA), 137, 326
Nasal congestion, cocaine and, 219
Nasal inhalation of cocaine, 216
National Association for Children of Alcoholics (NACOA), 327
National Cancer Institute, 335
National Clearinghouse for Alcohol and Drug Information (NCADI), 325
National Comorbidity Study, 3, 310
National Council on Alcoholism and Drug Dependence (NCADD), 334
National Federation of Parents for Drug-Free Youth (NFP), 325
National Household Survey on Drug Abuse
hallucinogens use in, 227
inhalant use in, 259–60
opiate use in, 244
National Institute of Mental Health Epidemiological Catchment Area, 309, 310
National Institute on Alcohol Abuse and Alcoholism (NIAAA), 334
Scientific Communications Branch, 334
National Institute on Drug Abuse, 333
publication of *Adolescent Assessment/Referral System (AARS) Manual,* 78
National Institute on Drug Use, initiative on club drugs, 263
National Network of Tobacco Prevention and Control Contacts, 335

Naxolone therapy for opiate use, 249
Negative parental modeling, 159–60
Neglected child, 176
Nembutal, 251
Neonatal abstinence syndrome, 293
Neonatal Behavioral Assessment
   Scale, 297
Neonatal neurobehavioral deficiencies,
   296–97
Neonatal withdrawal syndrome, 225,
   247–48
Neonates, cocaine-exposed, 220
Neuropsychologic tests of attention,
   204
Neurotoxic effect of marijuana, 205
NicoDerm CQ for tobacco cessation,
   198, 287
Nicotine, 194, 195, 279–81. *See also*
   Tobacco
   addiction to, 192, 198
   tolerance to, 194
   withdrawal from, 280
Nicotine patch therapy, 198, 288
Nicotine replacement therapy, 288
Nicotine transdermal systems for
   tobacco cessation, 287
Nicotrol for tobacco cessation, 198,
   287
Nightshade, 227
Nitrogen-phosphorus electron capture,
   116
Nitrous oxide, 259
Nonjudgmental health risk-based
   approach, 126
No-pass–no play rules in school
   athletics, 163*n*
Normative education, 150
   components of, 157–58
Nosology, issues of, in adolescent
   substance abuse, 307
Nystagmus, PCP as cause of, 233

O

Open-ended questions, need for, in
   interview on substance abuse,
   46–47
Opiate abstinence syndrome, 248
Opiates, 243–50
   dependence on, 206
   epidemiology, 243–44
   health consequences, 246–48
   immunoassay tests for, 107*t*
   laboratory evaluation, 248
   pharmacology, 244–46
   steroid use and, 242
   treatment considerations, 248–50
Opioids, immunoassays for, 115
Opisthotonic posturing, PCP as cause
   of, 233
Opisthotonos, PCP as cause of, 233
Opium, 243
Organic mental disorders, 315
Outpatient counseling for drug and
   alcohol abuse, minor consent to,
   49, 184
Outward Bound programs, 148
Oxandrolone (Oxandrin), 239
Oxycodone hydrochloride, 243
   immunoassays for, 115
Oxymetholone (Anadrol), 239
Oxymorphone hydrochloride,
   immunoassays for, 115

P

Pancreatitis, alcohol intoxication
   and, 212
Panic attacks, 229, 313
Pantydroppers, 256
Papaver sonmiferum, 243
Paradoxical reactions to benzodi-
   azepines, 258
Paranoia, cocaine use and, 219
Parens patriae, 187

Parental consent, 175, 179, 181–82,
184, 186, 187
Parenting skills, importance of good,
11
Parent Resources and Information for
Drug Education (PRIDE), 325
Parents
attitudes toward drugs, 34–35
concerns of, over substance abuse,
62
education programs for, 159–60
enabling behavior by, 125–26
involvement of, in outpatient
counseling for drug and alcohol
abuse, 49
presence of, at interview, 67
previous use of drugs as factor in
dealing with substance use of
children, 23
providing anticipatory guidance to,
23
referral of adolescents to drug
treatment programs, 32, 35–36
right to seek court order for
treatment, 187–88
in scheduling appointment for
evaluation of adolescent's
substance abuse, 47–48
Parent Teacher Association (PTA), 327
Parent-teacher organizations, advocacy
roles and opportunities in, 38
Parenting, styles of, and substance
abuse, 7
Parham v JR, 178
Parkinson disease, MPTP in
irreversible, 247
Paroxetine hydrochloride, 230
Partnership for a Drug-Free America,
drug prevention programs of,
165–66
Partying, 217

Passive inhalation of smoke, 195
Patient-to-staff ratio, 139
Patient-treatment matching, 127
PCP, 226, 231–34
clinical pharmacology, 231–32
epidemiology, 231
health consequences, 232–33
laboratory evaluation, 234
mixture of, with marijuana, 203
street names for, 231
treatment considerations, 234
Peace pill, 231
Peace weed, 231
Peer factors
in school-based prevention
programs, 151–52
in smoking, 193
in substance abuse, 9
Pentazocine, 243
Pentobarbital, 252
Pentobarbital sodium, 251
Perceived benefits scales, 61–62,
72–73
Percocet, 243
Percodan, 243
Perinatal exposure to maternal
substances of abuse, 5, 293–302
Peripheral nervous system, nicotine
in, 194
Personal competence, targeting,
154–59
Personal Experience Inventory (PEI),
56, 80, 82, 83
Personal Experience Inventory, Parent
Version (PEI-PV), 83–84
Personal Experience Screening
Questionnaire (PESQ), 73
Personal growth, promoting through
affective education, 147
Personal Involvement with Chemicals
Scale, 68–69

Personality disorders, 318–19

Peyote, 226

Pharmacodynamic tolerance, 252

Pharmacologic therapy for tobacco
cessation, 287, 288

Pharmacologic tolerance, marijuana
and, 206

Pharmacotherapy, 314
for cocaine dependence, 221

Pharyngitis, marijuana use in, 202

Phencyclidine hydrochloride, 231–32
immunoassay tests for, 107*t*

Phendimetrazine tartrate, 223

Phenobarbital, 252

Phenothiazines in treating lysergic
acid diethylamide (LSD)
intoxication, 230

1-(1-Phenycyclohexyl) piperidine
hydrochloride, 231–32

Phenylpropanolamine hydrochloride,
222, 224
immunoassays for, 115

Phenypropanolamine, 222

Physician-patient relationship, 187

Physicians, liability for nonnegligent
provision of care to minor
without parental consent, 182

Physostigmine in treating lysergic
acid diethylamide (LSD)
intoxication, 230

Plash, 221

Plasma and urine testing in detecting
barbiturates, 254

Pneumonia
heroin and, 247
smoking and, 195

Police power, 187–88

Polydrug use, 294

Poppers, 261

Positive consequences, 90

Positive drug history, confirmation of,
28–29

Post-traumatic stress disorder, 313–15
symptoms of, 314

Potassium nitrite, potential for
interference with testing, 112

Precontemplation stage, 89, 90, 92

Pregnancy
alcohol consumption in, 213, 293,
296, 298
amphetamine use in, 225, 294, 296
barbiturate use in, 254
benzodiazepine use and, 258
cocaine use in, 219–20, 293, 294,
295, 296, 298
failure to use contraception and
accidental, 213
heroin use in, 294, 298
LSD use in, 230
marijuana use in, 203, 293, 294, 295
maternal substances of abuse in,
293–302
opiate use in, 247–48, 294
PCP use in, 233
tobacco use in, 194, 195, 294, 296
tranquilizer use in, 258

Pregnant adolescents, special counseling
for, 31

Prenatal exposure to phenobarbital, 254

Preparation or determination stage, 89,
92

Preterm labor, 295

Prevention, 143–71
Adolescent Alcohol Prevention Trial,
154
alternatives in, 147–49
of cigarette smoking, 197
community programs for, 161–65
drinking and driving programs,
167–68
education programs in, 146–59, 283
effectiveness of, 152–54
family programs for, 159–61

implications of risk and protective
factors for the health care
professional, 1–12
increased prominence of, 144–45
indicated approaches to, 146
of marijuana use, 207
primary, 146
role of primary care physicians in,
34–36
school-based approaches in, 149–59
secondary, 146
selective approaches to, 146
social environment programs for,
165–67
social influences and general
personal competence in, 154–59
tertiary, 146
tobacco use and, 193–94, 283–85
types of, 145–46
universal approaches to, 146
Primary care physicians, 21–39
See also Health care professional,
barriers to involvement by, 21
in community action, 37–38
in consultation, 32–33
in diagnosis of substance abuse,
24–26, 123
in education, 36
in family support, 33–36
in identification of high-risk
pregnant woman, 300–302
in identifying patterns of substance
abuse, 27–31
in intervention and treatment,
21–22, 30*t*, 31
legal and ethical considerations for,
175–89
in prevention, 143–71
in providing anticipatory guidance,
22–23, 27–28
in referral process, 32–33, 123–40

Problem behavior syndrome, 241
Problem-Oriented Screening Instrument
for Parents (POSIP), 81
Problem-Oriented Screening Instrument
for Teenagers (POSIT), 68, 76,
79
validation of, 80
Problem-solving skills
effect of marijuana on, 204
tobacco cessation therapy and, 287
Procaine, 245
Project Adept, development of RAFFT
by, 69
Project Graduation, 167
Project STAR, 164–65
Propoxyphene hydrochloride, 243
immunoassay tests for, 107*t*
Prostate changes, steroid use and, 241
Prostep, 198
Protective factors in substance abuse,
10
Pseudoephedrine, 222
immunoassays for, 115
Psilocybin, 226, 227, 228, 231
Psychedelic drugs, 144
Psychiatric illness. *See also*
Comorbidity
coexistence of, with substance
abuse, 29, 45
involuntary commitment and
treatment for, 187
Psychiatrist, adolescent resistance to
consultation with, 32
Psychoactive drugs, 191, 200, 217
Psychologic inoculation, 149, 150
Psychologist, adolescent resistance to
consultation with, 32
Psychomotor performance, effects of
marijuana on, 204, 205

Psychosocial assessment, 53
   clinical screening interview in,
     63–66
   levels of assessment in, 55–56
   substantive areas of, 54*t*
Psychotherapists, Tarasoff rule and,
   183–84
Psychotic disorders, 310
Pulmonary abscesses, heroin and, 247
Pulmonary edema
   opiate use and, 248
   sedative-hypnotic drugs in, 253
Pychoses, LSD and, 229

Q

Quaaludes, 251
Questionnaires, 68–76. *See also*
   Interviews
   Achenbach Child Behavior
     Checklist, 77
   adolescent CAGE, 70–71
   Adolescent Diagnostic Interview
     (ADA), 83
   Adolescent Substance Abuse Subtle
     Screening Inventory (SASSI),
     75–76
   CAGE Adapted for Adolescents
     (CAGE-AA), 71
   Chemical Dependency Assessment
     Scale, 77
   Client Personal History
     Questionnaire, 81
   Comprehensive Assessment Battery
     (CAB), 81
   CRAFFT mnemonic tool, 68–69
   Diagnostic Interview Schedule for
     Children (DISC), 82
   Drug Use Screening Inventory
     (DUSI), 76, 77–78
   formal instruments, 66–68
   incorporation of, into evaluation
     protocol of adolescent patients'
     health status, 46
   mid-range evaluation instruments
     in, 82–84
   obtaining sensitive information
     with, 66–67
   perceived benefits scales in, 61–62,
     72–73
   Personal Experience Inventory
     (PEI), 56, 80, 82, 83–84
   Personal Experience Screening
     Questionnaire (PESQ), 73
   Personal Involvement with
     Chemicals Scale, 68–69
   Problem-Oriented Screening
     Instrument for Teenagers
     (POSIT), 68, 76, 79, 80
   RAFFT mnemonic tool, 68, 69–70
   Simple Screening Instrument for
     Alcohol and Other Drug Abuse
     (SSI-AOD), 73–75
   Symptom Checklist-90, 78
   Teen Addiction Severity Index
     (TASI), 56, 82, 84
   Youth Self Report (YSR), 82
Quicksilver, 261
Quinine, 245

R

R2s, 256
Radioimmunoassay, 114–15
   in detecting cocaine, 220
   techniques in detecting opiates, 248
RAFFT mnemonic tool, 68, 69–70
Rape
   alcohol and, 208
   club drugs and, 256
Raves, 235–36, 263
Reaction time, marijuana use and,
   203–4

Rebelliousness, substance abuse and, 6

Rebound dysphoria, cocaine use and, 218

Receptor desensitization, 252

Recurrent substance use, 87
  legal problems associated with, 87

Red devils, 251

Redisclosure, 137

Reds, 251

Referrals, 32–33, 123–40. *See also* Treatment
  adolescent placement criteria, 130–36*t*
  criteria for, of adolescent involved with substance abuse, 30*t*
  criteria for selection of treatment program, 138–39
  DSM-IV criteria for substance abuse, 127*t*
  DSM-IV criteria for substance dependence, 128*t*
  follow-up versus, 125–26
  managed care and, 129
  team approach in, 137

Refusal skills training, 150

Relapse, 137

Relaxation training for anxiety disorders, 314

Religiosity, substance abuse and low, 6

Residential treatment program, referral to, 35

Resistance skills training, 150, 151

Respiratory depression, opiate use and, 246, 248

Rhabdomyolysis
  amphetamines in, 224
  MDMA as cause of, 236
  PCP as cause of, 233

Rhinorrhea, cocaine and, 219

RIP, 256

Risk behavior theory, 279

Roches, 256, 258, 264*t*

Rohypnol, 256, 264*t*
  prevalance of use, ix

Roid rage, 241

Roofies, 264*t*

Rophies, 256, 264*t*

Ruffles, 256

Rush, 216, 261

S

Safe Rides, 167

Salicylates, spot tests for, 113

Saliva in drug testing, 111*t*

Schedule I drugs, 234–35

Schedule II drugs, 221, 251

Schedule III drugs, 238

Schizophrenia, 309, 315–16
  distinguishing from amphetamine psychosis and, 225
  PCP use and, 225

School-based approaches targeting social influences, 149–59
  adolescent alcohol prevention trial, 154
  competence enhancement approaches in, 165–67
  components, 150–51, 155–15
  effectiveness, 152–54, 156–57
  Life Skills Training Program as, 157–59
  peer leaders in, 151–52
  target population and program length, 152, 156

Schools
  advocacy roles and opportunities in, 38
  as factor in substance abuse, 8–9

Scientific issues in drug testing, 105–6, 107*t*, 108–12, 111*t*
  broadness of screen in, 108
  confirmation of immunoassay results, 106, 108

confirmation testing in, 106, 108
documentation of chain of custody
in, 109–10
hair testing in, 111*t*
nail testing in, 111*t*
potential for adulteration, 111–12
saliva testing in, 111*t*
sensitivity of screening procedure
in, 108–9
specificity of confirmatory
procedure, 109
sweat testing in, 111*t*
urine testing in, 110–12, 111*t*
variety of drugs being assayed,
106, 107*t*
Scopolamine, 227
adulteration of heroin, 245
Screen-only testing, potential for
false-negative result, 106
Seat belts, 167*n*
Secobarbital (Tubex), 251, 252
Second-hand smoke, 195
Sedative-hypnotic abstinence
syndrome, 254
Sedative-hypnotics, 251–56
epidemiology, 251–52
health consequences, 253–54
laboratory evaluation, 254
pharmacology, 252–53
steroid use and, 242
treatment considerations, 254–56
Seizures, PCP as cause of, 233
Selective prevention approaches, 146
Selective serotonin reuptake inhibitors,
LSD flashback syndrome and,
230
Self-disclosure, adolescent control
and, 50
Self-help and Advocacy Group
Resources, 325–28
Self-management skills, 158

Sensitive information, use of
questionnaire for obtaining,
66–67
Sernylan, 232
Serotonin, 227
Serotoninergic agents, 312
Serotoninergic neurodegeneration, 237
Serotonin reuptake inhibitors for
anxiety disorders, 314
Sertaline hydrochloride, 230
Settlement houses, 175
Sexual behavior, 2
Sexually transmitted diseases (STDs)
opiate use and, 247
right of minors to secure medical
care for, 181–82
Shooting up, 245
Short-term memory, effect of
marijuana on, 204, 205
Sickle cell disease, vulnerability to
substance abuse and, 44
Simple Screening Instrument for
Alcohol and Other Drug Abuse
(SSI-AOD), 73–75
Sinsemilla, 199
Sinus headaches, cocaine in, 219
Sinusitis, marijuana use in, 202
Skin abscesses, heroin in, 247
Skin popping, 245
Smokeless tobacco (SLT), 194, 287,
288
effects of, 282
prevalance of use, ix
products, 277
use of, 192
Smoking. *See* Tobacco
Smoking and Health, Office on, 335
Snorting, 245
of cocaine, 216
of heroin, 244, 245
of PCP, 233

Soapers, 251

Social bonding models, 163–64

Social environment, prevention programs based on, 160, 162–63, 165–67, 169, 287

Social influences, school-based approaches targeting, 149–59

Social isolation, vulnerability to substance abuse and, 44

Socialization deficits, 159

Social phobia, 313

Social skills component, 158

Society for Adolescent Medicine, 331

Society for General Internal Medicine (SGIM), 331

Society of Teachers of Family Medicine, 331

Specialized evaluation, 56

Special K, 264*t*

Speed, 221, 264*t*

Speedball, 216

Sperm counts, steroid use and, 241

Spinal cord injury, vulnerability to substance abuse and, 45

Spontaneous abortion, 294
 amphetamine and, 294
 cocaine and, 219, 294
 opiate use and, 247
 tobacco and, 294

Sports, steroid use and, 237–38, 239

Spot tests, 113

Stage change models of addiction, moving toward intervention, 89–91

Standardized instrument, advantages to using, 66

Stanozolol, 239

State-dependent learning, 204

Steroids. *See* Anabolic-androgenic steroids

Stigmatization, vulnerability to substance abuse and, 44

Stimulants. *See also* Amphetamines
 MDMA use and, 236

Street drugs, 221, 231
 purity of, 229

Strengthening Families program, 160–61

Students Against Drunk Driving (SADD), 328

Substance abuse
 in adolescents, viii, 2, 3, 4*f*
 adverse consequences associated with, 63
 association with other problems, 2
 child welfare and, 299–300
 clinical circumstances and problems meriting evaluation for, 45*t*
 coexistence of psychiatric disorder and, 29, 45, 307–19
 contextual factors in, 9–10
 continued, 87, 88
 criteria for selection of treatment program, 138–39
 criteria for treatment and referral of adolescent involved with, 30*t*
 diagnosis of, 24–26
 Diagnostic and Statistical Manual of Mental Disorders, Fourth Edition (DSM-IV) criteria for, 127*t*, 128*t*
 encouraging developments in area of, viii
 family factors in, 6–8
 fluctuation of, 3
 identifying patterns of, 27–31
 individual factors in, 5–6
 interplay between depression and, 311
 peer factors in, 9
 perinatal complications and, 5
 populations of adolescents with heightened vulnerability to, 44–45

predictors of, 29
prevalence of recent use, ix*t*
as preventable disorder, 1–2
protective factors in, 10
recurrent, 87
risk factors for, 5–11, 25*t*, 123
school factors in, 8–9
screening for as part of clinical
    preventive services, 44–45
societal costs of, viii–ix
strategies for interviewing
    adolescents for, 51–52
termination of, 137–38
testing for, 26*t*
treatment of, 145
Substance Abuse and Mental Health
Services Administration (SAMHSA),
    109
    in accrediting forensic laboratories,
    105
Substance dependence, 88
Substance-exposed infants, long-term
    outcome of, 297–99
Substance-induced dementia, 315
Substance-induced disorders, 87
Substance use history, 56–63, 59*t*
    adverse consequences in, 63, 64*t*
    confidentiality in obtaining reliable,
    33
    confirmation of positive, 28–29
    elements of, 59–62, 59*t*
    initial exploration in, 58
    maternal substances of abuse in, 300
    sequence of interview process,
    56–57
Sucrose, 245
Sudden infant death syndrome (SIDS),
    296, 301
    cocaine and, 296
    heroin and, 296
    tobacco and, 281–82, 296
Sugar, 264*t*

Suicide
    alcohol use and, 211, 212
    amphetamine use and, 225
    barbiturate use and, 254
    cocaine use and, 219
    depressive disorders and, 312
    LSD use and, 229
    risk of, 2
    shielding of patient and, 185
Super grass, 231
Sweat, in drug testing, 111*t*
Sympathomimetic amines, 115
Symptom Checklist-90, 78
Synesthesia, 228

T
Talking down, 230
Talwin, 243
Tarasoff rule, 183–84
Tars, 194–95
Teachers, enabling behavior by,
    125–26
Team approach, 137
Teen Addiction Severity Index (TASI),
    56, 82, 84
Teratogenicity of the drug, 233
Tertiary prevention, 146
Testicular atrophy, steroid use and, 241
Testing. *See also* Drug testing
    for alcohol, 214
Testosterone, 237
Testosterone cypionate (Depo-
    Testosterone), 239
Tetraethyl lead, toxic effects of, 263
Δ^9-Tetrahydrocannabinol
    (THC), 199–200, 231
Tetraper chloroethylene, 262
Therapeutic alliance, development of,
    between health care professional
    and adolescent, 46
Thin-layer chromatography, 113
    in detecting opiates, 248

Thiocyanate, 196
Thiopental sodium, 252
Thrombophlebitis, heroin and, 247
Thrust, 261
Tiered systems approaches to
    evaluation, 76–82
Time management approaches for
    formal assessment, 50–51
Time perception, marijuana in altering,
    203–4
Tobacco, 191–98, 277–89
    apnea and, 296
    cessation therapy for adolescents,
        287–88
    chewing, 191–92, 277
    clinical pharmacology, 194–95
    decrease in adolescent use of, viii
    epidemiology, 191–94
    health care professional's role in
        cessation efforts, 285–87
    health consequences, 195–96
    intrauterine growth retardation and,
        294–95
    laboratory evaluation, 196
    neonatal neurobehavioral
        deficiencies and, 296–97
    nicotine in, 279–81
    prevalance of use, ix
    prevention and the health care
        professional, 283–85
    risk factors for initiation of, 278–79
    role of health care professional in
        addressing, 282–83
    school-based preventive program
        for, 149
    scope of problem, 277–78, 277–89
    smokeless, ix, 192, 194, 277, 282,
        287, 288
    spontaneous abortion and, 294
    steroid use and, 242
    sudden infant death syndrome
        (SIDS) and, 296

toxic effects of, 281–82
    treatment, 197–98
Tolerance
    alcohol use and, 210
    amphetamine use and, 224
    barbiturate use and, 252
    cocaine use and, 218
    marijuana use and, 206
    measuring, 60–61
    nicotine use and, 194
    substance dependence and, 88
Toluene, 261
Toxic psychosis, 233
Toxoplasmosis, screening of mother
    for, 301
Tracking, marijuana in affecting,
    203–4
Traffic safety strategies in preventing
    drug use, 167, 168
Tranquilizers, 256–59
    epidemiology, 256
    health consequences, 257–58
    laboratory evaluation, 258
    pharmacology, 257
    prevalance of use, ix
    treatment considerations, 258–59
Transverse myelitis, heroin and, 247
Traumatic brain injury, vulnerability
    to substance abuse and, 45
Trazodone hydrochloride, for
    marijuana-induced insomnia, 206
Treatment. *See also* Referrals
    for alcohol use, 214–15
    for amphetamine use, 225–26
    for barbiturate use, 254–56
    for cigarette smoking, 197–98
    for cocaine use, 220–21
    costs of, 145
    for inhalant use, 262–63
    for LSD use, 230
    for marijuana use, 207
    for MDMA use, 237

for opiate use, 248–50
for PCP use, 234
referral to, 35
role of primary care physicians in,
30*t*, 31
for steroid use, 242
Trichloroethylene, 262
Trichloromethane, 262
Triglyceride levels, 240
True-positive results, 108
Tylox, 243
Typewriter correction fluid, 262

U

Universal prevention approaches, 146
Unruly child, defined, 176
Uppers, 221
Urine-specific gravity, 112
Urine testing, 110–12
for amphetamines, 225
for cocaine, 220
for marijuana, 207
for maternal substances of abuse,
300–301
for opiates, 248
for PCP, 231, 234
potential for adulteration, 112–13
for steroid use, 242
US Preventive Services Task Force,
recommendations on problem
drinking screening, 44

V

Valproic acid for bipolar disorder, 313
*Veronia School District 473 v Wayne
Action,* 178
Visual impairments, vulnerability to
substance abuse and, 44–45
Visual perception
effect of lysergic acid diethylamide
(LSD) on, 228
effect of marijuana on, 204

Visual-spatial memory, effect of
marijuana on, 204, 205
Vitamin K, 264*t*
Volatile nitrites, 260, 262
Voluntary screening, 26*t*

W

Wasting syndrome, anabolic-androgenic
steroids in testing, 237
Wernicke encephalopathy, chronic
alcoholism and, 212
White House Office on National Drug
Control Policy, 166
Wisconsin v Yoder, 178
Withdrawal
alchohol and, 210–11
from benzodiazepines, 258
from cocaine use, 218
from heroin use, 248
marijuana use and, 206
opiate dependence and, 206
substance dependence and, 88
Workplace drug testing, protocols for,
113

X

"X," 264*t*
XTC, 264*t*

Y

Yellow jackets, 251
Youth centers, establishment of, 148
Youth Risk Behavior Survey
steroid use in, 238–39, 241
tobacco use in, 192, 193, 197–98
Youth Self Report (YSR), 82